The Musculoskeletal Practitioner's Handbook

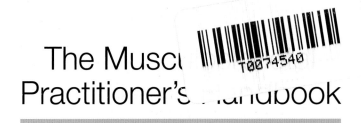

The Musculoskeletal Practitioner's Handbook

An Essential Guide for Clinical Practice

JONATHAN KENYON, MSc BSc (Hons) PGCert (NMP) MMACP MCSP

Pain Management Centre at National Hospital for Neurology and Neurosurgery, University College London Hospital, UK

GILES HAZAN, MBBS BSc MRCGP PGCert (MedEd) DipMSM

Sussex Partnership Foundation Trust, UK

ELSEVIER

Notices

Practitioners and researchers must always rely on their own experience and knowledge in evaluating and using any information, methods, compounds or experiments described herein. Because of rapid advances in the medical sciences, in particular, independent verification of diagnoses and drug dosages should be made. To the fullest extent of the law, no responsibility is assumed by Elsevier, authors, editors or contributors for any injury and/or damage to persons or property as a matter of products liability, negligence or otherwise, or from any use or operation of any methods, products, instructions, or ideas contained in the material herein.

ISBN: 978-0-7020-8491-1

Content Strategist: Andrae Akeh
Content Project Manager: Abdus Salam Mazumder
Design: Patrick C. Ferguson
Marketing Manager: Deborah Watkins

Printed in India

Last digit is the print number: 9 8 7 6 5 4 3 2 1

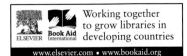

Working together
to grow libraries in
developing countries

www.elsevier.com • www.bookaid.org

CONTENTS

SECTION 4 *Systemic Conditions* *317*

PREFACE

We live in an age where information is readily available, and questions can be asked and answered with just a few taps on a keyboard. So, what made us think that clinicians needed a musculoskeletal handbook? The truth is that within a constantly evolving healthcare landscape and with the expansion of traditional clinical roles, clinical workloads are increasing and there's less time to plough through reams of information to find what's relevant and accurate. There is already a wealth of excellent textbooks out there, but it is not always possible to lug a dozen or so of them around with you on the off chance you'll need them. Also, and perhaps more importantly, we have found that none of them capture everything we are looking for in one book. Like most clinicians, we have accumulated a reasonable amount of knowledge and experience in our specialist areas but, more often than we would care to admit, we need to look stuff up – whether to remind ourselves of the features of a particular condition, check a blood value, read up on medication or simply review our anatomy. We have designed this handbook to contain key facts and figures that are easy to access and provide relevant information that can be used in day-to-day practice. Our hope is that it will act as a companion to help you navigate through the challenges of clinical practice.

Jonathan Kenyon, London, UK
Dr Giles Hazan, Eastbourne, UK

ACKNOWLEDGEMENTS

This book would not have been possible without the help of numerous clinicians who graciously gave their valuable time and expertise to read, suggest and query the initial drafts of this book and nudge us in the right direction. So, a huge thanks to Johan Holte, Jonathan Hearsey, Louise Warburton, Karen Kenyon, Mary McAllister, Georgia Aloof and Joanne Hall for their honest feedback and pointing out where we had gone wrong.

We would also like to thank the dedicated and extensive team at Elsevier who had so much faith in our initial idea and have kept the book on track through all the difficulties and delays posed by COVID. We appreciate all the help and support they brought to the project. In particular we would like to thank Poppy Garraway, Veronika Watkins, Chiara Giglio, Shravan Kumar, Abdus Salam Mazumder, Andrae Akeh and their teams.

We are fortunate to have worked with so many wonderful people over the years who have been a huge part of our clinical lives: GPs, consultants, physiotherapists, occupational therapists, nurse specialists, clinical psychologists, team leads and administrative staff. A special mention goes to our colleagues at Sussex MSK Partnership (East and Central), Sussex Partnership Foundation Trust and University College London Hospital who continue to inspire and motivate us and remind us when it is our turn to bring cake.

Dedications

To Karen
For being you – and making everything possible
JK

To Gemma, Grey and Beth.
For keeping me going and tolerating me burying
my head in the books, muttering to myself, over the years.
GH

Musculoskeletal Anatomy

Cardinal Planes

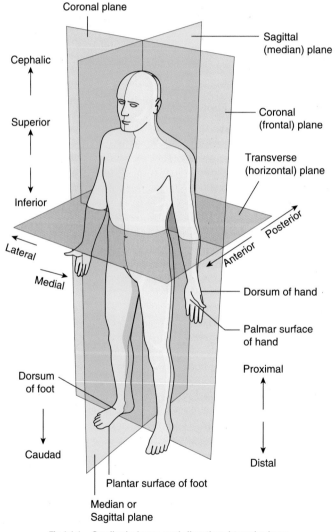

Coronal plane

Sagittal
(median) plane

Cephalic

Superior

Inferior

Lateral

Medial

Coronal
(frontal) plane

Transverse
(horizontal) plane

Posterior

Anterior

Dorsum of hand

Palmar surface
of hand

Proximal

Dorsum
of foot

Caudad

Distal

Plantar surface of foot

Median or
Sagittal plane

Fig 1.1.1   Cardinal planes and directional terminology

Joint Movements

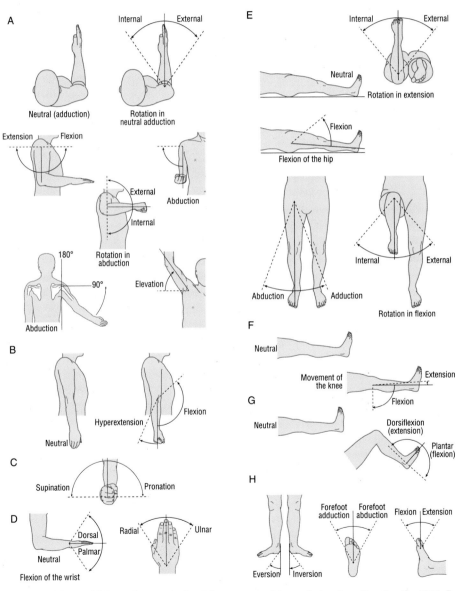

Fig 1.2.2 Joint positions and movements of the upper and lower limbs. From Douglas, G., Nicol, F., Robertson, C. (2013) MacLeod's Clinical Examination (13th ed). Elsevier.

Active Range of Joint Movement

Cervical Spine			Abduction	15°
Forward flexion	80–90°		Adduction	0°
Extension	70°		Thumb flexion	
Side flexion	25–45°		CMC	45–50°
Rotation	70–90°		MCP	50–55°
Thoracic Spine			IP	85–90°
Forward flexion	20–45°		Thumb extension	
Extension	25–45°		MCP	0°
Side flexion	20–40°		IP	0–5°
Rotation	35–50°		Thumb abduction	60–70°
Lumbar Spine			Thumb adduction	30°
Forward flexion	40–60°		***Hip***	
Extension	25–35°		Flexion	110–120°
Side flexion	15–20°		Extension	10–15°
Rotation	3–18°		Abduction	30–50°
Shoulder			Adduction	30°
Forward flexion	160–180°		Medial rotation	30–40°
Extension	50–60°		Lateral rotation	40–60°
Abduction	170–180°		***Knee***	
Adduction	50–75°		Flexion	0–135°
Medial rotation	60–100°		Extension	0–15°
Lateral rotation	80–90°		***Ankle***	
Elbow			Dorsiflexion	20°
Flexion	140–150°		Plantarflexion	50°
Extension	0–10°		Inversion	40–60°
Pronation	80–90°		Eversion	15–30°
Supination	90°		Toe extension (second to fifth toe)	
Wrist			MTP	40°
Flexion	80–90°		PIP	0°
Extension	70–90°		DIP	30°
Radial deviation	15°		Toe extension (great toe)	
Ulnar deviation	30–45°		MTP	70°
Hand			IP	0°
Finger flexion			Toe flexion (second to fifth toe)	
MCP	85–90°		MTP	40°
PIP	100–115°		PIP	35°
DIP	80–90°		DIP	60°
Finger extension			Toe flexion (great toe)	
MCP	30–45°		MTP	45°
PIP	0°		IP	90°
DIP	20–30°			

Normal ranges of movement vary greatly between individuals. The above figures represent average ranges of movement.

Close Packed Positions and Capsular Patterns for Selected Joints

Joint	Close Packed Position*	Capsular Pattern†
Cervical spine	Full extension	Side flexion and rotation equally limited, extension
Temporomandibular	Teeth tightly clenched	Limitation of mouth opening
Glenohumeral	Full abduction, lateral rotation	Lateral rotation, abduction, medial rotation
Acromioclavicular	90° abduction	Pain at extremes of ROM, especially horizontal adduction and full elevation
Sternoclavicular	Full elevation and protraction	Pain at extremes of ROM, especially horizontal adduction and full elevation
Ulnohumeral	Extension with supination	Flexion, extension
Radiohumeral	Elbow flexed to 90°, forearm supinated to 5°	Flexion, extension, supination, pronation
Superior radioulnar	5° of supination	Equal limitation of supination and pronation
Distal radioulnar	5° of supination	Full ROM, pain at extremes of rotation
Radiocarpal	Extension with radial deviation	Flexion and extension equally limited (works with midcarpal joints)
Intercarpal	Extension	None
Midcarpal	Extension with ulnar deviation	Equal limitation of flexion and extension (works with radiocarpal joints)
Carpometacarpal	Thumb, full opposition Fingers, full flexion	Thumb: abduction, extension Fingers: equal limitation in all directions
Metacarpophalangeal	Thumb, full opposition Fingers, full flexion	Flexion, extension
Interphalangeal	Full extension	Flexion, extension
Thoracic facet joints	Full extension	Slight flexion and rotation equally limited, extension
Lumbar	Full extension	Side flexion and rotation equally limited, extension
Hip	Full extension, medial rotation and abduction	Flexion, abduction and medial rotation (but in some cases, medial rotation is limited)
Tibiofemoral	Full extension, lateral rotation of the tibia	Flexion, extension
Tibiofibular	Maximum dorsiflexion	Pain when the joint is stressed
Talocrural	Maximum dorsiflexion	Plantarflexion, dorsiflexion
Subtalar	Supination	Limited ROM (varus, valgus)
Midtarsal	Supination	Dorsiflexion, plantarflexion, adduction, medial rotation
Tarsometatarsal	Supination	None
Metatarsophalangeal	Full extension	Big toe: extension, flexion Second to fifth toe: variable
Interphalangeal	Full extension	Flexion, extension

In the table above, movements are listed in order of restriction, from the most limited to the least limited.

*The close packed position: refers to the joint position in which articulating bones have their maximum area of contact with each other and are, therefore, at their most stable.

†The involvement of the entire joint capsule in certain pathological conditions limits the range of passive movement available within the joint in a particular pattern. This limitation in movement is unique to each joint and is called the capsular pattern.

Source: Data from Magee, D. J., Manske R. (2021). *Orthopedic physical assessment* (7th ed.). Elsevier.

Musculoskeletal Anatomy

Head and Neck

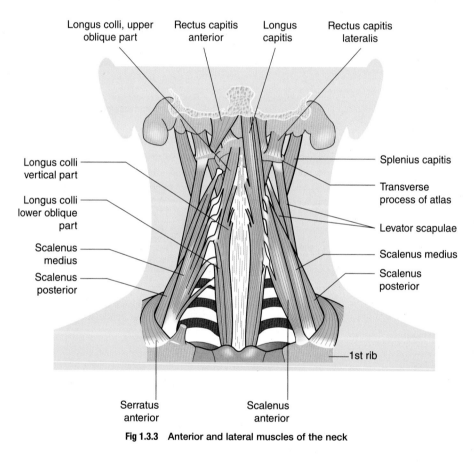

Longus colli, upper oblique part

Rectus capitis anterior

Longus capitis

Rectus capitis lateralis

Longus colli vertical part

Longus colli lower oblique part

Scalenus medius

Scalenus posterior

Splenius capitis

Transverse process of atlas

Levator scapulae

Scalenus medius

Scalenus posterior

1st rib

Serratus anterior

Scalenus anterior

Fig 1.3.3 Anterior and lateral muscles of the neck

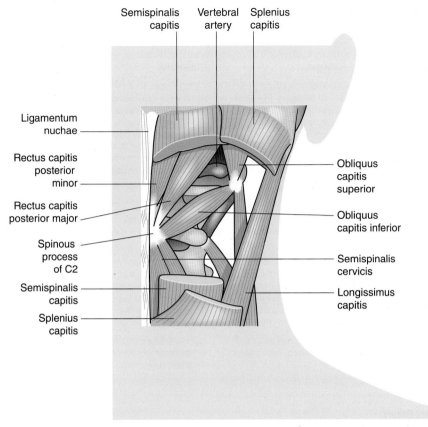

Fig 1.3.4   Posterior and lateral muscles of the neck

MUSCLES OF THE HEAD AND NECK

Flexors

Muscle	Origin	Insertion	Innervation
Longus colli	Inferior oblique part – front of bodies of T1–T2/3; vertical intermediate part – front of bodies of T1–T3 and C5–C7; superior oblique part – anterior tubercles of the transverse processes of C3–C5	Inferior oblique part – anterior tubercles of the transverse processes of C5 and C6; vertical intermediate part – front of bodies of C2–C4; superior oblique part – anterior tubercle of the atlas	Anterior primary rami (C2–C6)
Longus capitis	Occipital bone	Anterior tubercles of the transverse processes of C3–C6	Anterior primary rami (C1–C3)
Rectus capitis anterior	Anterior surface of the lateral mass of the atlas and root of its transverse process	Occipital bone	Anterior primary rami (C1, C2)
Sternocleidomastoid	Sternal head – the anterior surface of the manubrium sterni; clavicular head – the upper surface of the medial third of the clavicle	Mastoid process of the temporal bone, lateral half of the superior nuchal line of the occipital bone	Accessory nerve (XI)
Scalenus anterior	Anterior tubercles of the transverse processes of C3–C6	Scalene tubercle on the inner border of the first rib	Ventral rami (C4–C6)

Lateral Flexors

Muscle	Origin	Insertion	Innervation
Iliocostalis cervicis	Angles of the third to sixth ribs	Posterior tubercles of the transverse processes of C4–C6	Dorsal rami
Longissimus cervicis	Transverse processes of T1–T4/5	Transverse processes of C2–C6	Dorsal rami
Spinalis	*Spinalis capitis and spinalis cervicis are poorly developed and blend with adjacent muscles*		
Rectus capitis lateralis	Transverse process of the atlas	Jugular process of the occipital bone	Ventral rami (C1, C2)
Scalenus anterior	Anterior tubercles of the transverse processes of C3–C6	Scalene tubercle on the inner border of the first rib	Ventral rami (C4–C6)
Scalenus medius	Transverse processes of the atlas and axis, posterior tubercles of the transverse processes of C3–C7	Upper surface of the first rib	Ventral rami (C3–C8)
Scalenus posterior	Posterior tubercles of the transverse processes of C4–C6	Outer surface of the second rib	Ventral rami (C6–C8)

Lateral Flexors (Continued)

Muscle	Origin	Insertion	Innervation
Splenius cervicis	Spinous processes of T3–T6	Posterior tubercles of the transverse processes of C1–C3/4	Dorsal rami (C5–C7)
Splenius capitis	Lower half of the ligamentum nuchae, spinous processes of C7–T3/4 and their supraspinous ligaments	Mastoid process of the temporal bone, the lateral third of the superior nuchal line of the occipital bone	Dorsal rami (C3–C5)
Trapezius	Medial third of the superior nuchal line, external occipital protuberance, ligamentum nuchae, spinous processes and supraspinous ligaments of C7–T12	Upper fibres – posterior border of the lateral third of the clavicle; middle fibres – medial border of the acromion, the superior lip of the crest of the spine of scapula; lower fibres – tubercle at the medial end of the spine of scapula	Accessory nerve (XI), ventral rami (C3, C4)
Levator scapulae	Transverse processes of C1–C3/4	Medial border of the scapula between the superior angle and base of the spine	Ventral rami (C3, C4), dorsal scapular nerve (C5)
Sternocleidomastoid	Sternal head – the anterior surface of the manubrium sterni; clavicular head – the upper surface of the medial third of the clavicle	Mastoid process of the temporal bone, lateral half of the superior nuchal line of the occipital bone	Accessory nerve (XI)

Extensors

Muscle	Origin	Insertion	Innervation
Levator scapulae	Transverse processes of C1–C3/4	Medial border of the scapula between the superior angle and base of the spine	Ventral rami (C3, C4), dorsal scapular nerve (C5)
Splenius cervicis	Spinous processes of T3–T6	Posterior tubercles of the transverse processes of C1–C3/4	Dorsal rami (C5–C7)
Trapezius	Medial third of the superior nuchal line, external occipital protuberance, ligamentum nuchae, spinous processes and supraspinous ligaments of C7–T12	Upper fibres – posterior border of the lateral third of the clavicle; middle fibres – medial border of the acromion, the superior lip of the crest of the spine of scapula; lower fibres – tubercle at the medial end of the spine of scapula	Accessory nerve (XI), ventral rami (C3, C4)

Continued on following page

Extensors (Continued)

Muscle	Origin	Insertion	Innervation
Splenius capitis	Lower half of ligamentum nuchae, spinous processes of C7–T3/4 and their supraspinous ligaments	Mastoid process of the temporal bone, the lateral third of a superior nuchal line of the occipital bone	Dorsal rami (C3–C5)
Semispinalis capitis	Transverse processes of C7–T6/7, articular processes of C4–C6	Between superior and inferior nuchal lines of the occipital bone	Dorsal rami of the spinal nerves
Semispinalis cervicis	Transverse processes of T1–T5/6	Spinous processes of C2–C5	Dorsal rami of the spinal nerves
Superior oblique	Upper surface of the transverse process of the atlas	Superior and inferior nuchal lines of the occipital bone	Dorsal ramus (C1)
Sternocleidomastoid	Sternal head – the anterior surface of manubrium sterni; clavicular head – the upper surface of the medial third of the clavicle	Mastoid process of the temporal bone, lateral half of the superior nuchal line of the occipital bone	Accessory nerve (XI)
Iliocostalis cervicis	Angles of the third to sixth ribs	Posterior tubercles of the transverse processes of C4 to C6	Dorsal rami
Longissimus cervices	Transverse processes of T1–T4/5	Transverse processes of C2–C6	Dorsal rami
Spinalis cervicis and capitis	*Spinalis capitis and spinalis cervicis are poorly developed and blend with adjacent muscles*		
Rectus capitis posterior major	Spinous process of axis	Lateral part of the inferior nuchal line of the occipital bone	Dorsal ramus (C1)
Rectus capitis posterior minor	Posterior tubercle of the atlas	Medial part of the inferior nuchal line of the occipital bone	Dorsal ramus (C1)

Rotators

Muscle	Origin	Insertion	Innervation
Semispinalis capitis	Transverse processes of C7–T6/7, articular processes of C4–C6	Between the superior and inferior nuchal lines of the occipital bone	Dorsal rami of the spinal nerves
Semispinalis cervicis	Transverse processes of T1–T5/6	Spinous processes of C2–C5	Dorsal rami of the spinal nerves
Multifidus	Articular processes of the lower four cervical vertebrae	Spines of all vertebrae (deep layer attaches to vertebrae above; middle layer attaches to the second or third vertebrae above; outer layer attaches to the third or fourth vertebrae above)	Dorsal rami of the spinal nerves

Rotators (Continued)

Muscle	Origin	Insertion	Innervation
Scalenus anterior	Anterior tubercles of the transverse processes of C3–C6	Scalene tubercle on the inner border of the first rib	Ventral rami (C4–C6)
Sternoclei-domastoid	Sternal head – the anterior surface of manubrium sterni; clavicular head – the upper surface of the medial third of the clavicle	Mastoid process of the temporal bone, lateral half of the superior nuchal line of the occipital bone	Accessory nerve (XI)
Splenius cervicis	Spinous processes of T3–T6	Posterior tubercles of the transverse processes of C1–C3/4	Dorsal rami (C5–C7)
Splenius capitis	Lower half of the ligamentum nuchae, spinous processes of C7–T3/4 and their supraspinous ligaments	Mastoid process of the temporal bone, the lateral third of the superior nuchal line of the occipital bone	Dorsal rami (C3–C5)
Rectus capitis posterior major	Spinous process of axis	Lateral part of the inferior nuchal line of the occipital bone	Dorsal ramus (C1)
Inferior oblique	Lamina of the axis	Transverse process of the atlas	Dorsal ramus (C1)

Trunk

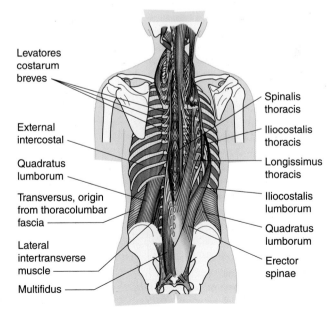

Levatores costarum breves

External intercostal

Quadratus lumborum

Transversus, origin from thoracolumbar fascia

Lateral intertransverse muscle

Multifidus

Spinalis thoracis

Iliocostalis thoracis

Longissimus thoracis

Iliocostalis lumborum

Quadratus lumborum

Erector spinae

Fig 1.3.5 Deep muscles of the back

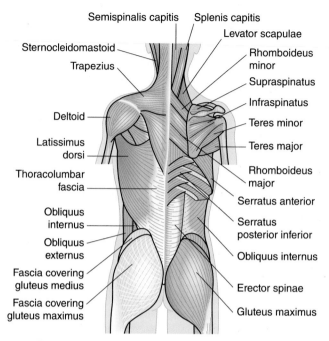

Fig 1.3.6　Superficial muscle of the back, neck and trunk

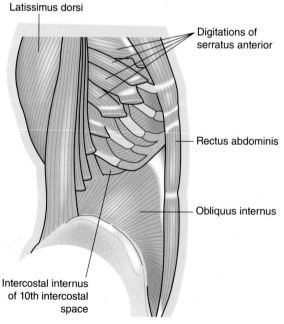

Fig 1.3.7　Muscles of the side of the trunk

MUSCLES OF THE TRUNK

Flexors

Muscle	Origin	Insertion	Innervation
Rectus abdominis	Symphysis pubis, pubic crest	Fifth to seventh costal cartilages, xiphoid process	Ventral rami of T6/7–T12
External oblique	Outer borders of the lower eight ribs and their costal cartilages	Outer lip of the anterior two-thirds of the iliac crest, abdominal aponeurosis to the linea alba stretching from the xiphoid process to symphysis pubis	Ventral rami of the lower six thoracic nerves (T7–T12)
Internal oblique	Lateral two-thirds of the inguinal ligament, anterior two-thirds of the intermediate line of the iliac crest, thoracolumbar fascia	Lower four ribs and their cartilages, the crest of pubis, abdominal aponeurosis to the linea alba	Ventral rami of the lower six thoracic nerves, first lumbar nerve
Psoas minor	Bodies of T12 and L1 vertebrae and intervertebral discs	Pecten pubis, iliopubic eminence, iliac fascia	Anterior primary ramus (L1)
Psoas major	Bodies of T12 and all lumbar vertebrae, bases of the transverse processes of all lumbar vertebrae, lumbar intervertebral discs	Lesser trochanter	Anterior rami of the lumbar plexus (L1–L3)
Iliacus	Superior two-thirds of the iliac fossa, inner lip of the iliac crest, ala of sacrum, anterior sacroiliac and iliolumbar ligaments	Blends with the insertion of psoas major into the lesser trochanter	Femoral nerve (L2, L3)

Lateral flexors

Muscle	Origin	Insertion	Innervation
Quadratus lumborum	Iliolumbar ligament, posterior part of the iliac crest	Lower border of the 12th rib, transverse processes of L1–L4	Ventral rami of T12 and L1–L3/4
Intertransversarii	Transverse processes of the cervical and lumbar vertebrae	Transverse process of the vertebra superior to the origin	Ventral and dorsal rami of the spinal nerves
External oblique	Outer borders of the lower eight ribs and their costal cartilages	Outer lip of the anterior two-thirds of the iliac crest, abdominal aponeurosis to the linea alba stretching from the xiphoid process to symphysis pubis	Ventral rami of the lower six thoracic nerves (T7–T12)
Internal oblique	Lateral two-thirds of the inguinal ligament, anterior two-thirds of the intermediate line of the iliac crest, thoracolumbar fascia	Lower four ribs and their cartilages, crest of pubis, abdominal aponeurosis to the linea alba	Ventral rami of the lower six thoracic nerves, first lumbar nerve

Continued on following page

Lateral flexors (Continued)

Muscle	Origin	Insertion	Innervation
Iliocostalis thoracis	Angles of the lower six ribs	Angles of the upper six ribs, transverse process of C7	Dorsal rami
Iliocostalis lumborum	Medial and lateral sacral crests; spines of T11, T12, and lumbar vertebrae and their supraspinous ligaments; the medial part of the iliac crest	Angles of the lower six or seven ribs	Dorsal rami
Longissimus thoracis	Transverse and accessory processes of the lumbar vertebrae and thoraco-lumbar fascia	Transverse processes of T1–T12 and the lower nine or 10 ribs	Dorsal rami
Spinalis Thoracis	Spinous processes of T11–L2	Spinous processes of the upper four to eight thoracic vertebrae	Dorsal rami
Multifidus	All thoracic transverse processes	Spines of all vertebrae (deep layer attaches to the vertebrae above; middle layer attaches to the second or third verte-brae above; outer layer attaches to the third or fourth vertebrae above)	Dorsal rami of the spinal nerves

Extensors

Muscle	Origin	Insertion	Innervation
Quadratus lumborum	Iliolumbar ligament, posterior part of the iliac crest	Lower border of the 12th rib, transverse processes of L1–L4	Ventral rami of T12 and L1–L3/4
Multifidus	All thoracic transverse processes	Spines of all vertebrae (deep layer attaches to vertebrae above; middle layer attaches to the second or third vertebrae above; outer layer attaches to the third or fourth vertebrae above)	Dorsal rami of the spinal nerves
Semispinalis thoracis	Transverse processes of T6–T10	Spinous processes of C6–T4	Dorsal rami of the spinal nerves
Iliocostalis thoracis	Angles of the lower six ribs	Angles of the upper six ribs, transverse process of C7	Dorsal rami
Iliocostalis lumborum	Medial and lateral sacral crests; spines of T11, T12, and lumbar vertebrae and their supraspinous liga-ments; the medial part of the iliac crest	Angles of the lower six or seven ribs	Dorsal rami

Extensors (Continued)

Muscle	Origin	Insertion	Innervation
Longissiumus thoracis	Transverse and accessory processes of the lumbar vertebrae and thoraco-lumbar fascia	Transverse processes of T1–T12 and the lower nine or 10 ribs	Dorsal rami
Spinalis thoracis	Spinous processes of T11–L2	Spinous processes of the upper four to eight thoracic vertebrae	Dorsal rami
Interspinales	Extend between adjacent spinous processes	Dorsal rami of the spinal nerves	
Rotatores	Transverse process of each vertebra	Lamina of the vertebra above	Dorsal rami of the spinal nerves

Rotators

Muscle	Origin	Insertion	Innervation
Multifidus	All thoracic transverse processes	Spines of all vertebrae (deep layer attaches to the vertebrae above; middle layer attaches to the second or third vertebrae above; outer layer attaches to the third or fourth vertebrae above)	Dorsal rami of the spinal nerves
Rotatores	Transverse process of each vertebra	Lamina of the vertebra above	Dorsal rami of the spinal nerves
External oblique	Outer borders of the lower eight ribs and their costal cartilages	Outer lip of the anterior two-thirds of the iliac crest, abdominal aponeurosis to the linea alba stretching from the xiphoid process to symphysis pubis	Ventral rami of the lower six thoracic nerves (T7–T12)
Internal oblique	Lateral two-thirds of the inguinal ligament, anterior two-thirds of the intermediate line of the iliac crest, thoracolumbar fascia	Lower four ribs and their cartilages, the crest of pubis, abdominal aponeurosis to the linea alba	Ventral rami of the lower six thoracic nerves, first lumbar nerve
Semispinalis thoracis	Transverse processes of T6–T10	Spinous processes of C6–T4	Dorsal rami of the spinal nerves

Shoulder, Scapula and Upper Arm

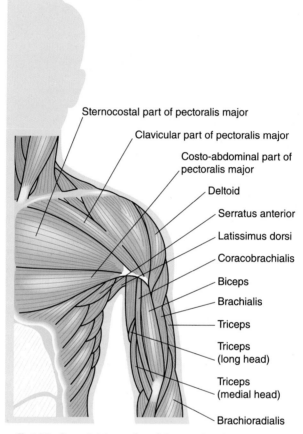

Sternocostal part of pectoralis major

Clavicular part of pectoralis major

Costo-abdominal part of pectoralis major

Deltoid

Serratus anterior

Latissimus dorsi

Coracobrachialis

Biceps

Brachialis

Triceps

Triceps (long head)

Triceps (medial head)

Brachioradialis

Fig 1.3.8   Superficial muscles of the anterior chest and arm

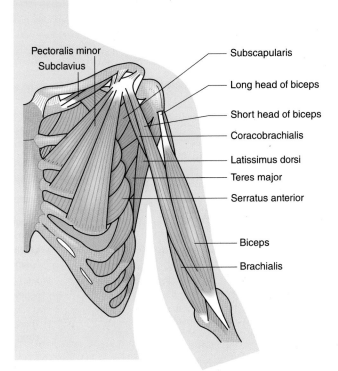

Fig 1.3.9   Deep muscles of the anterior chest and upper arm

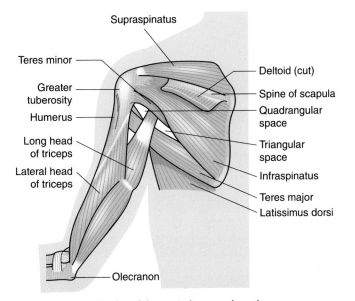

Fig 1.3.10   Muscles of the posterior scapula and upper arm

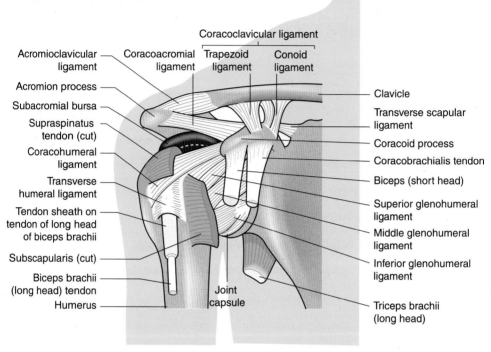

Fig 1.3.11   Ligaments of the glenohumeral joint

MUSCLES OF THE SHOULDER

Flexors

Muscle	Origin	Insertion	Innervation
Pectoralis major	Clavicular attachment – sternal half of the anterior surface of the clavicle; sternocostal attachment – anterior surface of the manubrium, body of the sternum, upper six costal cartilages, sixth rib, aponeurosis of the external oblique muscle	Lateral lip of the intertubercular sulcus of the humerus	Medial and lateral pectoral nerves (C5–T1)
Deltoid (anterior fibres)	Anterior border of the lateral third of the clavicle	Deltoid tuberosity of the humerus	Axillary nerve (C5, C6)
Biceps brachii (long head)	Long head – supraglenoid tubercle of the scapula and glenoid labrum; short head – the apex of coracoid process	Posterior part of the radial tuberosity, bicipital aponeurosis into the deep fascia over common flexor origin	Musculocutaneous nerve (C5, C6)
Coracobrachialis	Apex of coracoid process	Midway along the medial border of the humerus	Musculocutaneous nerve (C5–C7)

Extensors

Muscle	Origin	Insertion	Innervation
Latissimus dorsi	Spinous processes of the lower six thoracic and all lumbar and sacral vertebrae, intervening supra- and interspinous ligaments, outer lip of the iliac crest, outer surfaces of the lower three or four ribs, inferior angle of the scapula	Intertubercular sulcus of the humerus	Thoracodorsal nerve (C6–C8)
Teres major	Dorsal surface of the inferior scapular angle	Medial lip of the intertubercular sulcus of the humerus	Lower subscapular nerve (C5–C7)
Pectoralis major	Clavicular attachment – sternal half of the anterior surface of the clavicle; sternocostal attachment – anterior surface of the manubrium, body of the sternum, upper six costal cartilages, sixth rib, aponeurosis of the external oblique muscle	Lateral lip of the intertubercular sulcus of the humerus	Medial and lateral pectoral nerves (C5–T1)
Deltoid (posterior fibres)	Lower edge of crest of the spine of scapula	Deltoid tuberosity of the humerus	Axillary nerve (C5, C6)
Triceps (long head)	Infraglenoid tubercle of the scapula, shoulder capsule	Upper surface of the olecranon, deep fascia of forearm	Radial nerve (C6–C8)

Abductors

Muscle	Origin	Insertion	Innervation
Supraspina-tus	Medial two-thirds of the supraspi-nous fossa and supraspinous fascia	Capsule of the shoulder joint, greater tubercle of the humerus	Suprascapular nerve (C5, C6)
Deltoid (middle fibres)	Lateral margin of the acromion process	Deltoid tuberosity of the humerus	Axillary nerve (C5, C6)

Adductors

Muscle	Origin	Insertion	Innervation
Coracobrachialis	Apex of the coracoid process	Midway along the medial border of the humerus	Musculocutaneous nerve (C5–C7)
Pectoralis major	Clavicular attachment – sternal half of the anterior surface of the clavicle; sternocostal attachment – anterior surface of manubrium, body of the sternum, upper six costal cartilages, sixth rib, aponeurosis of the external oblique muscle	Lateral lip of the intertubercular sulcus of the humerus	Medial and lateral pectoral nerves (C5–T1)
Latissimus dorsi	Spinous processes of the lower six thoracic and all lumbar and sacral vertebrae, intervening supra- and interspinous ligaments, outer lip of the iliac crest, outer surfaces of the lower three or four ribs, inferior angle of the scapula	Intertubercular sulcus of the humerus	Thoracodorsal nerve (C6–C8)
Teres major	Dorsal surface of the inferior scapular angle	Medial lip of the intertubercular sulcus of the humerus	Lower subscapular nerve (C5–C7)

Medial Rotators

Muscle	Origin	Insertion	Innervation
Subscapularis	Medial two-thirds of the subscapular fossa and tendinous intramuscular septa	Lesser tubercle of the humerus, anterior capsule of the shoulder joint	Upper and lower subscapular nerves (C5, C6)
Teres major	Dorsal surface of the inferior scapular angle	Medial lip of the intertubercular sulcus of the humerus	Lower subscapular nerve (C5–C7)

Medial Rotators (Continued)

Muscle	Origin	Insertion	Innervation
Latissimus dorsi	Spinous processes of the lower six thoracic and all lumbar and sacral vertebrae, intervening supra- and interspinous ligaments, outer lip of the iliac crest, outer surfaces of the lower three or four ribs, inferior angle of the scapula	Intertubercular sulcus of the humerus	Thoracodorsal nerve (C6–C8)
Pectoralis major	Clavicular attachment – sternal half of the anterior surface of the clavicle; sternocostal attachment – anterior surface of the manubrium, body of the sternum, upper six costal cartilages, sixth rib, aponeurosis of the external oblique muscle	Lateral lip of the intertubercular sulcus of the humerus	Medial and lateral pectoral nerves (C5–T1)
Deltoid (anterior fibres)	Anterior border of the lateral third of the clavicle	Deltoid tuberosity of the humerus	Axillary nerve (C5, C6)

Lateral Rotators

Muscle	Origin	Insertion	Innervation
Teres minor	Upper two-thirds of the dorsal surface of the scapula	Lower facet on the greater tuberosity of the humerus, lower posterior surface of the capsule of the shoulder joint	Axillary nerve (C5, C6)
Infraspinatus	Medial two-thirds of the infraspinous fossa and infraspinous fascia	Middle facet on the greater tubercle of the humerus, posterior aspect of the capsule of the shoulder joint	Suprascapular nerve (C5, C6)
Deltoid (posterior fibres)	Lower edge of the crest of the spine of scapula	Deltoid tuberosity of the humerus	Axillary nerve (C5, C6)

MUSCLES OF THE SCAPULA

Retractors

Muscle	Origin	Insertion	Innervation
Rhomboid minor	Spines and supraspinous ligaments of C7–T1, the lower part of ligamentum nuchae	Medial end of the spine of scapula	Dorsal scapular nerve (C4, C5)
Rhomboid major	Spines and supraspinous ligaments of T2–T5	Medial border of the scapula between the root of the spine and the inferior angle	Dorsal scapular nerve (C4, C5)

Continued on following page

Retractors (Continued)

Muscle	Origin	Insertion	Innervation
Trapezius	Medial third of the superior nuchal line, external occipital protuberance, ligamentum nuchae, spinous processes and supraspinous ligaments of C7–T12	Upper fibres – posterior border of the lateral third of the clavicle; middle fibres – medial border of the acromion, superior lip of the crest of the spine of scapula; lower fibres – tubercle at the medial end of the spine of scapula	Accessory nerve (XI), ventral rami (C3, C4)
Levator scapulae	Transverse processes of C1–C3/4	Medial border of the scapula between the superior angle and base of the spine	Ventral rami (C3, C4), dorsal scapular nerve (C5)

Protractors

Muscle	Origin	Insertion	Innervation
Serratus anterior	Outer surfaces and superior borders of the upper eight, nine, or 10 ribs and intervening intercostal fascia	Costal surface of the medial border of the scapula	Long thoracic nerve (C5–C7)
Pectoralis minor	Outer surface of the third to fifth ribs and adjoining intercostal fascia	Upper surface and medial border of the coracoid process	Medial and lateral pectoral nerves (C5–T1)

Elevators

Muscle	Origin	Insertion	Innervation
Trapezius	Medial third of the superior nuchal line, external occipital protuberance, ligamentum nuchae, spinous processes and the supraspinous ligaments of C7–T12	Upper fibres – posterior border of the lateral third of the clavicle; middle fibres – medial border of the acromion, superior lip of the crest of the spine of scapula; lower fibres – tubercle at the medial end of the spine of scapula	Accessory nerve (XI), ventral rami (C3, C4)
Levator scapulae	Transverse processes of C1–C3/4	Medial border of the scapula between the superior angle and base of the spine	Ventral rami (C3, C4), dorsal scapular nerve (C5)

Depressors

Muscle	Origin	Insertion	Innervation
Trapezius	Medial third of the superior nuchal line, external occipital protuberance, ligamentum nuchae, spinous processes and supraspinous ligaments of C7–T12	Upper fibres – posterior border of the lateral third of the clavicle; middle fibres – medial border of the acromion, superior lip of the crest of the spine of scapula; lower fibres – tubercle at the medial end of the spine of scapula	Accessory nerve (XI), ventral rami (C3, C4)

Lateral Rotators

Muscle	Origin	Insertion	Innervation
Trapezius	Medial third of the superior nuchal line, external occipital protuberance, ligamentum nuchae, spinous processes and supraspinous ligaments of C7–T12	Upper fibres – posterior border of the lateral third of the clavicle; middle fibres – medial border of the acromion, superior lip of the crest of the spine of scapula; lower fibres – tubercle at the medial end of the spine of scapula	Accessory nerve (XI), ventral rami (C3, C4)
Serratus anterior	Outer surfaces and superior borders of the upper eight, nine, or 10 ribs and intervening intercostal fascia	Costal surface of the medial border of the scapula	Long thoracic nerve (C5–C7)

Medial Rotators

Muscle	Origin	Insertion	Innervation
Rhomboid minor	Spines and supraspinous ligaments of C7–T1, the lower part of the ligamentum nuchae	Medial end of the spine of scapula	Dorsal scapular nerve (C4, C5)
Rhomboid major	Spines and supraspinous ligaments of T2–T5	Medial border of the scapula between the root of the spine and the inferior angle	Dorsal scapular nerve (C4, C5)
Pectoralis minor	Outer surface of the third to fifth ribs and adjoining intercostal fascia	Upper surface and medial border of the coracoid process	Medial and lateral pectoral nerves (C5–T1)
Levator scapulae	Transverse processes of C1–C3/4	Medial border of the scapula between the superior angle and base of the spine	Ventral rami (C3, C4), dorsal scapular nerve (C5)

Elbow, Wrist and Hand

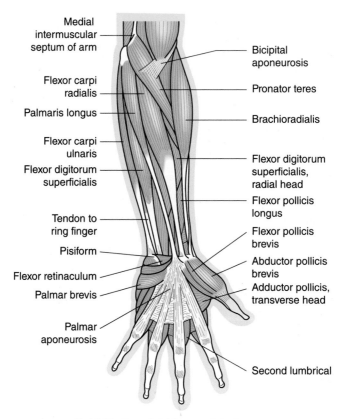

Fig 1.3.12 Superficial flexors of the forearm

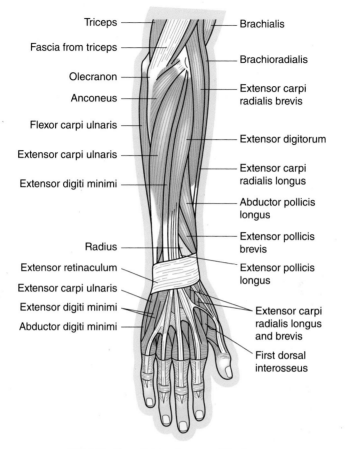

Triceps

Fascia from triceps

Olecranon

Anconeus

Flexor carpi ulnaris

Extensor carpi ulnaris

Extensor digiti minimi

Radius

Extensor retinaculum

Extensor carpi ulnaris

Extensor digiti minimi

Abductor digiti minimi

Brachialis

Brachioradialis

Extensor carpi radialis brevis

Extensor digitorum

Extensor carpi radialis longus

Abductor pollicis longus

Extensor pollicis brevis

Extensor pollicis longus

Extensor carpi radialis longus and brevis

First dorsal interosseus

Fig 1.3.13   Superficial extensors of the forearm

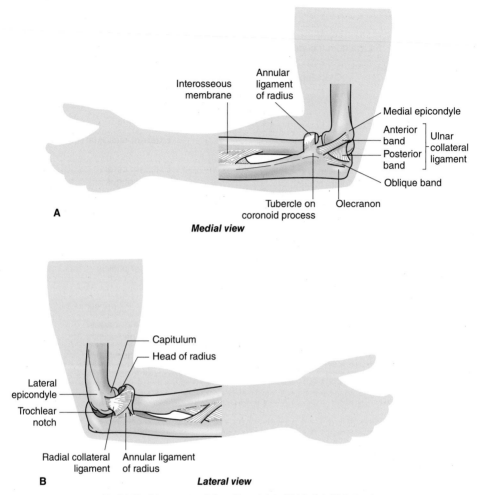

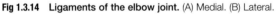

Fig 1.3.14　Ligaments of the elbow joint. (A) Medial. (B) Lateral.

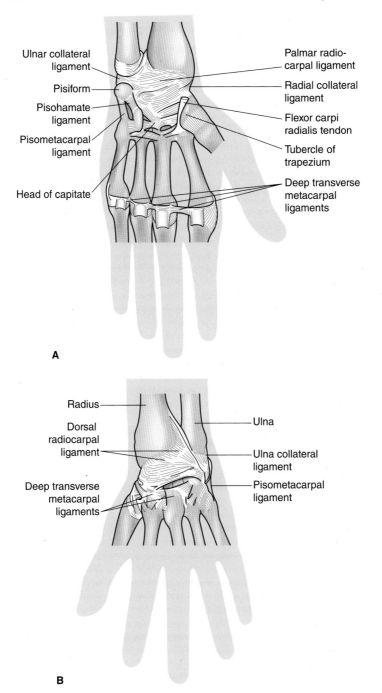

Fig 1.3.15 Ligaments of the wrist and hand. (A) Anterior. (B) Posterior.

MUSCLES OF THE ELBOW

Flexors

Muscle	Origin	Insertion	Innervation
Biceps brachii	Long head – supraglenoid tubercle of the scapula and glenoid labrum; short head – the apex of the coracoid process	Posterior part of the radial tuberosity, bicipital aponeurosis into the deep fascia over the common flexor origin	Musculocutaneous nerve (C5, C6)
Brachialis	Lower half of the anterior surface of the humerus, intermuscular septum	Coronoid process and tuberosity of the ulna	Musculocutaneous nerve (C5, C6), radial nerve (C7)
Brachioradi-alis	Upper two-thirds of the lateral supracondylar ridge of the humerus, lateral intermuscular septum	Lateral side of the radius above the styloid process	Radial nerve (C5, C6)
Pronator teres	Humeral head – medial epicondyle via the common flexor tendon, intermuscular septum, antebrachial fascia; ulnar head – medial part of the coronoid process	Middle of the lateral surface of the radius	Median nerve (C6, C7)

Extensors

Muscle	Origin	Insertion	Innervation
Triceps Bra-chii	Long head – infraglenoid tubercle of the scapula, shoulder capsule; lateral head – above and lateral to the spiral groove on the posterior surface of the humerus; medial head – below and medial to the spiral groove on the posterior surface of the humerus	Upper surface of the olecranon, deep fascia of the forearm	Radial nerve (C6–C8)
Anco-neus	Posterior surface of the lateral epicondyle of the humerus	Lateral surface of the olecranon, upper quarter of the posterior surface of the ulna	Radial nerve (C6–C8)

Pronators

Muscle	Origin	Insertion	Innervation
Pronator teres	Humeral head – medial epicondyle via the common flexor tendon, intermuscular septum, antebrachial fascia; ulnar head – medial part of the coronoid process	Middle of the lateral surface of the radius	Median nerve (C6, C7)
Pronator quadra-tus	Lower quarter of the anterior surface of the ulna	Lower quarter of the anterior surface of the radius	Anterior interosseous branch of the median nerve (C7, C8)

Supinators

Muscle	Origin	Insertion	Innervation
Supinator	Inferior aspect of the lateral epicondyle, radial collateral ligament, annular ligament, supinator crest and fossa of the ulna	Posterior, lateral and anterior aspects of the upper third of the radius	Posterior interosseous nerve (C6, C7)
Biceps brachii	Long head – supraglenoid tubercle of the scapula and glenoid labrum; short head – apex of the coracoid process	Posterior part of the radial tuberosity, bicipital aponeurosis into the deep fascia over the common flexor origin	Musculocutaneous nerve (C5, C6)

MUSCLES OF THE WRIST

Flexors

Muscle	Origin	Insertion	Innervation
Flexor carpi ulnaris	Humeral head – medial epicondyle via the common flexor tendon; ulnar head – medial border of the olecranon and upper two-thirds of the border of ulna	Pisiform, the hook of hamate and base of the fifth metacarpal	Ulnar nerve (C7–T1)
Flexor carpi radialis	Medial epicondyle via the common flexor tendon	Front of the base of the second and third metacarpal	Median nerve (C6, C7)
Palmaris longus	Medial epicondyle via the common flexor tendon	Flexor retinaculum, palmar aponeurosis	Median nerve (C7, C8)
Flexor digitorum superficialis	Humeroulnar head – medial epicondyle via common flexor tendon, the medial part of coronoid process of ulna, ulnar collateral ligament, intermuscular septa; radial head – upper two-thirds of the anterior border of the radius	Tendons divide and insert into the sides of the shaft of the middle phalanx of the second to fifth digits	Median nerve (C8, T1)
Flexor digitorum profundus	Medial side of the coronoid process of the ulna, upper three-quarters of the anterior and medial surfaces of the ulna, interosseous membrane	Base of the palmar surface of the distal phalanx of the second to fifth digits	Medial part – ulnar nerve (C8, T1); lateral part– anterior interosseous branch of the median nerve (C8, T1)
Flexor pollicis longus	Anterior surface of the radius, interosseous membrane	Palmar surface of the distal phalanx of the thumb	Anterior interosseous branch of the median nerve (C7, C8)

Extensors

Muscle	Origin	Insertion	Innervation
Extensor carpi radialis longus	Lower third of the lateral supracondylar ridge of the humerus, intermuscular septa	Posterior surface of the base of the second metacarpal	Radial nerve (C6, C7)
Extensor carpi radialis brevis	Lateral epicondyle via the common extensor tendon	Posterior surface of the base of the third metacarpal	Posterior interosseous branch of the radial nerve (C7, C8)
Extensor carpi ulnaris	Lateral epicondyle via the common extensor tendon	Medial side of the fifth metacarpal base	Posterior interosseous nerve (C7, C8)
Extensor digitorum	Lateral epicondyle via the common extensor tendon, intermuscular septa	Lateral and dorsal surfaces of the second to fifth digits	Posterior interosseous branch of the radial nerve (C7, C8)
Extensor indicis	Lower part of the posterior surface of the ulna, the interosseous membrane	Dorsal digital expansion on the back of the proximal phalanx of the index finger	Posterior interosseous nerve (C7, C8)
Extensor digiti minimi	Lateral epicondyle via the common extensor tendon, intermuscular septa	Dorsal digital expansion of the fifth digit	Posterior interosseous nerve (C7, C8)
Extensor pollicis longus	Middle third of the posterior surface of the ulna, interosseous membrane	Dorsal surface of the distal phalanx of the thumb	Posterior interosseous nerve (C7, C8)
Extensor pollicis brevis	Posterior surface of the radius, interosseous membrane	Dorsolateral base of the proximal phalanx of the thumb	Posterior interosseous nerve (C7, C8)

Ulnar Deviation

Muscle	Origin	Insertion	Innervation
Flexor carpi ulnaris	Humeral head – medial epicondyle via the common flexor tendon; ulnar head – medial border of the olecranon and upper two-thirds of the border of the ulna	Pisiform, the hook of hamate and base of the fifth metacarpal	Ulnar nerve (C7–T1)
Extensor carpi ulnaris	Lateral epicondyle via the common extensor tendon	Medial side of the fifth metacarpal base	Posterior interosseous nerve (C7, C8)

Radial Deviation

Muscle	Origin	Insertion	Innervation
Flexor carpi radialis	Medial epicondyle via the common flexor tendon	Front of the base of the second and third metacarpal	Median nerve (C6, C7)
Extensor carpi radialis longus	Lower third of the lateral supra-condylar ridge of the humerus, intermuscular septa	Posterior surface of the base of the second metacarpal	Radial nerve (C6, C7)
Extensor carpi radialis brevis	Lateral epicondyle via the common extensor tendon	Posterior surface of the base of the third metacarpal	Posterior interos-seous branch of the radial nerve (C7, C8)
Abductor polli-cis longus	Upper part of the posterior surface of the ulna, middle third of the posterior surface of the radius, interosseous membrane	Radial side of the first metacarpal base, trapezium	Posterior interos-seous nerve (C7, C8)
Extensor polli-cis longus	Middle third of the posterior surface of the ulna, interosse-ous membrane	Dorsal surface of the distal phalanx of the thumb	Posterior interos-seous nerve (C7, C8)
Extensor polli-cis brevis	Posterior surface of the radius, interosseous membrane	Dorsolateral base of the proximal phalanx of the thumb	Posterior interos-seous nerve (C7, C8)

MUSCLES OF THE FINGERS

Flexors

Muscle	Origin	Insertion	Innervation
Flexor digito-rum superfi-cialis	Humeroulnar head – medial epicondyle via the common flexor tendon, medial part of the coronoid process of the ulna, ulnar collateral ligament, intermuscular septa; radial head – upper two-thirds of the anterior border of the radius	Tendons divide and insert into the sides of the shaft of the middle phalanx of the second to fifth digits	Median nerve (C8, T1)
Flexor digito-rum profun-dus	Medial side of the coronoid process of the ulna, upper three-quarters of the ante-rior and medial surfaces of the ulna, interosseous membrane	Base of the palmar surface of the distal phalanx of the second to fifth digits	Medial part – ulnar nerve (C8, T1); lateral part – anterior inter-osseous branch of the median nerve (C8, T1)

Continued on following page

Flexors (Continued)

Muscle	Origin	Insertion	Innervation
Lumbricals	Tendons of the flexor digitorum profundus	Lateral margin of the dorsal digital expansion of the extensor digitorum	First and second – median nerve (C8, T1); third and fourth – ulnar nerve (C8, T1)
Flexor digiti minimi brevis	Hook of hamate, flexor retinaculum	Ulnar side of the base of the proximal phalanx of the little finger	Ulnar nerve (C8, T1)

Extensors

Muscle	Origin	Insertion	Innervation
Extensor digitorum	Lateral epicondyle via the common extensor tendon, intermuscular septa	Lateral and dorsal surfaces of the second to fifth digits	Posterior interosseous branch of the radial nerve (C7, C8)
Extensor digiti minimi	Lateral epicondyle via the common extensor tendon, intermuscular septa	Dorsal digital expansion of the fifth digit	Posterior interosseous nerve (C7, C8)
Extensor indicis	Lower part of the posterior surface of the ulna, interosseous membrane	Dorsal digital expansion on the back of the proximal phalanx of the index finger	Posterior interosseous nerve (C7, C8)
Dorsal interossei	Adjacent sides of two metacarpal bones (four bipennate muscles)	Bases of the proximal phalanges and dorsal digital expansions (first attaches laterally to the index finger; second and third attach to both sides of the middle finger; fourth attaches medially to the ring finger)	Ulnar nerve (C8, T1)
Lumbricals	Tendons of the flexor digitorum profundus	Lateral margin of the dorsal digital expansion of the extensor digitorum	First and second – median nerve (C8, T1); third and fourth – ulnar nerve (C8, T1)

Abductors

Muscle	Origin	Insertion	Innervation
Dorsal interossei	Adjacent sides of two metacarpal bones (four bipennate muscles)	Bases of the proximal phalanges and dorsal digital expansions (first attaches laterally to the index finger; second and third attach to both sides of the middle finger; fourth attaches medially to the ring finger)	Ulnar nerve (C8, T1)
Abductor digiti minimi	Pisiform, tendon of the flexor carpi ulnaris, pisohamate ligament	Ulnar side of the base of the proximal phalanx of the little finger	Ulnar nerve (C8, T1)
Opponens digiti minimi	Hook of hamate, flexor retinaculum	Medial border of the fifth metacarpal	Ulnar nerve (C8, T1)

Adductors

Muscle	Origin	Insertion	Innervation
Palmar interossei	Shaft of the metacarpal of the digit on which it acts	Dorsal digital expansion and base of the proximal phalanx of the same digit	Ulnar nerve (C8, T1)

MUSCLES OF THE THUMB

Flexors

Muscle	Origin	Insertion	Innervation
Flexor pollicis longus	Anterior surface of the radius, interosseous membrane	Palmar surface of the distal phalanx of the thumb	Anterior interosseous branch of the median nerve (C7, C8)
Flexor pollicis brevis	Flexor retinaculum, tubercle of the trapezium, capitate, trapezoid	Base of the proximal phalanx of the thumb	Median nerve (C8–T1). Sometimes also supplied by the ulnar nerve (C8–T1)

Extensors

Muscle	Origin	Insertion	Innervation
Extensor pollicis longus	Middle third of the posterior surface of the ulna, interosseous membrane	Dorsal surface of the distal phalanx of the thumb	Posterior interosseous nerve (C7, C8)
Extensor pollicis brevis	Posterior surface of the radius, interosseous membrane	Dorsolateral base of the proximal phalanx of the thumb	Posterior interosseous nerve (C7, C8)
Abductor pollicis longus	Upper part of the posterior surface of the ulna, middle third of the posterior surface of the radius, interosseous membrane	Radial side of the first metacarpal base, trapezium	Posterior interosseous nerve (C7, C8)

Abductors

Muscle	Origin	Insertion	Innervation
Abductor pollicis longus	Upper part of the posterior surface of the ulna, middle third of the posterior surface of the radius, interosseous membrane	Radial side of the first metacarpal base, trapezium	Posterior interosseous nerve (C7, C8)
Abductor pollicis brevis	Flexor retinaculum, tubercles of the scaphoid and trapezium, tendon of the abductor pollicis longus	Radial side of the base of the proximal phalanx of the thumb	Median nerve (C8, T1)

Adductors

Muscle	Origin	Insertion	Innervation
Adductor pollicis	Oblique head – palmar ligaments of the carpus, flexor carpi radialis tendon, base of the second to fourth metacarpals, capitate; transverse head – palmar surface of the third metacarpal	Base of the proximal phalanx of the thumb	Ulnar nerve (C8, T1)

Opposition

Muscle	Origin	Insertion	Innervation
Opponens pollicis	Flexor retinaculum, tubercles of the scaphoid and trapezium, abductor pollicis longus tendon	Radial side of the base of the proximal phalanx of the thumb	Median nerve (C8, T1)

Pelvis and Hip

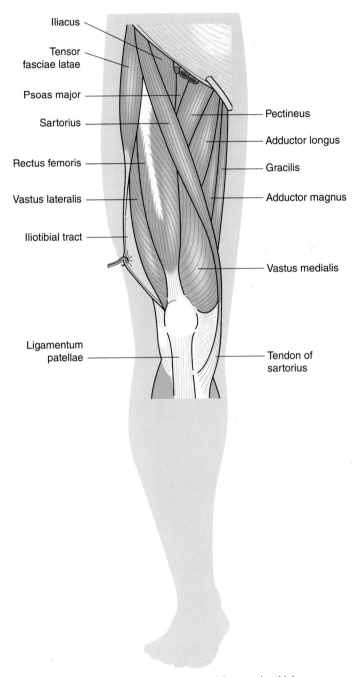

Iliacus

Tensor
fasciae latae

Psoas major

Sartorius

Rectus femoris

Vastus lateralis

Iliotibial tract

Ligamentum
patellae

Pectineus

Adductor longus

Gracilis

Adductor magnus

Vastus medialis

Tendon of
sartorius

Fig 1.3.16 Superficial muscles of the anterior thigh

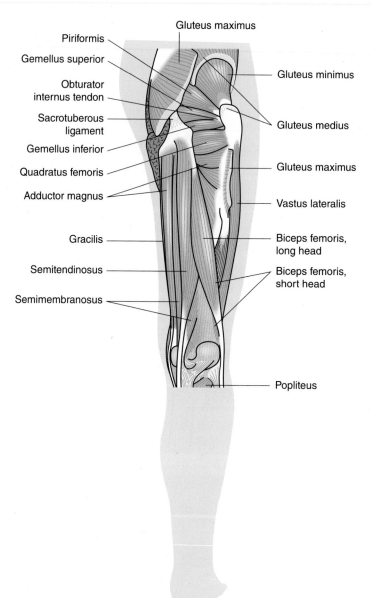

Piriformis

Gemellus superior

Obturator
internus tendon

Sacrotuberous
ligament

Gemellus inferior

Quadratus femoris

Adductor magnus

Gracilis

Semitendinosus

Semimembranosus

Gluteus maximus

Gluteus minimus

Gluteus medius

Gluteus maximus

Vastus lateralis

Biceps femoris,
long head

Biceps femoris,
short head

Popliteus

Fig 1.3.17 Muscles of the posterior thigh

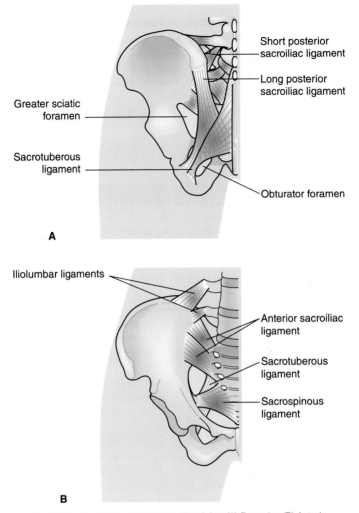

Short posterior
sacroiliac ligament

Long posterior
sacroiliac ligament

Greater sciatic
foramen

Sacrotuberous
ligament

Obturator foramen

A

Iliolumbar ligaments

Anterior sacroiliac
ligament

Sacrotuberous
ligament

Sacrospinous
ligament

B

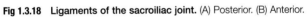

Fig 1.3.18   Ligaments of the sacroiliac joint. (A) Posterior. (B) Anterior.

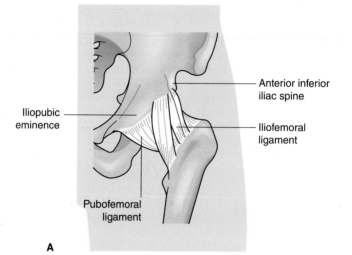

Iliopubic eminence

Anterior inferior iliac spine

Iliofemoral ligament

Pubofemoral ligament

A

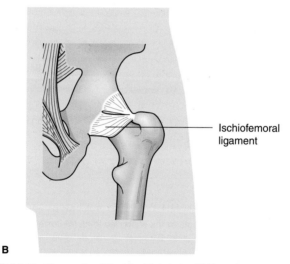

Ischiofemoral ligament

B

Fig 1.3.19   Ligaments of the hip. (A) Anterior. (B) Posterior.

MUSCLES OF THE HIP

Flexors

Muscle	Origin	Insertion	Innervation
Psoas major	Bodies of T12 and all lumbar vertebrae, bases of the transverse processes of all lumbar vertebrae, lumbar intervertebral discs	Lesser trochanter	Anterior rami of the lumbar plexus (L1–L3)
Iliacus	Superior two-thirds of the iliac fossa, inner lip of the iliac crest, ala of the sacrum, anterior sacroiliac and iliolumbar ligaments	Blends with the insertion of the psoas major into the lesser trochanter	Femoral nerve (L2, L3)
Rectus femoris	Straight head – anterior inferior iliac spine; reflected head – area above acetabulum, capsule of the hip joint	Base of the patella, then forms part of the patellar ligament	Femoral nerve (L2–L4)
Sartorius	Anterior superior iliac spine and area just below	Upper part of the medial side of the tibia	Femoral nerve (L2, L3)
Pectineus	Pecten pubis, iliopectineal eminence, pubic tubercle	Along a line from the lesser trochanter to the linea aspera	Femoral nerve (L2, L3), occasionally accessory obturator (L3)

Extensors

Muscle	Origin	Insertion	Innervation
Gluteus maximus	Posterior gluteal line of the ilium, posterior border of the ilium and adjacent part of the iliac crest, aponeurosis of the erector spinae, posterior aspect of the sacrum, side of the coccyx, sacrotuberous ligament, gluteal aponeurosis	Iliotibial tract of the fascia lata, gluteal tuberosity of the femur	Inferior gluteal nerve (L5–S2)
Semitendinosus	Ischial tuberosity	Upper part of the medial surface of the tibia	Tibial division of the sciatic nerve (L5–S2)
Semimembranosus	Ischial tuberosity	Posterior aspect of the medial tibial condyle	Tibial division of the sciatic nerve (L5–S2)
Biceps femoris	Long head – ischial tuberosity, sacrotuberous ligament; short head – the lower half of lateral lip of linea aspera, lateral supracondylar line of the femur, lateral intermuscular septum	Head of the fibula, lateral tibial condyle	Sciatic nerve (L5–S2). Long head – tibial division; short head – common peroneal division

Abductors

Muscle	Origin	Insertion	Innervation
Gluteus maximus	Posterior gluteal line of the ilium, posterior border of the ilium and adjacent part of the iliac crest, aponeurosis of the erector spinae, posterior aspect of the sacrum, side of the coccyx, sacrotuberous ligament, gluteal aponeurosis	Iliotibial tract of the fascia lata, gluteal tuberosity of the femur	Inferior gluteal nerve (L5–S2)
Gluteus medius	Gluteal surface of the ilium between the posterior and anterior gluteal lines	Superolateral side of the greater trochanter	Superior gluteal nerve (L4–S1)
Gluteus minimus	Gluteal surface of the ilium between the anterior and inferior gluteal lines	Anterolateral ridge on the greater trochanter	Superior gluteal nerve (L4–S1)
Tensor fascia lata	Outer lip of the iliac crest between the iliac tubercle and anterior superior iliac spine	Iliotibial tract	Superior gluteal nerve (L4–S1)
Sartorius	Anterior superior iliac spine and area just below	Upper part of the medial side of the tibia	Femoral nerve (L2, L3)
Piriformis	Front of the second to fourth sacral segments, the gluteal surface of the ilium, pelvic surface of the sacrotuberous ligament	Medial side of the greater trochanter	Anterior rami of the sacral plexus (L5–S2)

Adductors

Muscle	Origin	Insertion	Innervation
Adductor magnus	Inferior ramus of the pubis, conjoined ischial ramus, inferolateral aspect of the ischial tuberosity	Linea aspera, proximal part of the medial supracondylar line	Obturator nerve and tibial division of the sciatic nerve (L2–L4)
Adductor longus	Front of the pubis	Middle third of the linea aspera	Anterior division of the obturator nerve (L2–L4)
Adductor brevis	External aspect of the body and inferior ramus of the pubis	Upper half of the linea aspera	Obturator nerve (L2, L3)
Gracilis	Lower half of the body and inferior ramus of the pubis, adjacent ischial ramus	Upper part of the medial surface of the tibia	Obturator nerve (L2, L3)
Pectineus	Pecten pubis, iliopectineal eminence, pubic tubercle	Along a line from the lesser trochanter to linea aspera	Femoral nerve (L2, L3), occasionally accessory obturator (L3)

Medial Rotators

Muscle	Origin	Insertion	Innervation
Gluteus medius	Gluteal surface of the ilium between the posterior and anterior gluteal lines	Superolateral side of the greater trochanter	Superior gluteal nerve (L4–S1)
Gluteus minimus	Gluteal surface of the ilium between the anterior and inferior gluteal lines	Anterolateral ridge on the greater trochanter	Superior gluteal nerve (L4–S1)
Tensor fascia lata	Outer lip of the iliac crest between the iliac tubercle and anterior superior iliac spine	Iliotibial tract	Superior gluteal nerve (L4–S1)

Lateral Rotators

Muscle	Origin	Insertion	Innervation
Gluteus maximus	Posterior gluteal line of the ilium, posterior border of the ilium and adjacent part of the iliac crest, aponeurosis of the erector spinae, posterior aspect of the sacrum, side of the coccyx, sacrotuberous ligament, gluteal aponeurosis	Iliotibial tract of the fascia lata, gluteal tuberosity of the femur	Inferior gluteal nerve (L5–S2)
Piriformis	Front of the second to fourth sacral segments, gluteal surface of the ilium, pelvic surface of the sacrotuberous ligament	Medial side of the greater trochanter	Anterior rami of the sacral plexus (L5–S2)
Obturator internus	Internal surface of the obturator membrane and the surrounding bony margin	Medial surface of the greater trochanter	Nerve to the obturator internus (L5, S1)
Gemellus superior	Gluteal surface of the ischial spine	With the obturator internus tendon into the medial surface of the greater trochanter	Nerve to the obturator internus (L5, S1)
Gemellus inferior	Upper part of the ischial tuberosity	With the obturator internus tendon into the medial surface of the greater trochanter	Nerve to the quadratus femoris (L5, S1)
Quadratus femoris	Ischial tuberosity	Quadrate tubercle midway down the intertrochanteric crest	Nerve to the quadratus femoris (L5, S1)
Obturator externus	Outer surface of the obturator membrane and adjacent bone of the pubic and ischial rami	Trochanteric fossa of the femur	Posterior branch of the obturator nerve (L3, L4)
Sartorius	Anterior superior iliac spine and area just below	Upper part of the medial side of the tibia	Femoral nerve (L2, L3)

Knee, Foot and Ankle

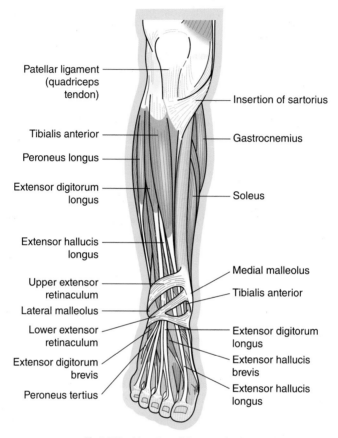

Patellar ligament (quadriceps tendon)

Insertion of sartorius

Tibialis anterior

Gastrocnemius

Peroneus longus

Extensor digitorum longus

Soleus

Extensor hallucis longus

Upper extensor retinaculum

Medial malleolus

Tibialis anterior

Lateral malleolus

Lower extensor retinaculum

Extensor digitorum longus

Extensor hallucis brevis

Extensor digitorum brevis

Peroneus tertius

Extensor hallucis longus

Fig 1.3.20   Muscles of the anterior leg

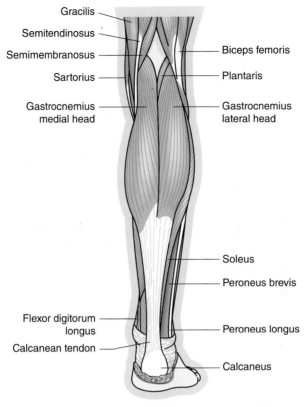

Fig 1.3.21 Superficial muscles of the posterior calf

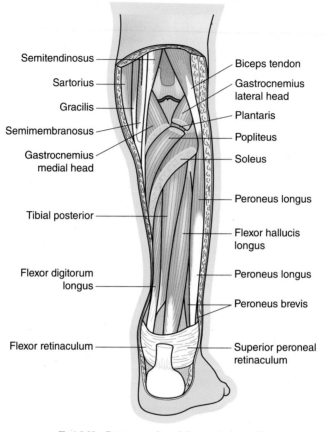

Semitendinosus

Sartorius

Gracilis

Semimembranosus

Gastrocnemius
medial head

Tibial posterior

Flexor digitorum
longus

Flexor retinaculum

Biceps tendon

Gastrocnemius
lateral head

Plantaris

Popliteus

Soleus

Peroneus longus

Flexor hallucis
longus

Peroneus longus

Peroneus brevis

Superior peroneal
retinaculum

Fig 1.3.22   Deep muscles of the posterior calf

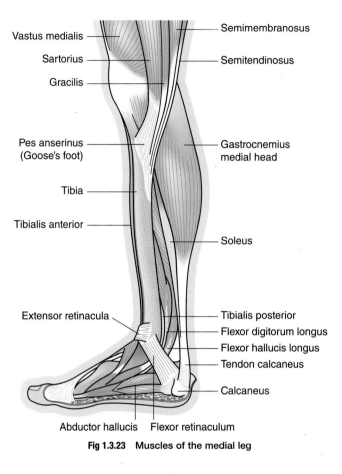

Fig 1.3.23 **Muscles of the medial leg**

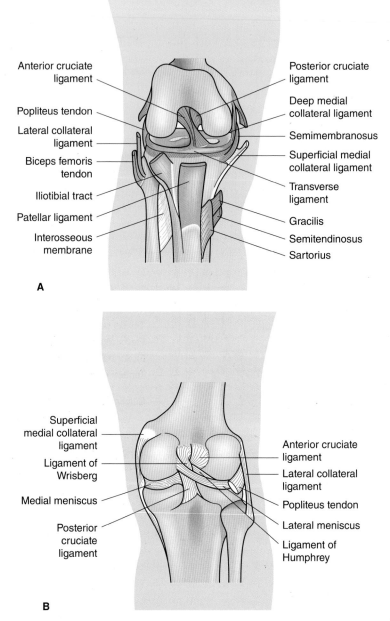

Fig 1.3.24 Ligaments of the knee joint. (A) Anterior. (B) Posterior.

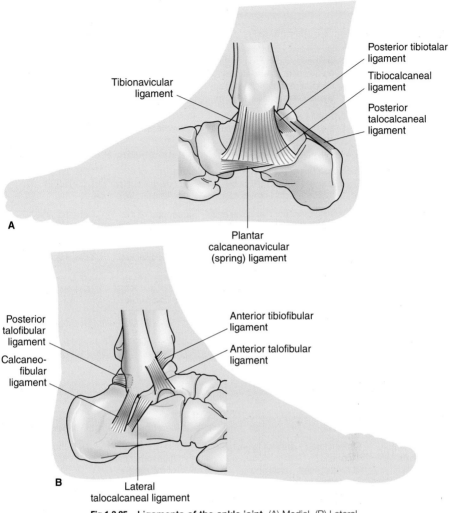

Fig 1.3.25 **Ligaments of the ankle joint.** (A) Medial. (B) Lateral.

MUSCLES OF THE KNEE

Flexors

Muscle	Origin	Insertion	Innervation
Semitendinosus	Ischial tuberosity	Upper part of the medial surface of the tibia	Tibial division of the sciatic nerve (L5–S2)
Semimembranosus	Ischial tuberosity	Posterior aspect of the medial tibial condyle	Tibial division of the sciatic nerve (L5–S2)

Continued on following page

Flexors (Continued)

Biceps femoris	Long head – ischial tuberosity, sacrotuberous ligament Short head – lateral lip of the linea aspera, lateral supra-condylar line of the femur, lateral intermuscular septum	Head of the fibula, lateral tibial condyle	Sciatic nerve (L5–S2)
Gastrocnemius	Medial head – posterior part of the medial femoral condyle Lateral head – lateral surface of the lateral femoral condyle	Posterior surface of the calcaneus	Tibial nerve (S1, S2)
Gracilis	Lower half of the body and inferior ramus of the pubis, adjacent ischial ramus	Upper part of the media surface of the tibia	Obturator nerve (L2, L3)
Sartorius	Anterior superior iliac spine and area just below	Upper part of the medial side of the tibia	Femoral nerve (L2, L3)
Plantaris	Lateral supracondylar ridge, oblique popliteal ligament	Tendon calcaneus	Tibial nerve (S1, S2)
Popliteus	Outer surface of the lateral femoral condyle	Posterior surface of the tibia above the soleal line	Tibial nerve (L4–S1)

Extensors

Muscle	Origin	Insertion	Innervation
Rectus femoris	Straight head – anterior inferior iliac spine Reflected head – area above acetabulum, capsule of the hip joint	Base of the patella, then forms part of the patellar ligament	Femoral nerve (L2-L4)
Vastus lateralis	Intertrochanteric line, greater trochanter, gluteal tuberosity, lateral lip of the linea aspera	Tendon of the rectus femoris, lateral border of the patella	Femoral nerve (L2–L4)
Vastus medialis	Intertrochanteric line, spiral line, medial lip of the linea aspera, medial supracondylar line, medial intermuscular septum, tendons of the adductor longus and adductor magnus	Tendon of the rectus femoris, medial border of the patella, medial tibial condyle	Femoral nerve (L2–L4)
Vastus intermedius	Upper two-thirds of the anterior and lateral surfaces of the femur, lower part of the lateral intermuscular septum	Deep surface of the quadriceps tendon, lateral border of the patella, lateral tibial condyle	Femoral nerve (L2–L4)
Tensor fascia lata	Outer lip of the iliac crest between the iliac tubercle and anterior superior iliac spine	Iliotibial tract	Superior gluteal nerve (L4–S1)

Tibial Lateral Rotators

Muscle	Origin	Insertion	Innervation
Biceps femoris	Long head – ischial tuberosity, sacrotuberous ligament Short head – lateral lip of the linea aspera, lateral supracondylar line of the femur, lateral intermuscular septum	Head of the fibula, lateral tibial condyle	Sciatic nerve (L5–S2)

Tibial Medial Rotators

Muscle	Origin	Insertion	Innervation
Semitendinosus	Ischial tuberosity	Upper part of the medial surface of the tibia	Tibial division of the sciatic nerve (L5–S2)
Semimembranosus	Ischial tuberosity	Posterior aspect of the medial tibial condyle	Tibial division of the sciatic nerve (L5–S2)
Gracilis	Lower half of the body and inferior ramus of the pubis, adjacent ischial ramus	Upper part of the media surface of the tibia	Obturator nerve (L2, L3)
Sartorius	Anterior superior iliac spine and area just below	Upper part of the medial side of the tibia	Femoral nerve (L2, L3)
Popliteus	Outer surface of the lateral femoral condyle	Posterior surface of the tibia above the soleal line	Tibial nerve (L4–S1)

MUSCLES OF THE ANKLE

Plantar Flexors

Muscle	Origin	Insertion	Innervation
Gastrocnemius	Medial head – posterior part of the medial femoral condyle; lateral head – lateral surface of the lateral femoral condyle	Posterior surface of the calcaneus	Tibial nerve (S1, S2)
Soleus	Soleal line and middle third of the medial border of the tibia, posterior surface of the head and upper quarter of the fibula, fibrous arch between the tibia and fibula	Posterior surface of the calcaneus	Tibial nerve (S1, S2)
Plantaris	Lateral supracondylar ridge, oblique popliteal ligament	Tendon calcaneus	Tibial nerve (S1, S2)
Peroneus longus	Lateral tibial condyle, upper two-thirds of the lateral surface of the fibula, intermuscular septa	Lateral side of the base of the first metatarsal, medial cuneiform	Superficial peroneal nerve (L5, S1)

Continued on following page

Plantar Flexors (Continued)

Muscle	Origin	Insertion	Innervation
Tibialis posterior	Lateral aspect of the posterior surface of the tibia below the soleal line, interosseous membrane, upper half of the posterior surface of the fibula, deep transverse fascia	Tuberosity of the navicular, medial cuneiform, sustentaculum tali, intermediate cuneiform, the base of the second to fourth metatarsals	Tibial nerve (L4, L5)
Flexor digitorum longus	Medial part of the posterior surface of the tibia, deep transverse fascia	Plantar aspect of the base of the distal phalanges of the second to fifth toes	Tibial nerve (L5–S2)
Flexor hallucis longus	Lower two-thirds of the posterior surface of the fibula, interosseous membrane, intermuscular septum	Plantar surface of the base of the distal phalanx of the great toe	Tibial nerve (L5–S2)
Peroneus brevis	Lower two-thirds of the lateral surface of the fibula, intermuscular septa	Lateral side of the base of the fifth metatarsal	Superficial peroneal nerve (L5, S1)

Dorsiflexors

Muscle	Origin	Insertion	Innervation
Tibialis anterior	Lateral tibial condyle and upper two-thirds of the lateral surface of the tibia, interosseous membrane	Medial and inferior surface of the medial cuneiform, the base of the first metatarsal	Deep peroneal nerve (L4, L5)
Extensor digitorum longus	Upper three-quarters of the medial surface of the fibula, interosseous membrane, lateral tibial condyle	Middle and distal phalanges of four lateral toes	Deep peroneal nerve (L5, S1)
Extensor hallucis longus	Middle half of the medial surface of the fibula, interosseous membrane	Base of the distal phalanx of the great toe	Deep peroneal nerve (L5)
Peroneus tertius	Distal third of the medial surface of the fibula, interosseous membrane, intermuscular septum	Medial aspect of the base of the fifth metatarsal	Deep peroneal nerve (L5, S1)

Invertors

Muscle	Origin	Insertion	Innervation
Tibialis anterior	Lateral tibial condyle and the upper two-thirds of the lateral surface of the tibia, interosseous membrane	Medial and inferior surface of the medial cuneiform, the base of the first metatarsal	Deep peroneal nerve (L4, L5)
Tibialis posterior	Lateral aspect of the posterior surface of the tibia below the soleal line, interosseous membrane, the upper half of the posterior surface of the fibula, deep transverse fascia	Tuberosity of the navicular, medial cuneiform, sustentaculum tali, intermediate cuneiform, the base of the second to fourth metatarsals	Tibial nerve (L4, L5)

Evertors

Muscle	Origin	Insertion	Innervation
Peroneus longus	Lateral tibial condyle, upper two-thirds of the lateral surface of the fibula, intermuscular septa	Lateral side of the base of the first metatarsal, medial cuneiform	Superficial peroneal nerve (L5, S1)
Peroneus tertius	Distal third of the medial surface of the fibula, interosseous membrane, intermuscular septum	Medial aspect of the base of the fifth metatarsal	Deep peroneal nerve (L5, S1)
Peroneus brevis	Lower two-thirds of the lateral surface of the fibula, intermuscular septa	Lateral side of the base of the fifth metatarsal	Superficial peroneal nerve (L5, S1)

MUSCLES OF THE TOES

Flexors

Muscle	Origin	Insertion	Innervation
Flexor digitorum longus	Medial part of the posterior surface of the tibia, deep transverse fascia	Plantar aspect of the base of distal phalanges of the second to fifth toes	Tibial nerve (L5–S2)
Flexor digitorum accessorius	Medial head – medial tubercle of the calcaneus; lateral head – lateral tubercle of the calcaneus and long plantar ligament	Flexor digitorum longus tendon	Lateral plantar nerve (S1–S3)
Flexor digitorum brevis	Calcaneal tuberosity, plantar aponeurosis, intermuscular septa	Tendons divide and attach to both sides of the base of the middle phalanges of the second to fifth toes	Medial plantar nerve (S1, S2)
Flexor hallucis longus	Lower two-thirds of the posterior surface of the fibula, interosseous membrane, intermuscular septum	Plantar surface of the base of the distal phalanx of the great toe	Tibial nerve (L5–S2)

Continued on following page

Flexors (Continued)

Muscle	Origin	Insertion	Innervation
Flexor hallucis brevis	Medial side of the plantar surface of the cuboid, lateral cuneiform	Medial and lateral sides of the base of the proximal phalanx of the great toe	Medial plantar nerve (S1, S2)
Flexor digiti minimi brevis	Plantar aspect of the base of the fifth metatarsal, sheath of the peroneus longus tendon	Lateral side of the base of the proximal phalanx of the fifth toe	Lateral plantar nerve (S2, S3)
Dorsal interossei (metatarsophalangeal joints)	Proximal half of the sides of adjacent metatarsals	Bases of the proximal phalanges and dorsal digital expansion (first attaches medially to the second toe; second, third, and fourth attach laterally to the second, third, and fourth toes, respectively)	Lateral plantar nerve (S2, S3)
Plantar interossei (metatarsophalangeal joints of the lateral three toes)	Base and medial side of the lateral three toes	Medial side of the base of the proximal phalanx of the same toes and dorsal digital expansions	Lateral plantar nerve (S2, S3)
Lumbricals	Tendons of the flexor digitorum longus	Medial side of the extensor hood and base of the proximal phalanx of the lateral four toes	First lumbrical – medial plantar nerve (S2, S3); lateral three lumbricals – lateral plantar nerve (S2, S3)
Abductor hallucis	Flexor retinaculum, calcaneal tuberosity, plantar aponeurosis, intermuscular septum	Medial side of the base of the proximal phalanx of the great toe	Medial plantar nerve (S1, S2)

Extensors

Muscle	Origin	Insertion	Innervation
Extensor hallucis longus	Middle half of the medial surface of the fibula, the interosseous membrane	Base of the distal phalanx of the great toe	Deep peroneal nerve (L5)
Extensor digitorum longus	Upper three-quarters of the medial surface of the fibula, interosseous membrane, lateral tibial condyle	Middle and distal phalanges of the four lateral toes	Deep peroneal nerve (L5, S1)

Extensors (Continued)

Muscle	Origin	Insertion	Innervation
Extensor digitorum brevis	Superolateral surface of the calcaneus, inferior extensor retinaculum, interosseous talocalcaneal ligament	Base of the proximal phalanx of the great toe, lateral side of the dorsal hood of the adjacent three toes	Deep peroneal nerve (L5, S1)
Lumbricals	Tendons of the flexor digitorum longus	Medial side of the extensor hood and base of the proximal phalanx of the lateral four toes	First lumbrical – medial plantar nerve (S2, S3); lateral three lumbricals – lateral plantar nerve (S2, S3)

Abductors

Muscle	Origin	Insertion	Innervation
Abductor hallucis	Flexor retinaculum, calcaneal tuberosity, plantar aponeurosis, intermuscular septum	Medial side of the base of the proximal phalanx of the great toe	Medial plantar nerve (S1, S2)
Abductor digiti minimi	Calcaneal tuberosity, plantar aponeurosis, intermuscular septum	Lateral side of the base of the proximal phalanx of the fifth toe	Lateral plantar nerve (S1–S3)
Dorsal interossei	Proximal half of the sides of the adjacent metatarsals	Bases of the proximal phalanges and dorsal digital expansion (first attaches medially to the second toe; second, third, and fourth attach laterally to the second, third, and fourth toes, respectively)	Lateral plantar nerve (S2, S3)

Adductors

Muscle	Origin	Insertion	Innervation
Abductor hallucis	Flexor retinaculum, calcaneal tuberosity, plantar aponeurosis, intermuscular septum	Medial side of the base of the proximal phalanx of the great toe	Medial plantar nerve (S1, S2)
Plantar interossei (adduct third to fifth toes)	Base and medial side of the lateral three toes	Medial side of the base of the proximal phalanx of the same toes and dorsal digital expansions	Lateral plantar nerve (S2, S3)

Bones of the Hand and Foot

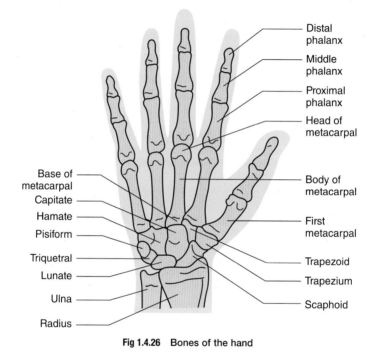

Distal phalanx

Middle phalanx

Proximal phalanx

Head of metacarpal

Base of metacarpal

Capitate

Hamate

Pisiform

Triquetral

Lunate

Ulna

Radius

Body of metacarpal

First metacarpal

Trapezoid

Trapezium

Scaphoid

Fig 1.4.26 Bones of the hand

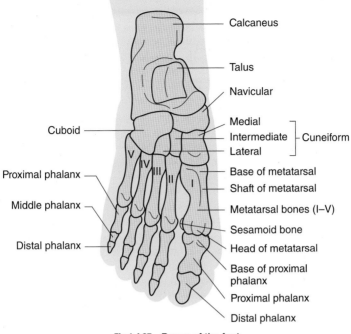

Calcaneus

Talus

Navicular

Cuboid

Medial
Intermediate — Cuneiform
Lateral

Proximal phalanx

Base of metatarsal

Shaft of metatarsal

Middle phalanx

Metatarsal bones (I–V)

Sesamoid bone

Distal phalanx

Head of metatarsal

Base of proximal
phalanx

Proximal phalanx

Distal phalanx

Fig 1.4.27   Bones of the foot

1.5

Muscle Innervation Chart

Muscle Innervation Chart

Upper Limb

C1	C2	C3	C4	C5	C6	C7	C8	T1
Inferior and superior oblique								
Rectus capitis posterior major and minor								
Rectus capitis anterior and lateralis								
Longus capitis								
	Longissimus cervicis							
	Longus colli							
		Levator scapulae						
		Trapezius						
		Diaphragm						
		Splenius capitis						
		Scalenus medius						
			Rhomboid major					
			Rhomboid minor					
			Scalenus anterior					
			Longissimus capitis					
				Biceps brachii				
				Brachioradialis				
				Deltoid				
				Infraspinatus				
				Subscapularis				
				Supraspinatus				
				Teres minor				
				Brachialis				

Muscle Innervation Chart (Continued)

C1	C2	C3	C4	C5	C6	C7	C8	T1
				Coracobrachialis				
				Serratus anterior				
				Splenius cervicis				
				Teres major				
				Pectoralis major				
				Pectoralis minor				
					Extensor carpi radialis longus			
					Flexor carpi radialis			
					Pronator teres			
					Supinator			
					Anconeus			
					Latissimus dorsi			
					Scalenus posterior			
					Triceps brachii			
						Abductor pollicis longus		
						Extensor carpi radialis brevis		
						Extensor carpi ulnaris		
						Extensor digiti minimi		
						Extensor digitorum		
						Extensor indicis		
						Extensor pollicis brevis		
						Extensor pollicis longus		
						Flexor pollicis longus		
						Palmaris longus		
						Pronator quadratus		
						Flexor carpi ulnaris		
							Abductor digiti minimi	
							Abductor pollicis brevis	
							Adductor pollicis	
							Dorsal interossei	

Continued on following page

Muscle Innervation Chart (Continued)

C1	C2	C3	C4	C5	C6	C7	C8	T1
							Flexor digiti minimi brevis	
							Flexor digitorum profundus	
							Flexor digitorum superficialis	
							Flexor pollicis brevis	
							Lumbricals	
							Opponens digiti minimi	
							Opponens pollicis	
							Palmar interossei	

Lower Limb

T12	L1	L2	L3	L4	L5	S1	S2	S3
Quadratus lumborum								
	Psoas minor							
	Psoas major							
		Adductor brevis						
		Gracilis						
		Iliacus						
		Pectineus						
		Sartorius						
		Adductor longus						
		Adductor magnus						
		Rectus femoris						
		Vastus intermedius						
		Vastus lateralis						
		Vastus medialis						
			Obturator externus					
			Gluteus medius					
			Gluteus minimus					
			Popliteus					
				Tibialis anterior				
				Tibialis posterior				
				Tensor fascia lata				

Muscle Innervation Chart (Continued)

T12	L1	L2	L3	L4	L5	S1	S2	S3
					Extensor hallucis longus			
					Extensor digitorum brevis			
					Extensor digitorum longus			
					Gemellus inferior			
					Gemellus superior			
					Obturator internus			
					Peroneus brevis			
					Peroneus longus			
					Peroneus tertius			
					Quadratus femoris			
					Biceps femoris			
					Flexor digitorum longus			
					Flexor hallucis longus			
					Gluteus maximus			
					Piriformis			
					Semimembranosus			
					Semitendinosus			
						Abductor hallucis		
						Flexor digitorum brevis		
						Flexor hallucis brevis		
						Gastrocnemius		
						Plantaris		
						Soleus		
						Abductor digiti minimi		
						Flexor digitorum accessorius		
							Adductor hallucis	
							Dorsal interossei	
							Flexor digiti minimi brevis	
							Lumbricals	
							Plantar interossei	

Source: Data compiled from Standring, S. (2021). *Gray's anatomy: the anatomical basis of clinical practice* (42nd ed). Elsevier.

Musculoskeletal Assessment

Dermatomes

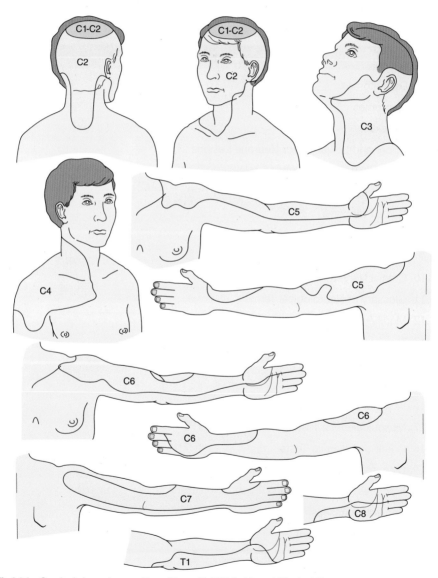

Fig 2.1.1 Cervical dermatomes. From Olson, K. (2021). *Manual Physical Therapy of the Spine.* (3rd Ed) Elsevier.

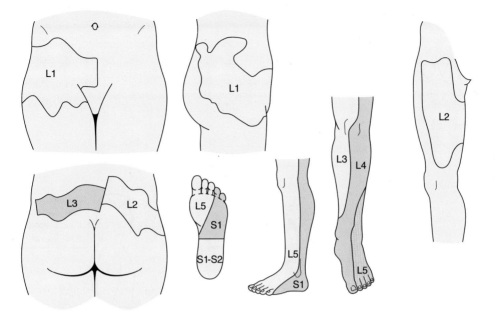

Fig 2.1.2 Lumbar dermatomes. From Olson, K. (2021). *Manual Physical Therapy of the Spine.* (3rd Ed) Elsevier.

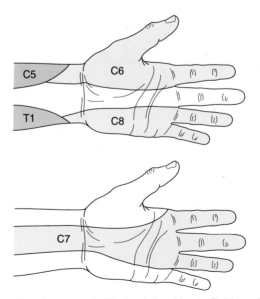

Fig 2.1.3 Dermatomes on the palmar aspect of the hand. From Manske, R., Magee, D. J. (2021). *Orthopedic Physical Assessment* (7th Ed). Elsevier.

Myotomes

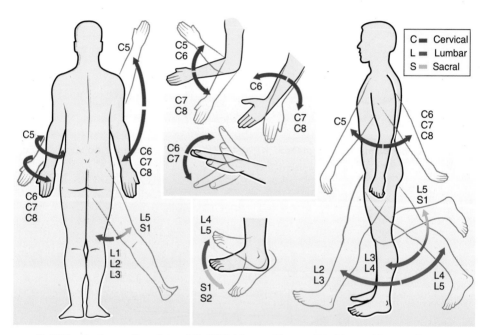

Fig 2.2.4 **Myotomes.** From Salvo, S.G. 2011. Massage Therapy: Principles and Practice. Elsevier.

Joint Movements with the Strongest Association with Each Myotome

Root	Joint Action
C1–C2	Cervical flexion
C3	Cervical lateral flexion
C4	Shoulder girdle elevation
C5	Shoulder abduction
C6	Elbow flexion and/or wrist extension
C7	Elbow extension and/or wrist flexion
C8	Thumb extension and/or ulnar deviation
T1	Finger abduction/adduction
T2–L1	No muscle test
L2	Hip flexion
L3	Knee extension
L4	Ankle dorsiflexion
L5	Great toe extension
S1	Ankle eversion/hip extension/ankle plantar flexion
S2	Knee flexion

Reflexes

Deep Tendon Reflex	Root	Nerve
Biceps jerk	C5–C6	Musculocutaneous
Brachioradialis jerk	C5–C6	Radial
Triceps jerk	C7–C8	Radial
Knee jerk	L3–L4	Femoral
Ankle jerk	S1–S2	Tibial

Testing the Deep Tendon Reflexes in Supine

BICEPS REFLEX

Place the arm in a neutral position between flexion and extension. Place your thumb over the biceps tendon with your fingers curled around the elbow (to locate the tendon, you can ask the patient to resist elbow flexion). Tap the thumb over the tendon briskly. The forearm should flex at the elbow.

TRICEPS REFLEX

Place the arm in a neutral position between flexion and extension. Support the patient's forearm. Locate the triceps insertion on the olecranon. Tap the tendon briskly just above the point where it inserts. The forearm should extend.

BRACHIORADIALIS REFLEX

The brachioradialis tendon is located at the base of the styloid process of the radius. Tap the tendon briskly. The forearm should flex and supinate.

KNEE JERK

Support the knee in a neutral position between flexion and extension. Tap the patellar tendon briskly. The knee should extend, and the quadriceps should contract.

ANKLE JERK

The patient should lie in supine with the leg externally rotated and the knee slightly bent. Grip the patient's forefoot and dorsiflex it slightly. Tap the Achilles tendon briskly just above its insertion on the calcaneus. The foot should plantarflex.

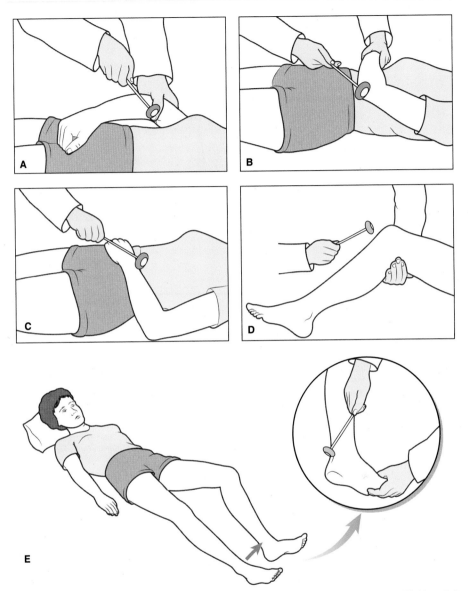

Fig 2.3.5 Testing for reflexes. (A) Biceps jerk. (B) Triceps jerk. (C) Brachioradialis jerk. (D) Knee jerk. (E) Ankle jerk. From Purcell, D. (2017). *Minor Injuries*. Elsevier. (3rd Ed). Elsevier.

Reinforcement Manoeuvres

If a reflex cannot be elicited, a reinforcement manoeuvre can be used to facilitate a stronger response. These can include asking the patient to:

- Clench their teeth or fist
- Hook together the flexed fingers of their right and left hand and pull them apart as forcefully as possible (Jendrassik's manoeuvre)
- Cross the legs at the ankle and push one ankle against the other

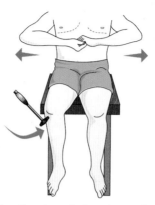

Fig 2.3.6 **Jendrassik's manoeuvre.** From Gesenhues, S., Gesenhues, A. (2020). *Praxisleitfaden Allgemeinmedizin.* (9th Ed). Elsevier.

Other Reflexes

Other Reflexes	Method	Normal Response	Abnormal Response (Indicating Possible Upper Motor Neurone Lesion)
Plantar (superficial reflex)	Run a blunt object over the lateral border of the sole of the foot from the heel up toward the little toe and across the foot pad	Flexion of toes	Extension of the big toe and fanning of other toes (Babinski response)
Clonus (tone)	Apply sudden and sustained dorsiflexion to the ankle	Oscillatory beats may occur, but they are not rhythmic or sustained	More than three rhythmic contractions of the plantarflexors
Hoffman reflex	Flick the distal phalanx of the third or fourth finger downward	No movement of the thumb	Reflex flexion of distal phalanx of thumb

Documenting Reflexes

Reflexes may be recorded using the National Institute of Neurological Disorders and Stroke myotatic reflex scale, noting any asymmetry (Hallet, 1993).

 0 = no response; always abnormal
 1+ = a slight but definitely present response; may or may not be normal
 2+ = a brisk response; normal
 3+ = a very brisk response; may or may not be normal
 4+ = a tap elicits a repeating reflex (clonus); always abnormal

Upper and Lower Motor Neurone Lesions

Key Features of Upper and Lower Motor Neurone Lesions

	Upper Motor Neurone	Lower Motor Neurone
Muscle tone	Increased	Decreased
Clonus	Present	Absent
Muscle fasciculation	Absent	Present
Tendon reflexes	Increased	Depressed or absent
Plantar response	Extensor (Babinski's sign)	Flexor (normal)
Distribution	Extensor weakness in the upper limb and flexor weakness in the lower limb Whole limb(s) involved	Weakness of muscle groups innervated by affected spinal segment/root, plexus, or peripheral nerve

Medical Research Council Scale

The Medical Research Council Scale for Muscle Power

Grade	Response
0	No contraction
1	Flicker or trace of contraction
2	Active movement with gravity eliminated
3	Active movement against gravity
4	Active movement against gravity and resistance
5	Normal strength

In addition, Grade 4 movements may be subdivided into:
4- Movement against slight resistance
4   Movement against moderate resistance
4+ Movement against strong resistance

Source: Medical Research Council. (1976). *Aids to the investigation of peripheral nerve injuries.*
London: HMSO. Used with the kind permission of the Medical Research Council.

Peripheral Nerve Sensory Innervation

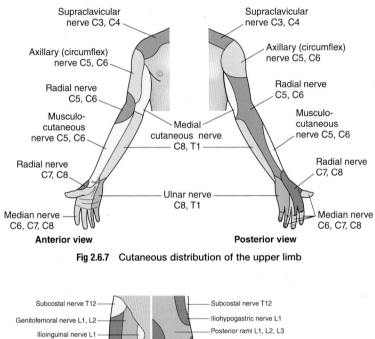

Fig 2.6.7   Cutaneous distribution of the upper limb

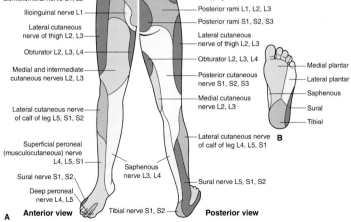

Fig 2.6.8   **Cutaneous distribution of** (A) the lower limb and (B) the foot

Nerve Pathways

Upper Limb

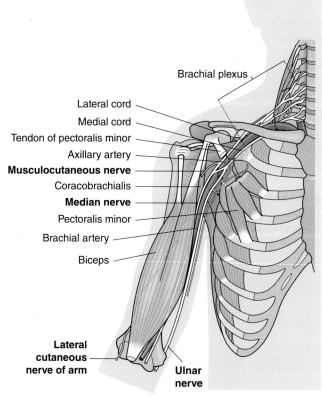

Brachial plexus

Lateral cord

Medial cord

Tendon of pectoralis minor

Axillary artery

Musculocutaneous nerve

Coracobrachialis

Median nerve

Pectoralis minor

Brachial artery

Biceps

Lateral cutaneous nerve of arm

Ulnar nerve

Fig 2.7.9   Brachial plexus and musculocutaneous nerve

MUSCULOCUTANEOUS NERVE

Origin: Large terminal branch of the lateral cord (C5–C7).
Course:

- Descends from the lower border of pectoralis minor, lateral to the axillary artery
- Pierces the coracobrachialis and descends diagonally between the biceps and brachialis to the lateral side of the arm
- Pierces the deep fascia of the antecubital fossa and continues as the lateral cutaneous nerve of the forearm
- Divides into the anterior and posterior branches

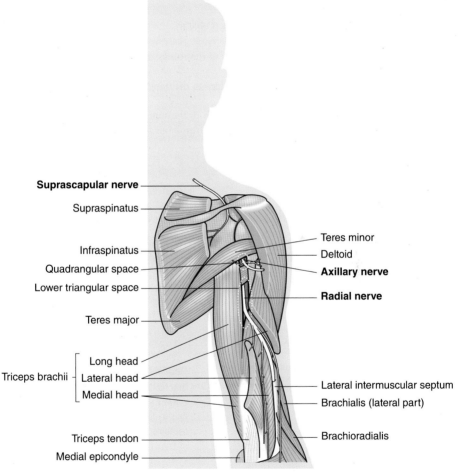

Fig 2.7.10   Axillary and suprascapular nerve

AXILLARY NERVE

Origin: Posterior cord (C5–C6).
Course:

■ Descends laterally posterior to the axillary artery and anterior to the subscapularis
■ Passes posteriorly at the lower border of the subscapularis together with the posterior circumflex humeral vessels via the quadrangular space
■ Divides into the anterior and posterior branches. The anterior branch winds around the surgical neck of the humerus and supplies the anterior deltoid. The posterior branch supplies the teres minor and posterior deltoid. Continues as the upper lateral cutaneous nerve of the arm after passing around the deltoid

SUPRASCAPULAR NERVE

Origin: Superior trunk of the brachial plexus (C5, C6).
Course:

■ Descends inferolaterally above and parallel to the trunks of the brachial plexus and passes through the posterior triangle of the neck
■ Traverses through the suprascapular notch deep to the trapezius and enters the supraspinous fossa of the scapula
■ At the supraspinous fossa, it gives off a branch to the supraspinatus muscle and continues through the spinoglenoid notch to reach the infraspinous fossa
■ It terminates within the infraspinatus muscle

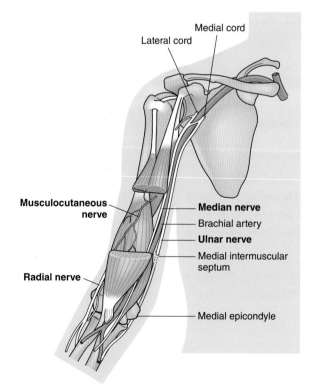

Fig 2.7.11   Median and musculocutaneous nerve

MEDIAN NERVE

Origin: Lateral cord (C5–C7) and medial cord (C8, T1).
Course:

- The two cords unite anterior to the third part of the axillary artery at the inferior margin of the teres major
- Descends lateral to the brachial artery and posterior to the biceps passing medial and anterior to the brachial artery at the insertion of coracobrachialis
- Crosses in front of the elbow lying on the brachialis and deep to the bicipital aponeurosis
- Dives between the two heads of pronator teres and descends through the flexor digitorum superficialis and profundus
- Becomes superficial near the wrist, passing between the tendons of the flexor carpi radialis (lateral) and flexor digitorum superficialis (medial), deep to the palmaris longus
- Passes through the carpal tunnel
- Divides into the medial and lateral branches

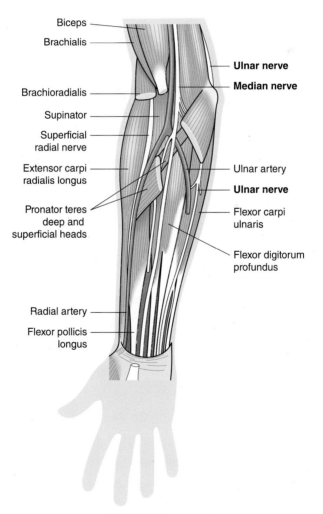

Fig 2.7.12   Ulnar nerve

ULNAR NERVE

Origin: Large terminal branch of the medial cord (C7, C8, T1).

Course:

- Descends medial to the brachial artery and anterior to the triceps as far as the insertion of the coracobrachialis
- Penetrates the medial intermuscular septum and enters the posterior compartment to continue descent anterior to the medial head of the triceps
- Passes posteriorly to the medial epicondyle
- Enters the anterior compartment between the humeral and ulnar heads of the flexor carpi ulnaris
- Descends medially, anterior to the flexor digitorum profundus and posterior to the flexor carpi ulnaris
- Pierces the deep fascia lateral to the flexor carpi ulnaris and proximal to the flexor retinaculum
- Passes anterior to the flexor retinaculum and lateral to the pisiform
- Crosses the hook of hamate
- Divides into the superficial and deep branches

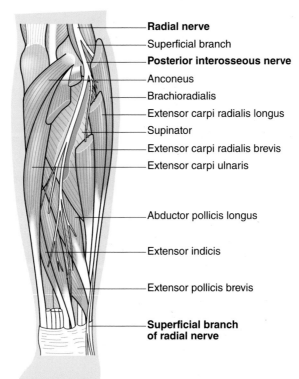

Radial nerve
Superficial branch
Posterior interosseous nerve
Anconeus
Brachioradialis
Extensor carpi radialis longus
Supinator
Extensor carpi radialis brevis
Extensor carpi ulnaris

Abductor pollicis longus

Extensor indicis

Extensor pollicis brevis

Superficial branch of radial nerve

Fig 2.7.13 Radial nerve and posterior interosseous nerve

RADIAL NERVE

Origin: Posterior cord (C5–C8 (T1)).
Course:

- Descends posterior to the axillary and brachial arteries and anterior to the tendons of the subscapularis, latissimus dorsi and teres major
- Enters the posterior compartment via the lower triangular space together with the profunda brachii artery
- Descends obliquely towards the lateral humerus along the spiral groove, lying between the lateral and medial head of the triceps
- Enters the anterior compartment via the lateral intermuscular septum to lie between the brachialis and brachioradialis
- Divides into the superficial radial nerve (sensory) and posterior interosseous nerve (motor) anterior to the lateral epicondyle

POSTERIOR INTEROSSEOUS NERVE

Course:

- Enters the posterior compartment between the two heads of the supinator
- Descends between the deep and superficial groups of the extensors
- Ends in flattened expansion on the interosseous membrane

Lower Limb

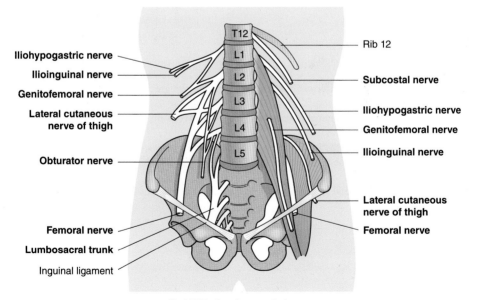

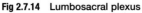

Fig 2.7.14 Lumbosacral plexus

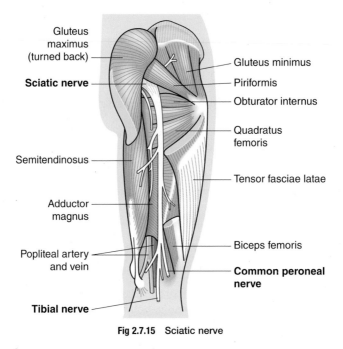

Gluteus maximus (turned back)

Sciatic nerve

Semitendinosus

Adductor magnus

Popliteal artery and vein

Tibial nerve

Gluteus minimus

Piriformis

Obturator internus

Quadratus femoris

Tensor fasciae latae

Biceps femoris

Common peroneal nerve

Fig 2.7.15   Sciatic nerve

SCIATIC NERVE

Origin: Ventral rami L4–S3.

Course:

- Forms anterior to piriformis. Leaves the pelvis via the greater sciatic foramen below the piriformis
- Enters the gluteal region approximately midway between the ischial tuberosity and greater trochanter
- Descends on top of the superior gemellus, obturator internus, inferior gemellus, quadratus femoris and adductor magnus and under the gluteus maximus and long head of the biceps femoris
- Divides into the tibial and common peroneal nerves at approximately the distal third of the thigh

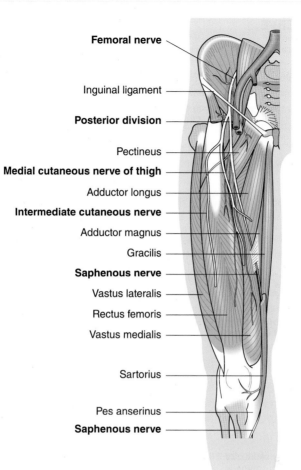

Femoral nerve

Inguinal ligament

Posterior division

Pectineus

Medial cutaneous nerve of thigh

Adductor longus

Intermediate cutaneous nerve

Adductor magnus

Gracilis

Saphenous nerve

Vastus lateralis

Rectus femoris

Vastus medialis

Sartorius

Pes anserinus

Saphenous nerve

Fig 2.7.16 Femoral nerve

FEMORAL NERVE

Origin: Posterior divisions of L2–L4.

Course:

- Posterior divisions unite in the psoas major
- Emerges from the lower lateral border of the psoas major
- Descends in the groove between the psoas major and iliacus, deep to the iliac fossa
- Passes posterior to the inguinal ligament and lateral to the femoral artery
- Enters the femoral triangle
- Divides into a number of anterior and posterior branches

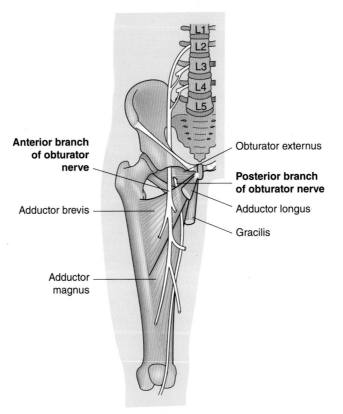

Fig 2.7.17   Obturator nerve

OBTURATOR NERVE

Origin: Anterior divisions of L2–L4.

Course:
- Anterior divisions unite in the psoas major
- Emerges from the psoas major on the lateral aspect of the sacrum
- Crosses the sacroiliac joint and obturator internus
- Enters the obturator canal below the superior pubic rami
- Exits the obturator canal above the obturator externus in the medial compartment of the thigh
- Divides into the anterior and posterior branches (separated by the obturator externus and adductor brevis)

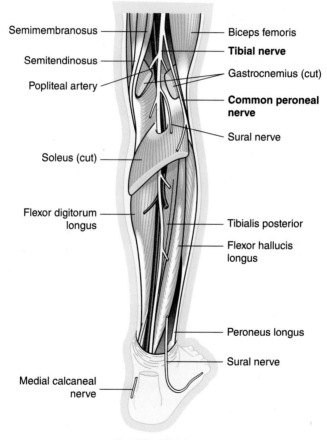

Semimembranosus

Semitendinosus

Popliteal artery

Soleus (cut)

Flexor digitorum longus

Medial calcaneal nerve

Biceps femoris

Tibial nerve

Gastrocnemius (cut)

Common peroneal nerve

Sural nerve

Tibialis posterior

Flexor hallucis longus

Peroneus longus

Sural nerve

Fig 2.7.18   Tibial nerve

TIBIAL NERVE

Origin: Medial terminal branch of sciatic nerve (L4–S3).

Course:

- Descends through the popliteal fossa, passing laterally to medially across the popliteal vessels
- Passes under the tendinous arch of soleus
- Descends inferomedially under the soleus and gastrocnemius, lying on the tibialis posterior and between the flexor digitorum longus and flexor hallucis longus
- Passes through the tarsal tunnel (formed by the flexor retinaculum, which extends from the medial malleolus to the medial calcaneus)
- Enters the plantar aspect of the foot
- Divides into the medial and lateral plantar nerves

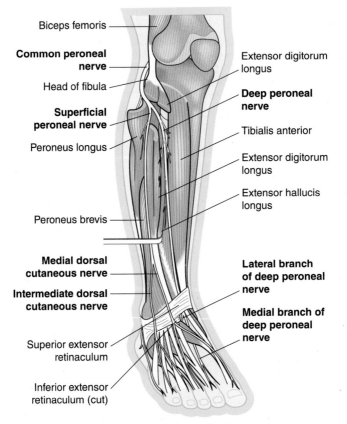

Fig 2.7.19   Common, deep and superficial peroneal nerves

COMMON PERONEAL NERVE

Origin: Lateral terminal branch of the sciatic nerve (L4–S3).

Course:

- Descends along the lateral side of the popliteal fossa between the biceps femoris and lateral head of the gastrocnemius
- Passes anteriorly by winding around the neck of the fibula, deep to the peroneus longus
- Divides into the superficial and deep peroneal nerves

DEEP PERONEAL NERVE

Course:

- Passes inferomedially into the anterior compartment deep to the extensor digitorum longus
- Descends on the interosseous membrane deep to the extensor hallucis longus and superior extensor retinaculum
- Crosses ankle deep to the inferior extensor retinaculum and tendon of the extensor hallucis longus and medial to the tibialis anterior
- Enters the dorsum of the foot between the tendons of the extensor hallucis and digitorum longus
- Divides into the medial and lateral branches

SUPERFICIAL PERONEAL NERVE

Course:

- Descends between the extensor digitorum longus and peroneus longus, anterior to the fibula
- Pierces the deep fascia halfway down the leg to become superficial
- Divides into the medial and intermediate dorsal cutaneous nerves, which enter the foot via the anterolateral aspect of the ankle

2.8

Neurological Tests

Test	Procedure	Possible Pathologies
Finger–nose test	Hold your finger about an arm's length from the patient Ask the patient to touch your finger with their index finger, and then touch their nose, repeating the movement back and forth Patients may demonstrate past pointing (missing your finger) or intention tremor	Cerebellar dysfunction
Heel–shin test	With the patient lying down, ask them to place one heel on the opposite knee, and then run the heel down the tibial shaft toward the ankle and back again Patients may demonstrate intention tremor, an inability to keep the heel on the shin or uncoordinated movements	Cerebellar dysfunction
Dysdiadochoki-nesis (Rapidly alternating movement)	Ask the patient to hold one hand palm up, and then alternately slap it with the palmar and dorsal aspect of the fingers of the other hand Where there is a loss of rhythm and fluency, it is referred to as dysdiadochokinesia For the lower limbs, ask the patient to tap first one foot on the floor and then the other	Cerebellar dysfunction
Hoffman reflex	Flick the distal phalanx of the patient's third or fourth finger. Look for any reflex flexion of the patient's thumb	Upper motor neurone lesion
Joint position sense	Test the most distal joint of the limb (i.e., distal phalanx of the index finger or the interphalangeal joint of the hallux). With the patient's eyes open, demonstrate the movement To test, ask the patient to close their eyes Hold the joint to be tested at the sides between two fingers, and move it up and down Ask the patient to identify the direction of movement, ensuring that you are not moving more proximal joints or brushing against the neighbouring toes or fingers If there is impairment, test more proximal joints	Loss of proprioception
Light touch	Use a wisp of cotton wool. With the patient's eyes open, demonstrate what you are going to do. To test, ask the patient to close their eyes. Stroke the patient's skin with the cotton wool at random points, asking them to indicate every time they feel the touch	Altered touch sensation

Test	Procedure	Possible Pathologies
Pinprick	Use a disposable neurological pin that has a sharp end and a blunt end With the patient's eyes open, demonstrate what you are going to do To test, ask the patient to close their eyes Test various areas of the limb randomly using sharp and blunt stimuli, and ask the patient to tell you which sensation they feel	Altered pain sensation
Plantar reflex (Babinski)	Apply a firm pressure along the lateral aspect of the sole of the foot and across the base of the toes, observing the big toe If the big toe flexes, the response is normal If the big toe extends and the other toes spread, it indicates a positive Babinski's sign	Upper motor neurone lesion
Romberg's test	The patient stands with feet together and eyes open Ask the patient to close their eyes (ensuring that you can support them if they fall) Note any excessive postural sway or loss of balance	Proprioceptive or vestibular deficit if they fall only when they close their eyes
Temperature sense	A quick test involves using a cold object such as a tuning fork and asking the patient to describe the sensation when applied to various parts of the body For more formal testing, two test tubes are filled with cold and warm water, and patients are asked to distinguish between the two sensations	Altered temperature sensation
Two-point discrimination	Requires a two-point discriminator, a device similar to a pair of blunted compasses With the patient's eyes open, demonstrate what you are going to do Ask the patient to close their eyes Alternately touch the patient with either one prong or two Reduce the distance between the prongs until the patient can no longer discriminate between being touched by one or two prongs Varies according to skin thickness, but normal young patients can distinguish a separation of approximately 5 mm in the index finger and approximately 4 cm in the legs Compare left to right	Impaired sensory function
Vibration sense	Use a 128-Hz tuning fork Ask the patient to close their eyes. Place the tuning fork on a bony prominence or the fingertips or toes The patient should report feeling the vibration and not simply the contact of the tuning fork If in doubt, apply the tuning fork and then stop its vibration suddenly by pinching it between your fingers, and see if the patient can correctly identify when it stops vibrating	Altered vibration sense

Neurodynamic Tests

Upper Limb Neurodynamic Test 1: Median Nerve Bias

Upper limb neurodynamic test 1 (Fig 2.9.20) consists of:

- Neutral position of the patient on a couch in supine
- Fixing the shoulder to prevent shoulder elevation during abduction [1]
- Shoulder joint abduction [2]
- Wrist and finger extension [3]
- Forearm supination [3]
- Shoulder lateral rotation [4]
- Elbow extension [5]

Sensitising test: cervical lateral flexion away from the symptomatic side [6].
Desensitising test: cervical lateral flexion towards the symptomatic side.

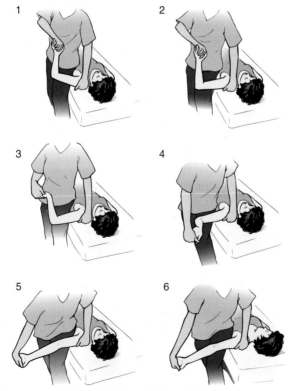

Fig 2.9.20 (1-6) Upper limb neurodynamic test 1

Upper Limb Neurodynamic Test 2a: Median Nerve Bias

Upper limb neurodynamic test 2a (Fig 2.9.21) consists of:

- Neutral position of the patient on a couch in supine
- Shoulder girdle depression [1, 2]
- Elbow extension [3]
- Lateral rotation of the whole arm [4]
- Wrist, finger and thumb extension [5]
- Abduction of the shoulder [6]

Sensitising test: cervical lateral flexion away from the symptomatic side.

Desensitising tests: cervical lateral flexion toward the symptomatic side or release of the shoulder girdle depression.

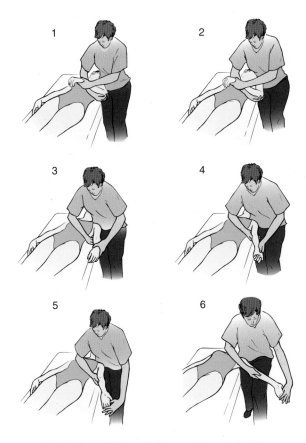

Fig 2.9.21   (1-6) Upper limb neurodynamic test 2a

Upper Limb Neurodynamic Test 2b: Radial Nerve Bias

Upper limb neurodynamic test 2b (Fig 2.9.22) consists of:
- Neutral position of the patient on a couch in supine
- Shoulder girdle depression [1]
- Elbow extension [2]
- Medial rotation of the whole arm [3]
- Wrist, finger and thumb flexion [4]
- Shoulder abduction

Sensitising test: cervical lateral flexion away from the symptomatic side.

Desensitising tests: cervical lateral flexion toward the symptomatic side or release of the shoulder girdle depression.

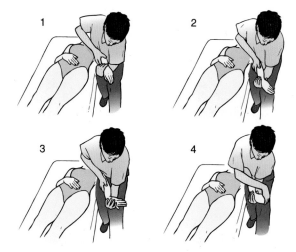

Fig 2.9.22   (1-4) Upper limb neurodynamic test 2b

Upper Limb Neurodynamic Test 3: Ulnar Nerve Bias

Upper limb neurodynamic test 3 (Fig 2.9.23) consists of:
- Neutral position of the patient on a couch in supine
- Shoulder girdle stabilised [1]
- Wrist and finger extension [1]
- Forearm pronation [2]
- Elbow flexion [3]
- Shoulder lateral rotation [4]
- Shoulder abduction [5]

Sensitising test: cervical lateral flexion away from the symptomatic side.

Desensitising tests: cervical lateral flexion toward the symptomatic side or release of the shoulder girdle depression.

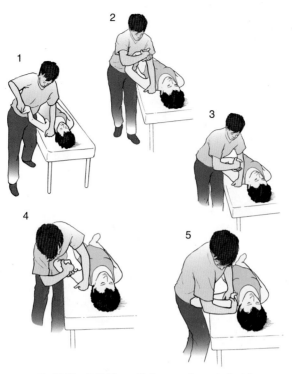

Fig 2.9.23   (1-5) Upper limb neurodynamic test 3

Slump Test

Starting position: patient sits upright with the knee crease at the edge of the plinth and hands behind their back [1].

The slump test (Fig 2.9.24) consists of:

- Spinal slump [2]
- Cervical flexion [3]
- Knee extension [4]
- Release neck flexion [5]

The steps can be performed in any order.

Additional movements: add dorsiflexion or plantarflexion with knee extension, bilateral knee extension [6], hip abduction (obturator nerve bias), hip medial rotation and hip flexion.

Positive test: development of pain or discomfort in the mid-thoracic area, behind the knees or in the hamstrings; restriction of knee extension while slumped with the neck flexed; restriction of dorsiflexion while slumped with the neck flexed.

Release of neck flexion decreases pain or increases the range of knee extension and/or dorsiflexion.

Desensitising test: a decrease in pain or increase in range of knee extension and/or dorsiflexion with cervical extension.

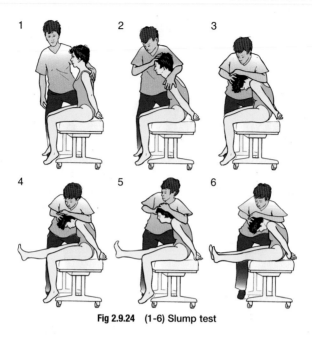

Fig 2.9.24   (1-6) Slump test

Straight Leg Raise

Starting position: the patient lies supine. The test consists of passive hip flexion with the knee in extension.

Normal response: a feeling of stretch or tingling in the posterior leg. Altered responses can be determined by comparing one side with the other.

Sensitising tests: dorsiflexion, hip adduction, hip medial rotation, neck flexion and trunk lateral flexion.

Additional sensitising tests: add ankle dorsiflexion and forefoot eversion (tibial nerve bias), ankle plantarflexion and forefoot inversion (common peroneal nerve bias), dorsiflexion and inversion (sural nerve bias).

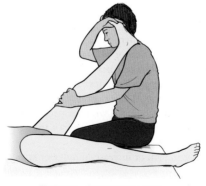

Fig 2.9.25   Straight leg raise

Passive Neck Flexion

Starting position: the patient lies supine. The test consists of passive neck flexion.
Normal response: full, pain-free movement.
Sensitising tests: straight leg raise, upper limb neurodynamic tests.

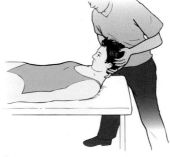

Fig 2.9.26   Passive neck flexion

Femoral Nerve Slump Test

Starting position: patient side-lying with the symptomatic side uppermost. Holds bottom knee
   to chest and flexes neck.
Sensitising tests: the uppermost knee is passively flexed and the hip extended.
Positive test: reproduction of symptoms in the anterior thigh.
Desensitising test: cervical extension reduces symptoms.
Additional sensitising tests: hip medial or lateral rotation and/or hip abduction/adduction.

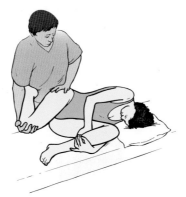

Fig 2.9.27   Femoral nerve slump test

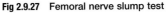

2.10

Cranial Nerves

Cranial nerves arise from the brainstem and have motor and/or sensory roles, including vision, smell and sensation. They also supply the muscles involved in facial expression and eye, jaw and shoulder movements.

Their function can be affected by a range of pathologies, from tumours and space-occupying lesions within the skull and brain to infection, inflammation and demyelinating diseases.

Examination may be prompted when faced with symptoms such as headache, dizziness, visual disturbance and balance problems, especially in the context of neck pain. Symptoms may be transient (as in transient ischaemic attacks) or more persistent.

Examination of Cranial Nerves

Cranial Nerve (Number)	Cranial Nerve (Name)	Function	Test	Pathologies
I	Olfactory	Smell	Identify a familiar odour (e.g., coffee, mint, or orange)	Common • Nasal congestion/infections affect smell (not from olfactory nerve lesion) Rare • Head injury • Skull base tumours • Parkinson's disease • Huntington's disease

II	Optic	Visual acuity	• Acuity
			  • use a Snellen chart
			• Visual field testing
			  • detect an object brought into their field of vision with the other eye closed
				Visual field defects and loss of acuity (e.g., bitemporal hemianopia [lesion at the optic chasm], pituitary tumour

III	Occulomotor	• Eye and eyelid movement (all movements except abduction and looking down when adducted)
		• Pupil constriction
		• Lens accommodation
			• Eye movements
			  • tracking an object moving in an H pattern in front of them whilst keeping the head in a neutral position
			• Pupillary reaction to light and accommodation
				• Third nerve palsy causes ptosis and loss of movements (eye tends to be left looking down and outward)
				May be caused by:
				  • tumours
				  • brainstem lesions
				  • aneurysm
				  • infarction
				  • trauma
				• Horner's syndrome
				• Myasthenia gravis

IV	Trochlear	• Eye movement
		  • downward and inward
			• Eye movements
			  • tracking an object moving in an H pattern in front of them, keeping the head in a neutral position
				• Diplopia and eye drifting upward
				• Rare: caused by lesions within the midbrain

Continued on following page

Examination of Cranial Nerves (Continued)

Cranial Nerve (Number)	Cranial Nerve (Name)	Function	Test	Pathologies

V	Trigeminal
	There are three branches:
	1. Ophthalmic (V1)
	2. Maxillary (V2)
	3. Mandibular (V3)
		• Sensation to the face and mouth
		• Muscles in the jaw for chewing
			• Sensory component
			  • check facial sensation: fine touch throughout all three territories
			• Motor component
			  • direct patient to clench teeth (palpate masseter/temporalis muscles for tone and symmetry)
			  • open jaw and test movement of jaw side to side against resistance and assess strength
				• Pain (trigeminal neuralgia)
				• Loss of ability to chew
				• Loss of sensation in the face
				• May be caused by:
				  • facial or sinus cancer
				  • shingles (herpes zoster)
				  • facial fractures

VI	Abducens	• Eye movement
		  • lateral gaze
			• Eye movements
			  • tracking an object moving in an H pattern in front of them whilst keeping their head in a neutral position
				• Loss of lateral movement with double vision
				• Caused by:
				  • cancers
				  • trauma
				  • cerebrovascular accident
				  • diabetes
				  • mastoid and middle ear infections (children)

VII	Facial	• Motor fibres to muscles involved in facial expression
		• Parasympathetic fibres to the tear and salivary glands
			• Test facial muscles
			  • raise eyebrows
			  • screw up eyes and resist opening
			  • smile
			  • ow out cheeks
				• Bell's palsy (lower motor neurone)
				  • cannot raise eyebrows/wrinkle forehead: distinguishes from upper motor neurone lesions where this is preserved
				  • Loss of taste
				  • Ramsay-Hunt syndrome
				• lower motor nerve palsy associated with shingles
				• Upper motor neurone palsy due to:
				  • stroke
				  • tumour
				  • multiple sclerosis (unilateral)
				  • trauma

	Nerve	Function	Examination	Clinical features
VIII	Vestibulocochlear	• Hearing • Balance	• Rub fingers together near the patient's ear on one side of the head (whilst holding fingers on the other ear still) ◦ ask the patient to identify the side where they can hear the noise • Whisper numbers into one ear and ask the patient to repeat • Audiometry is required for formal testing	• Hearing loss • Tinnitus • Vertigo and balance problems • May be caused by: ◦ infection ◦ tumours (acoustic neuroma) ◦ brainstem lesions ◦ Meniere's disease ◦ diabetes ◦ hypothyroidism ◦ Paget's disease ◦ age-related loss (presbyacusis or otosclerosis)
IX	Glossopharyngeal	• Sensation and taste for the posterior third of the tongue • Swallow • Salivation • Regulation of blood pressure	• Swallow • Evoke the gag reflex by touching the back of the throat with a tongue depressor	• Loss of tongue sensation and taste • Reduced salivation • Dysphagia • Rarely affected in isolation • May be caused by: ◦ skull base tumours ◦ fracture
X	Vagus	• Motor and sensation for heart, lungs, digestive tract, and diaphragm • Secretion of digestive fluids • Taste • Swallow • Hiccups	As for glossopharyngeal	• Vocal cord paralysis • Dysphagia • Loss of sensation from internal organs • Bilateral X nerve palsy • Causes include: ◦ motor neurone disease ◦ cerebrovascular disease (stroke) ◦ multiple sclerosis
XI	Accessory	Motor function to the soft palate, larynx, pharynx, trapezius, and sternocleidomastoid	• Rotate neck to one side and resist flexion (i.e., contract sternocleidomastoid) • Shrug shoulders against resistance	• Paralysis of innervated muscles • May occur due to: ◦ surgery to the neck (posterior triangle) ◦ trauma ◦ local tumours
XII	Hypoglossal	Control of tongue and strap muscles of the neck	• Stick out the tongue • Push the tongue into the left and right sides of the cheek	• Dysphagia • Dysarthria • Difficulty masticating • May be seen alongside lesions in IX, X, and XI nerves in motor neurone disease (bulbar palsy)

Glossary of Neurological Terms

Acalculia	Inability to calculate
Agnosia	Inability to interpret sensations such as sounds (auditory agnosia), three-dimensional objects by touch (tactile agnosia) or symbols and letters (visual agnosia)
Agraphia	Inability to write
Akinesia	Loss of the ability to initiate movement and episodes of "freezing" during movement
Alexia	Inability to read
Allodynia	A painful response to a non-noxious stimulus
Amnesia	Total or partial loss of memory
Amusia	Impaired recognition of music
Aneurysm	A bulge in a blood vessel (usually an artery) caused by a weakness in the vessel wall
Anomia	Inability to name objects
Anosmia	Loss of ability to smell
Anosognosia	Denial of ownership or the existence of a hemiplegic limb
Aphasia	Inability to generate and understand language, whether verbal or written
Apraxia	A motor planning disorder characterised by an inability to perform learned movements despite intact power, sensation, coordination, perception and understanding. Different forms include ideomotor (inability to carry out motor commands but able to perform movements under different circumstances) and ideational (inability to carry out a sequence of movements, each of which can be performed separately), constructional (inability to build, assemble or draw objects), oculomotor (impaired voluntary eye movement), dressing and gait
Astereognosis	Inability to recognise objects by touch alone, despite intact sensation
Ataxia	Shaky and uncoordinated voluntary movements that may be associated with cerebellar or posterior column disease
Athetosis	Involuntary writhing movements affecting the face, tongue and hands
Ballismus	Sudden, involuntary violent flinging movements of limbs, usually unilateral (hemiballismus)
Bradykinesia	Slowness of movement
Bulbar	Relating to or involving the medulla oblongata
Chorea	Irregular, jerky, involuntary movement
Clonus	More than three rhythmic contractions of the plantarflexors in response to sudden passive dorsiflexion

Decorticate rigidity	Characterised by bent arms held in toward the chest, clenched fists and extended lower limbs. Associated with disinhibition of the red nucleus (midbrain) and disruption of the lateral corticospinal tract
Decerebrate rigidity	Characterised by extended and internally rotated upper and lower limbs, with the wrists in flexion, the ankles in plantarflexion and the head in extension. Usually indicates damage to the brainstem, specifically lesions in the midbrain and cerebellum
Diplopia	Double vision
Dysaesthesia	Perverted response to sensory stimuli producing an abnormal and sometimes unpleasant sensation
Dysarthria	Difficulty articulating speech
Dysdiadochokinesia	Clumsiness in performing rapidly alternating movements
Dyskinesia	Involuntary movements (e.g. tremor, chorea, dystonia, myoclonus)
Dysmetria	Under- or overshooting while reaching toward a target
Dysphagia	Difficulty or inability to swallow
Dysphasia	Difficulty understanding language (receptive dysphasia) or generating language (expressive dysphasia)
Dysphonia	Difficulty in producing the voice
Dyssynergia	Clumsy, uncoordinated movements
Dystonia	Hypertonia associated with abnormal postural movements caused by the co-contraction of agonists and antagonists, usually at an extreme flexion or extension
Extrapyramidal signs	Refers to the neural network (principally the basal ganglia) located outside the pyramids of the medulla that modulates and regulates pyramidal function (i.e. movement)
Fasciculation	Small, local involuntary muscle contraction (twitching)
Graphanaesthesia	Inability to recognise numbers or letters traced onto the skin with a blunt object
Hemianopia	Loss of half the normal visual field
Hemiparesis	Weakness affecting one side of the body
Hemiplegia	Paralysis affecting one side of the body
Homonymous	Affecting the same side (i.e. homonymous diplopia)
Hyperacusis	Increased sensitivity to sound
Hyperaesthesia	Increased sensitivity to any stimulus
Hyperalgesia	Increased sensitivity to a noxious stimulus
Hyperreflexia	Increased reflexes
Hypertonia	Increase in normal muscle tone
Hypertrophy	Abnormal increase in tissue size
Hypoaesthesia	Reduced sensitivity to any stimulus
Hypokinesia	Slowness in the initiation of movement
Hypotonia	Reduced muscle tone
Kinaesthesia	Perception of body position and movement
Miosis	Pupil constriction

Continued on following page

Monoparesis	Weakness affecting one limb
Monoplegia	Paralysis affecting one limb
Myoclonus	Brief, involuntary, shock-like jerks of a muscle/group of muscles
Myotonia	Persistent muscle contraction after cessation of voluntary contraction
Nystagmus	Involuntary, repetitive, oscillatory movement of the eye in one direction, alternating with a slower movement in the opposite direction
Paraesthesia	Tingling sensation often described as 'pins and needles'
Paraphasia	Insertion of inappropriate or incorrect words in a person's speech
Paraplegia	Paralysis of both legs
Paresis	Muscle weakness
Photophobia	Intolerance to light
Prosopagnosia	Inability to recognise faces
Ptosis	Drooping of the upper eyelid
Pyramidal signs	Refers to the corticospinal tract that travels from the motor cortex to the brainstem and spinal cord via the pyramids of the medulla. Injuries to the corticospinal tract show characteristics of an upper motor neurone lesion
Rigidity	Hypertonia, associated with increased resistance to passive stretch at very low speeds of movement, is not velocity-dependent and can simultaneously affect agonists and antagonists and movements in both directions. Subtypes are "cog-wheel" (increased resistance that gives way in little jerks) and "lead-pipe" (sustained resistance throughout the whole range of movement)
Quadrantanopia	Loss of a quarter of the normal visual field
Quadriparesis	Weakness of all four limbs
Quadriplegia	Paralysis of all four limbs
Spasticity	Hypertonia associated with exaggerated deep tendon reflexes and a velocity-dependent increase in muscle resistance in response to passive stretch that varies with the direction of joint movement. Subtypes are "clasp-knife" (initial increased resistance to stretch that suddenly gives way) and "clonus" (repetitive rhythmic contractions in response to a maintained stretch)
Stereognosis	Ability to identify common objects by touch alone
Tetraplegia	Another term for quadriplegia
Tetraparesis	Another term for quadriparesis

Modified Ashworth Scale

Grade	Description
0	Normal tone, no increase in muscle tone
1	Slight increase in muscle tone, manifested by a catch and release or by minimal resistance at the end of the range of motion (ROM) when the affected part(s) is moved in flexion or extension
1 +	Slight increase in muscle tone, manifested by a catch, followed by minimal resistance throughout the remainder (less than half) of the ROM
2	A more marked increase in muscle tone through most of the ROM but the affected part(s) easily moved
3	Considerable increase in muscle tone, passive movement difficult
4	Affected part(s) rigid in flexion or extension

Trigger Points

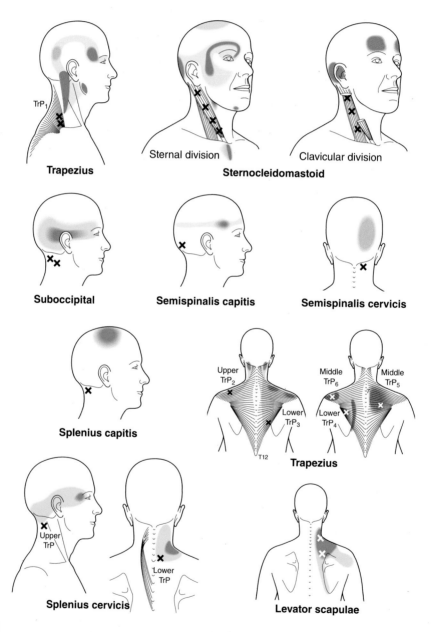

Trapezius

TrP₁

Sternal division Clavicular division

Sternocleidomastoid

Suboccipital

Semispinalis capitis

Semispinalis cervicis

Splenius capitis

Upper TrP₂ Middle TrP₆ Middle TrP₅

Lower TrP₃ Lower TrP₄

T12

Trapezius

Upper TrP

Lower TrP

Splenius cervicis

Levator scapulae

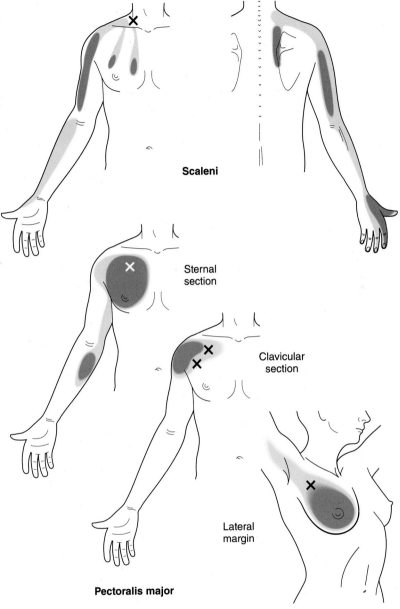

Scaleni

Sternal
section

Clavicular
section

Lateral
margin

Pectoralis major

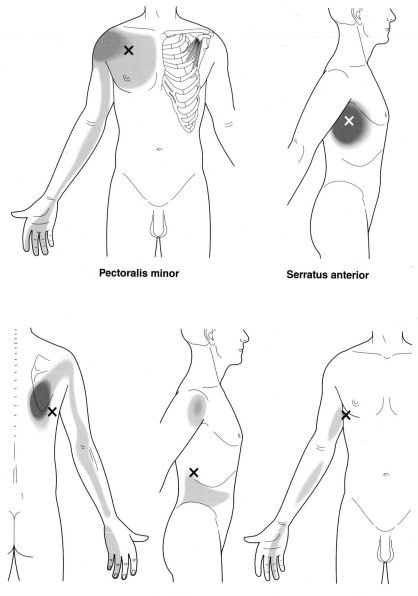

Pectoralis minor

Serratus anterior

Latissimus dorsi

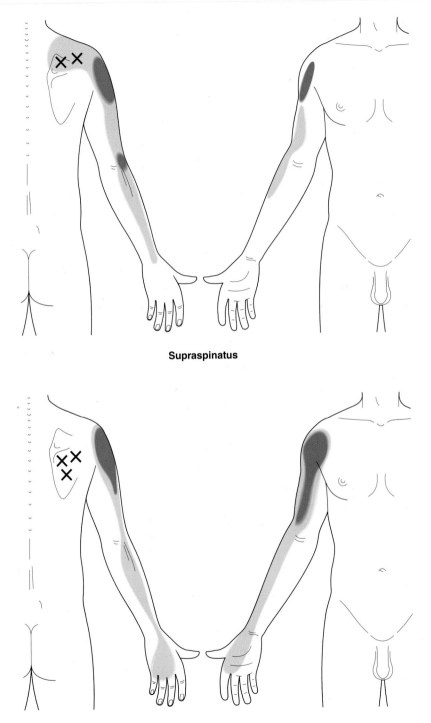

Supraspinatus

Infraspinatus

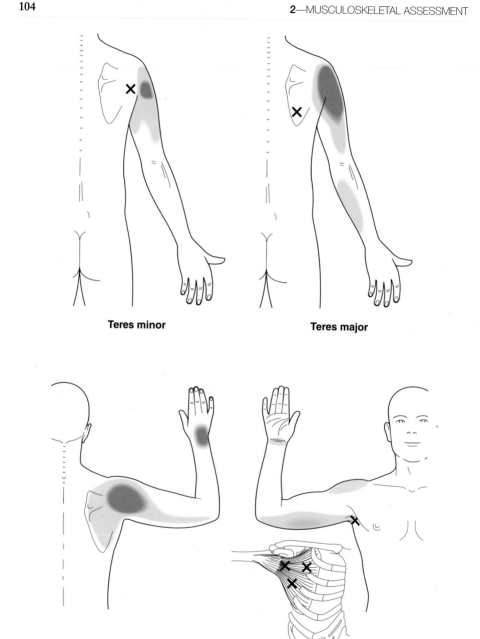

Teres minor

Teres major

Subscapularis

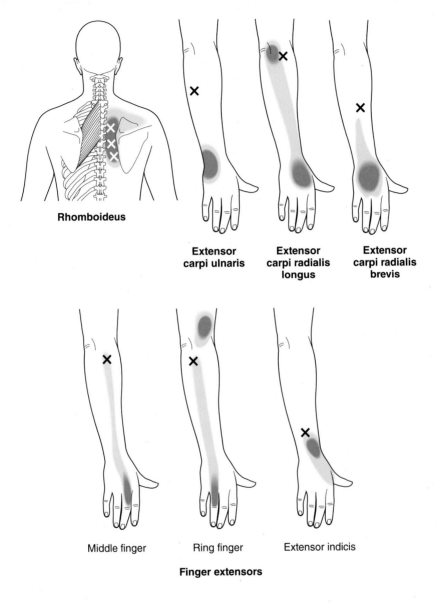

Rhomboideus

Extensor carpi ulnaris

Extensor carpi radialis longus

Extensor carpi radialis brevis

Middle finger

Ring finger

Extensor indicis

Finger extensors

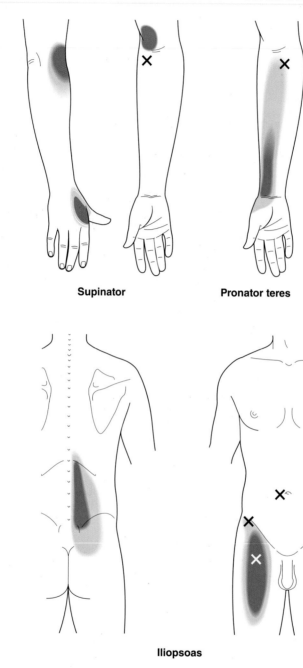

Supinator   **Pronator teres**

Iliopsoas

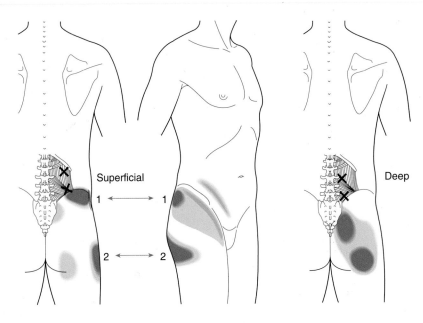

Quadratus lumborum

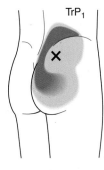

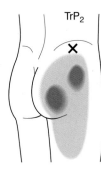

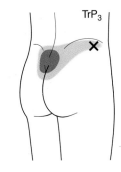

Gluteus medius

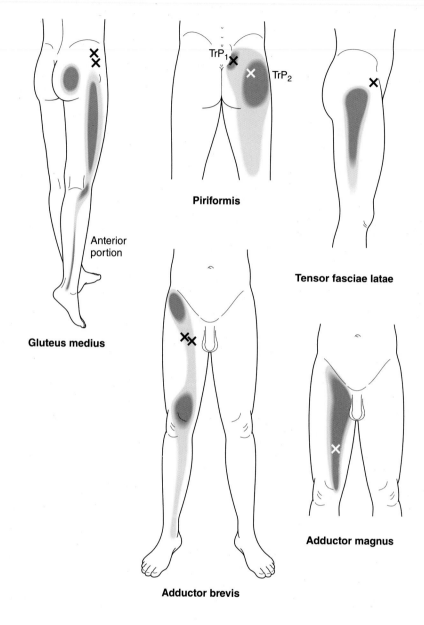

Gluteus medius

Anterior
portion

Piriformis

Tensor fasciae latae

Adductor brevis

Adductor magnus

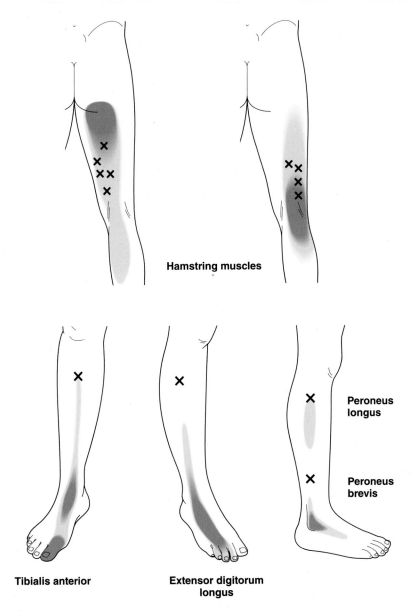

Hamstring muscles

Tibialis anterior

Extensor digitorum longus

Peroneus longus

Peroneus brevis

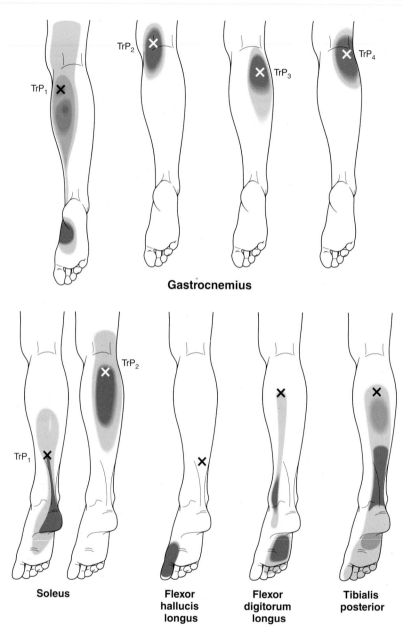

Gastrocnemius

Soleus

Flexor hallucis longus

Flexor digitorum longus

Tibialis posterior

Visceral Referral Patterns

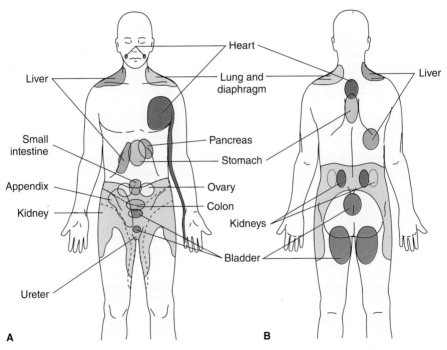

Fig 2.14.29 Sites of referred pain. (A) Front. (B) Back. From Harding, M. M., et al. (2020). *Lewis's medical-surgical nursing: Assessment and management of clinical problems* (11th ed.). St. Louis, MO: Elsevier.

Flags in Back Pain

Flag	Domain	Examples
Red[1]	Signs of serious pathology	Cancer • History of cancer – especially those that metastasise to bone • Unexplained weight loss (5-10% over a 3-6 month period) • Constant, progressive pain – not responding to treatment • Night pain (an inability to lie flat)
		Infection • History of immunosuppression • Intravenous drug use • History of TB – in or from an area where TB is endemic • Fever • Night sweats • Systemically unwell
		Fracture • Thoracic back pain • History of osteoporosis • History of corticosteroid use >5 mg/day for > 3 months • History of previous spinal fracture • History of severe trauma (e.g. fall from height; five stairs or 3 feet) • Increased age and female sex
		Cauda equina syndrome • Saddle anaesthesia • Bladder disturbance • Bowel disturbance • Back and/or nerve pain (especially if alternating leg pain or progressive from unilateral to bilateral leg pain) • Loss of sexual function
Orange[6,2,7]	Psychiatric features	• Depression • Anxiety, irritability, distress • Substance misuse

Flag	Domain	Examples
Yellow[7,5-6]	Beliefs	• Pain = Harm • Pain must go before returning to activity • Pain is uncontrollable • There is nothing that can be done
	Emotions	• Fear of pain • Depression • Anxiety, irritability, distress • Fear of movement • Learned helplessness
	Behaviours	• Extended time off • Withdrawal from activities • Activity intolerance/avoidance • Poor compliance • Reliance on aids/appliances
Blue[7,6,3]	Occupational	• Belief that work will make the pain worse/cause injury • Perceived lack of support from co-workers/boss
Black[6,7]	System or contextual factors	• History of compensation claims/ongoing claims • Ill health retirement benefit issues • Overprotective partner • Lack of support • Cultural beliefs/behaviours
	Healthcare related[4,8]	• Conflicting opinions/advice • Unhelpful language • Over investigation • Prolonged use of passive treatments • Advice to stop activities

References

1. Finucane, L. M., et al. (2020). International framework for red flags for potential serious spinal pathologies. *The Journal of Orthopaedic and Sports Physical Therapy, 50*(7), 350–372.
2. Glattacker, M., Heyduck, K., Jakob, T. (2018). Yellow flags as predictors of rehabilitation outcome in chronic low back pain. *Rehabilitation Psychology, 63*(3), 408–417.
3. Gray, H., Adefolarin, A. T., Howe, T. E. (2011). A systematic review of instruments for the assessment of work-related psychosocial factors (Blue Flags) in individuals with non-specific low back pain. *Manual Therapy, 16*(6), 531–543.
4. Kouyanou, K., Pither, C.E. and Wessely, S., 1997. Iatrogenic factors and chronic pain. *Psychosomatic Medicine*, 59(6), pp.597-604.
5. Hallner, D., Hasenbring, M. (2004). Classification of psychosocial risk factors (yellow flags) for the development of chronic low back and leg pain using artificial neural network. *Neuroscience Letters, 361*(1-3), 151–154.
6. Hayden, J. A., et al. (2010). What is the prognosis of back pain? *Best Practice & Research. Clinical Rheumatology*, 24, 167–179.
7. Nicholas, M. K., Linton, S. J., Watson, P. J., Main, C. J. (2011). "Decade of the flags" working group. Early identification and management of psychological risk factors ("yellow flags") in patients with low back pain: a reappraisal. *Physical Therapy*, 91(5):737–753.
8. Wippert, P. M., Fliesser, M., Krause, M. (2017). Risk and protective factors in the clinical rehabilitation of chronic back pain. *Journal of Pain Research*, 10, 1569–1579.

Vascular Assessment

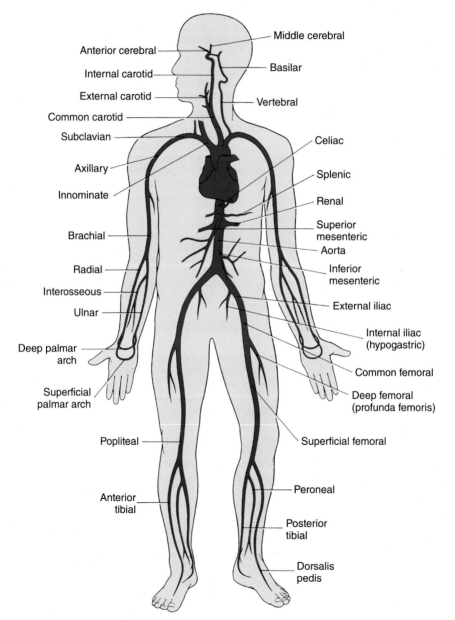

Fig 2.16.30 Anatomy of the major arteries. From Fahey, V. A. 2004. *Vascular Nursing* (4th ed). Philadelphia: Saunders.

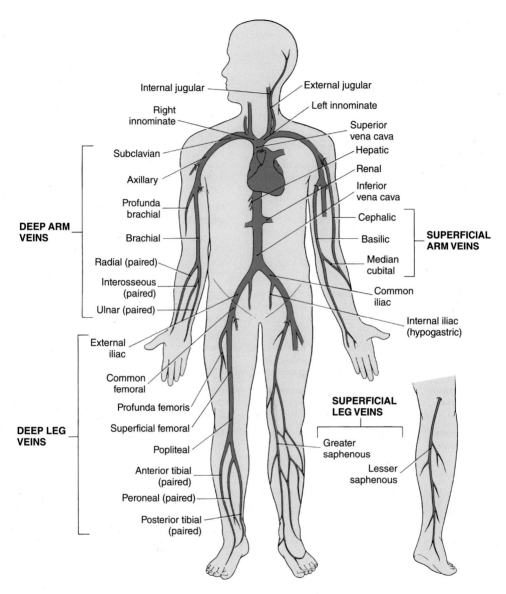

Fig 2.16.31 Anatomy of the major veins. From Fahey, V. A. 2004. *Vascular Nursing* (4th ed). Philadelphia: Saunders.

Pulse Sites

Pulse	Site	Notes
Radial	**Wrist** • Below the thumb and lateral to the flexor tendons (flexor carpi radialis)	• Feel both radial arteries together – if they are out of sync, this may imply aortic dissection or subclavian artery stenosis • Palpate whilst lifting the arm to detect a 'collapsing pulse' (sign of aortic regurgitation)
Brachial	**Antecubital fossa** • Medial to the biceps tendon	• The brachial pulse may be used in preference to other pulse sites to assess the volume and character of the peripheral pulse
Carotid	**Neck** • At the angle of the jaw, anterior to the sternomastoid	• Auscultation of the carotid artery for bruits may suggest carotid artery stenosis (useful if features of transient ischemic attack/cerebrovascular accident)
Axillary	**Axilla** • Lateral wall of the axilla in the groove behind the coracobrachialis	• May be a site of compression or occlusion relating to thoracic outlet syndrome
Femoral	**Groin** • Below the inguinal ligament at the mid-inguinal point	• Can be felt in conjunction with radial pulse and, if out of sync, may suggest coarctation of the aorta*
Popliteal	**Popliteal fossa** • Lies deep in the midline at the level of the knee crease	• A pulsatile mass here would imply a popliteal aneurysm, whilst a pulseless mass would suggest a Baker's cyst
Anterior tibial	**Ankle** • Above the level of the ankle joint, between the tibialis anterior and extensor hallucis longus tendons	• Useful to assess for peripheral arterial disease
Posterior tibial	**Medial aspect of the ankle** • 2 cm below and behind the medial malleolus	• Useful to assess for peripheral arterial disease
Dorsalis Pedis	**Forefoot** • At the proximal end of the groove between the first and second metatarsals	• Useful to assess for peripheral arterial disease

*Coarctation of the aorta is when there is a congenital narrowing of the aorta normally just after it becomes the left subclavian artery of varying severity and consequence that may cause radio-femoral delay, hypertension and heart failure.

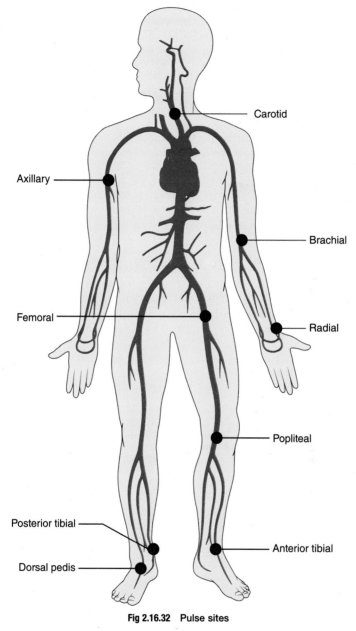

Fig 2.16.32 Pulse sites

Pulse Assessment

RATE

The adult resting heart rate is usually 60–100 bpm (though in very fit people, this may be as low as 40 bpm).

- Bradycardia <60 bpm
- Tachycardia >100 bpm

RHYTHM

Normal (sinus rhythm)
- There is sometimes a subtle speeding up and slowing down of the pulse on inspiration and expiration called sinus arrhythmia

Pulsus paradoxus
- Slowing down of the pulse on inspiration – may be caused by chronic lung disease or pneumothorax

Irregular
- Regularly irregular (e.g. hyperthyroid, anaemia, fever)
- Irregularly irregular (e.g. atrial fibrillation, atrial or ventricular extra beats)

CHARACTER AND VOLUME

Low volume (weak, thready) pulse
- May be a sign of heart failure or loss of volume (e.g. trauma, bleeding)

Bounding
- Fuller or easier to feel than normal (e.g. fever, hyperthyroidism, anxiety)

Collapsing
- Rapidly falling pulse, which is more obvious at the wrist when the arm is raised. May indicate aortic regurgitation

Slow rising
- May indicate aortic stenosis

Pulse Changes

Causes of a Fast Pulse (Tachycardia) >100 bpm

Regular	Irregular
Exercise	Atrial flutter
Emotion	Atrial fibrillation
Fever	Ventricular tachycardia
Infection	Supraventricular tachycardia
Anaemia	
Pregnancy	
Hyperthyroidism	
Medication (e.g. adrenaline, atropine)	
Myocardial infarction	

Causes of a Slow Pulse (Bradycardia) <60 bpm

Regular	Irregular
Physical training (being very fit)	Heart block
Hypothyroidism	Sick sinus syndrome
Hypothermia	Carotid sinus hypersensitivity
Medication (e.g. beta-blockers, digoxin, diltiazem)	
Post myocardial infarction	

Ankle-Brachial Pressure Index (ABPI)

Ankle-brachial pressure index is a test to assess for peripheral vascular disease using a Doppler ultrasound probe to assess systolic pressure at the pedal pulse(s) (either postural tibial artery [PTA] or dorsalis pedis [DP]) compared to systolic pressure at the brachial artery.

- Measured as a ratio (highest pressure of either left PTA or DP) ÷ (highest brachial pressure)
  - Normal ratio is around 1
  - Reduced <1 is consistent with peripheral arterial disease (claudication typically at <0.8 and critical ischaemia <0.4)
  - Raised >1 may be found in calcified and incompressible veins

2.17

Musculoskeletal Tests

Shoulder

ACTIVE COMPRESSION TEST (O'BRIEN)

Purpose
- Superior labrum anterior posterior (SLAP) or superior labral tears; acromioclavicular joint pathology

Procedure
- Patient standing with their elbow in extension. Flex the shoulder to 90° and add 10-15° adduction and medial rotation so that the thumb points downward. Stand behind the patient and apply a downward force to the arm. Repeat with the arm in lateral rotation

Positive Sign
- Pain or clicking is produced with the arm in medial rotation but decreased with the arm in lateral rotation
- Deep pain inside the glenohumeral joint may indicate a labral lesion while superficial pain over the acriomioclavicular indicates acromioclavicular abnormality

ANTERIOR DRAWER TEST

Tests
- Anterior shoulder stability

Procedure
- Patient supine. Place the shoulder in 80-120° abduction, 0-20° forward flexion, and 0-30° lateral rotation and place the patient's hand in your axilla. With the other hand, stabilise the scapula with the index and middle fingers on the scapular spine and the thumb on the coracoid. With the hand that is supporting the arm, grasp the upper arm and draw the humerus anteriorly

Positive Sign
- Click and/or apprehension

ANTERIOR SLIDE TEST

Tests
- Labral pathology

Procedure
- Patient upright with hands on hips and thumbs facing posteriorly. Stand behind the patient and stabilise the scapula and clavicle with one hand. With the other hand, apply

an anterosuperior force to the elbow while instructing the patient to gently push back against the force

Positive Sign
- Pain/reproduction of symptoms/click

APPREHENSION AND RELOCATION TEST

Tests
- Glenohumeral joint stability

Procedure
- Patient supine. Abduct the shoulder to 90° and slowly move it into lateral rotation. If the movement is well tolerated, apply a posteroanterior force to the humeral head to further test the stability of the shoulder
- At the point where the patient feels pain or apprehension, apply an anteroposterior force to the humeral head

Positive Sign
- Decrease in pain or apprehension and increased lateral rotation when the posteroanterior force is applied to the humeral head

APPREHENSION TEST ANTERIOR RELEASE METHOD

Tests
- Glenohumeral joint stability

Procedure
- Patient supine. Abduct the shoulder to 90° and flex the elbow to 90°. Apply anteroposterior force to the humeral head and rotate the arm laterally to the end of the available range. Release pressure slowly

Positive Sign
- Signs of apprehension or pain when the pressure on the humerus is released

APPREHENSION TEST FULCRUM METHOD

Tests
- Glenohumeral joint stability.

Procedure
- Patient supine. Abduct the shoulder to 90° and flex the elbow to 90°. Support the arm with one hand, and place the other hand under the posterior shoulder to act as a fulcrum. Rotate the arm laterally

Positive Sign
- Signs of apprehension or pain as the arm is laterally rotated

BICEPS LOAD TEST

Tests
- Superior labral pathology

Procedure
- Patient standing. Shoulder abducted and laterally rotated, elbow in 90° flexion and forearm supinated. Laterally rotate the shoulder until the patient becomes apprehensive. Maintain this position. Resist elbow flexion

Positive Sign
- Pain/apprehension remains unchanged or increases during resisted elbow flexion

BICEPS TENSION TEST

Tests
- Superior labral pathology

Procedure
- Patient supine. Shoulder abducted and laterally rotated to 90°, elbow extended, and forearm supinated. Apply an adduction force to the arm

Positive Sign
- Reproduction of symptoms

CLUNK TEST

Tests
- Glenoid labrum tear

Procedure
- Patient supine. Abduct shoulder over patient's head. Apply anterior force to the posterior aspect of the humeral head while rotating the humerus laterally

Positive Sign
- A clunk or grinding sound and/or apprehension if anterior instability is present

LABRAL CRANK TEST

Tests
- Labral pathology

Procedure
- Patient sitting or supine. Shoulder in 160° flexion in the scapular plane. Hold the elbow with one hand, and apply a longitudinal compressive force to the humerus while the other hand rotates it medially and laterally

Positive Sign
- Pain/reproduction of symptoms, with or without click, usually during lateral rotation

DROP ARM TEST (CODMAN'S TEST)

Tests
- Complete or partial tear in rotator cuff complex

Procedure
- Patient standing. Abduct shoulder to 90°. Patient slowly lowers their arm to the side

Positive Sign
- Inability to lower the arm slowly (i.e. it drops) or severe pain during the movement

EXTERNAL ROTATION LAG SIGN

Tests
- Infraspinatus and supraspinatus integrity

Procedure
- Patient upright with shoulder passively elevated to 20° abduction (in the scapular plane) with the elbow in 90° flexion. Passively move the shoulder into full lateral rotation. Support the elbow, and ask the patient to hold that position

Positive Sign
- Patient unable to maintain lateral rotation, and there is a lag, or the arm drops back to the starting position

HAWKINS-KENNEDY IMPINGEMENT TEST

Tests
- Impingement and supraspinatus tendon integrity

Procedure
- Patient sitting or standing. Forward flex the shoulder to 90°, and flex the elbow to 90°. Apply passive medial rotation

Positive Sign
- Reproduction of symptoms

HORNBLOWER'S TEST

Tests
- Teres minor integrity

Procedure
- Patient sitting or standing with arms by their side. Patient lifts their hands to their mouth

Positive Sign
- Inability to lift their hand to their mouth without abducting the arm first

INTERNAL ROTATION RESISTANCE STRENGTH TEST

Tests
- Presence of primary or internal impingement following Neer's test

Procedure
- Patient standing. Place the arm in 90° abduction and 80°-85° lateral rotation with the elbow flexed to 90°. Apply isometric resistance to lateral rotation, and then apply isometric resistance to medial rotation

Positive Sign
- Weakness of medial rotation compared to lateral rotation indicates an internal impingement. If medial rotation is stronger than lateral rotation, primary impingement may be indicated

JERK TEST

Tests
- Posterior shoulder stability

Procedure
- Patient sitting. Place the shoulder in 90° forward flexion and medial rotation. Hold the patient's elbow and, while applying a longitudinal cephalad force to the humerus, move the arm into horizontal adduction

Positive Sign
- Sudden jerk or clunk

LIFT-OFF TEST

Tests
- Subscapularis integrity

Procedure
- Patient upright with arm medially rotated behind back and the back of the hand resting on their lower back. Lift the patient's hand away from their back. Instruct the patient to hold the position as you release their arm

Positive Sign
- Inability to maintain the position, and the arm springs back toward the spine

LOAD AND SHIFT TEST

Tests
- Anterior and posterior shoulder stability

Procedure
- Patient sitting. Stabilise the scapula by fixing the coracoid process and the spine of the scapula with one hand. Grasp the humeral head with the other, and apply a medial, compressive force to seat it in the glenoid fossa (load). Glide the humeral head anteriorly and posteriorly (shift)

Positive Sign
- Increased anterior or posterior glide indicates anterior or posterior instability

NEER'S TEST

Tests
- Impingement of supraspinatus tendon and/or biceps tendon

Procedure
- Patient sitting or standing. Passively elevate the arm through forward flexion and medial rotation

Positive Sign
- Reproduction of symptoms

NORWOOD STRESS TEST

Tests
- Posterior shoulder instability

Procedure
- Patient supine. Abduct the arm to 60-100°, and rotate laterally to 90° with the elbow flexed to 90°, so the arm is horizontal. Stabilise the scapular with the thumb on the anterior shoulder and the fingers positioned posteriorly. With the other hand, hold the forearm, and adduct the arm until it is vertical while feeling for posterior translation with the fingers

Positive Sign
- Humeral head slips posteriorly
- Familiar sensation of instability or pain when the arm is adducted
- When the arm is returned to its starting position, it may be accompanied by a click as the head of the humerus glides over the glenoid rim

PAINFUL ARC TEST

Tests
- Shoulder impingement and rotator cuff integrity

Procedure
- Patient standing. Their arm is slowly raised to 180° abduction or as far as possible

Positive Sign
- Pain between 60-120° abduction. Pain often decreases between 120-170° abduction

PATTE TEST

Tests
- Infraspinatus and teres minor integrity

Procedure
- Patient sitting. Place the shoulder in 90° flexion in the scapular plane and the elbow in 90° flexion. Patient rotates their arm laterally against resistance

Positive Sign

- Resistance with pain indicates tendinopathy
- Inability to resist with a gradual lowering of the arm or forearm indicates tendon rupture

POSTERIOR DRAWER TEST

Tests

- Posterior shoulder stability

Procedure

- Patient supine. Place the shoulder in 100-120° abduction and 20-30° forward flexion with the elbow flexed to 120° while grasping the forearm with one hand. With the other hand, stabilise the scapula with the index and middle fingers on the scapular spine and the thumb on the coracoid. Medially rotate and forward flex the shoulder between 60° and 80° while pushing the head of the humerus posteriorly

Positive Sign

- Significant posterior displacement and/or patient apprehension

SCARF TEST (CROSSED-ARM ADDUCTION TEST)

Tests

- Acromioclavicular joint pathology

Procedure

- Patient upright. Horizontally adduct the arm as far as possible

Positive Sign

- Localised pain around the acromioclavicular joint

SHEAR TEST

Tests

- Acromioclavicular joint pathology

Procedure

- Patient sitting. Place the heel of your hand on the clavicle with your fingers pointing upward and the other hand on the spine of the scapula. Interlace your fingers together over the top of the shoulder, cupping the anterior and posterior deltoid muscles. Squeeze the heels of your hands together

Positive

- Localised acromioclavicular pain or abnormal movement of the acromioclavicular joint

SLAP PREHENSION TEST

Tests

- Glenoid labrum tear (SLAP lesion)

Procedure

■ Patient sitting or standing. Abduct the shoulder to 90°, extend the elbow, and pronate the forearm. Patient horizontally adducts their arm. Repeat movement with the forearm supinated

Positive Sign

■ The patient feels pain in the bicipital groove when the arm is pronated, but the pain lessens or goes away when the arm is supinated

SPEED'S TEST

Tests

■ Biceps tendon pathology

Procedure

■ Patient sitting or standing. Forward flex the shoulder, supinate the forearm, and extend the elbow. Resist patient's attempts to flex their shoulder

Positive Sign

■ Increased pain in the bicipital groove

SULCUS SIGN

Tests

■ Inferior shoulder stability

Procedure

■ Patient standing or sitting, arm by the side. Grip the arm below the elbow and pull distally

Positive Sign

■ Reproduction of symptoms and/or appearance of a sulcus under the acromion

SUPRASPINATUS (EMPTY CAN OR JOBE) TEST (CHECK TEST)

Tests

■ Supraspinatus tendon pathology
■ Suprascapular nerve neuropathy

Procedure

■ Patient sitting or standing. Abduct the shoulder to 90° with the palm of the hand facing downward. Resist patient's attempt to abduct
■ Medially rotate shoulder and angle forward 30° so thumbs point downward (empty can position) in the scapular plane. Resist patient's attempt to abduct

Positive Sign

■ Reproduction of pain or weakness when the arm is in the empty can position

YERGASON'S TEST

Tests

■ Subluxation of the biceps tendon out of the bicipital groove
■ Biceps tendon pathology

Procedure
- Patient sitting or standing with the elbow in 90° flexion and forearm pronated. Resist supination while the patient laterally rotates their arm against resistance

Positive Sign
- Biceps tendon will "pop out" of the bicipital groove if the humeral ligament is torn
- Increased pain in the bicipital groove without subluxation indicates a tendon pathology

YOCUM'S TEST

Tests
- Shoulder impingement and rotator cuff integrity

Procedure
- Patient upright. Place the patient's hand on the opposite shoulder. Elevate the patient's elbow

Positive Sign
- Reproduction of symptoms

Elbow

ELBOW FLEXION TEST

Tests
- Integrity of the ulnar nerve at the cubital tunnel

Procedure
- Patient standing or sitting. Fully flex elbows with the wrist supinated and wrists extended. Hold for 3 min

Positive Sign
- Tingling or paraesthesia in the ulnar nerve distribution

RESISTED TENNIS ELBOW TEST

Tests
- Tendinopathy of the wrist extensors involving the common extensor origin at the lateral epicondyle

Procedure
- Patient sitting or standing with the shoulder in 90° of flexion, elbow in full extension and wrist in full flexion and pronation. Resist patient's attempts to extend their wrist while supporting their arm under the elbow

Positive Sign
- Reproduction of symptoms

PASSIVE TENNIS ELBOW TEST

Tests
- Tendinopathy of the wrist extensors involving the common extensor origin at the lateral epicondyle

Procedure
- Patient sitting or standing with their shoulder flexed to 90°. Passively extend the elbow, pronate the forearm, and flex the wrist and fingers, applying a stretch on the common extensor origin at the lateral epicondyle

Positive Sign
- Reproduction of symptoms

LATERAL EPICONDYLITIS TEST

Tests
- Tendinopathy of the wrist extensors involving the common extensor origin at the lateral epicondyle

Procedure
- Resist extension of the middle finger distal to the proximal interphalangeal joint

Positive Sign
- Reproduction of symptoms

ISOMETRIC TENNIS ELBOW TEST

Tests
- Tendinopathy of the wrist extensors involving the common extensor origin at the lateral epicondyle

Procedure
- Patient sitting or standing with their shoulder flexed to 90°, elbow in full extension and wrist in neutral. Resist wrist extension

Positive Sign
- Reproduction of symptoms

RESISTED GOLFER'S ELBOW TEST

Tests
- Tendinopathy of the wrist flexors involving the common flexor origin at the medial epicondyle

Procedure
- Patient sitting or standing with their shoulder in 90° flexion, elbow in full extension and wrist in full extension and pronation. Resist patient's attempts to flex their wrist while supporting the arm under the elbow

Positive Sign
- Reproduction of symptoms

PASSIVE GOLFER'S ELBOW TEST

Tests
- Tendinopathy of the wrist flexors involving the common flexor origin at the medial epicondyle

Procedure
- Patient sitting or standing with their shoulder in 90° flexion. Passively extend the elbow, supinate the forearm, and extend the wrist and fingers, applying a stretch at the common flexor origin

Positive Sign
- Reproduction of symptoms

ISOMETRIC GOLFER'S ELBOW TEST

Tests
- Tendinopathy of the wrist flexors involving the common flexor origin at the medial epicondyle

Procedure
- Patient sitting or standing with their shoulder in 90° flexion, elbow in extension and wrist in neutral. Resist wrist flexion

Positive Sign
- Reproduction of symptoms

PINCH GRIP TEST

Tests
- Anterior interosseous branch of the median nerve entrapment

Procedure
- Patient pinches tips of index finger and thumb together

Positive Sign
- Inability to pinch tip to tip

POSTEROLATERAL PIVOT SHIFT TEST

Tests
- Posterolateral rotatory instability of the elbow and the integrity of the lateral collateral ligament

Procedure
- Patient supine with affected arm overhead (around 160°) and elbow flexed 20° and supinated. Stabilise the forearm distal to the elbow, and apply a longitudinal compressive force to the radius and ulna. With the other hand, hold the patient's wrist, and apply valgus stress to the forearm while maintaining supination

Positive Sign
- Apprehension and pain

TINEL'S TEST (AT ELBOW)

Tests
- Point of regeneration of the sensory fibres of the ulnar nerve (cubital tunnel syndrome)

Procedure
- Tap the ulnar nerve in the groove between the olecranon and medial epicondyle

Positive Sign
- Tingling sensation in the ulnar distribution of the forearm and hand (little finger, ulnar half of the ring finger and medial aspect of the hand)

VARUS STRESS TEST

Tests
- Integrity of lateral collateral ligament

Procedure
- Patient sitting or standing. Stabilise the upper arm with the elbow in 20-30° flexion and the humerus in full medial rotation. Apply adduction/varus force to the forearm

Positive Sign
- Excessive laxity or reproduction of symptoms

VALGUS STRESS TEST (JOBE'S TEST)

Tests
- Integrity of the medial collateral ligament

Procedure
- Patient sitting or standing. Stabilise the upper arm with the elbow in 20-30° flexion and fully supinated. Apply abduction/valgus force to the forearm

Positive Sign
- Increased laxity or reproduction of symptoms

Wrist and Hand

CARPAL COMPRESSION TEST

Tests
- Aids diagnosis of carpal tunnel syndrome

Procedure
- Patient sitting with the elbow in extension and supination. Place your thumb over the course of the median nerve, just distal to the wrist crease, and press firmly for up to 30 seconds

Positive Sign
- Paraesthesia and pain in the median nerve distribution

FINKELSTEIN TEST

Tests
- Tenosynovitis of abductor pollicis longus and extensor pollicis brevis tendons (de Quervain's tenosynovitis)

Procedure
- Patient makes a fist with their thumb inside. Passively move their wrist into ulnar deviation

Positive Sign
- Reproduction of symptoms in the radial aspect of the wrist

FROMENT'S 'PAPER' SIGN

Tests
- Integrity of the ulnar nerve

Procedure
- Patient grips a piece of paper between their index finger and thumb. Pull the paper away

Positive Sign
- Flexion of the terminal phalanx of the thumb as the paper is pulled away

HAND ELEVATION TEST

Tests
- Aids diagnosis of carpal tunnel syndrome

Procedure
- Patient sitting with their arm elevated as high above their head as possible. Hold for up to 1 min

Positive Sign
- Reproduction of symptoms (paraesthesia and/or pain) within a minute

LIGAMENTOUS INSTABILITY TEST FOR THE FINGERS

Tests
- Stability of the collateral ligaments

Procedure
- Apply valgus and varus force to the proximal interphalangeal or distal interphalangeal joint

Positive Sign
- Increased laxity compared to unaffected hand

LUNOTRIQUETRAL BALLOTTEMENT (REAGAN'S) TEST

Tests
- Stability of the lunotriquetral ligament

Procedure
- Stabilise the lunate and apply a posterior and anterior glide to the triquetrum and pisiform

Positive Sign
- Reproduction of symptoms, crepitus, or laxity

PHALEN'S (WRIST FLEXION) TEST

Tests
- Median nerve pathology
- Carpal tunnel syndrome

Procedure
- Patient sitting. Place the dorsal aspect of the hands together with the wrists flexed. Hold for 1 min

Positive Sign
- Tingling in the distribution of the median nerve

REVERSE PHALEN'S TEST

Tests
- Median nerve pathology

Procedure
- Place the palms of hands together with wrists extended. Hold for 1 min

Positive Sign
- Tingling in the distribution of the median nerve

SCAPHOID SHIFT (WATSON'S) TEST

Tests
- Stability of the scaphoid

Procedure
- Hold the wrist in full ulnar deviation and slight extension. With the other hand, apply pressure to the scaphoid tubercle (palmar aspect), and move the wrist into radial deviation and slight flexion

Positive Sign
- Pain and/or subluxation of scaphoid

SITTING HANDS TEST (PRESS TEST)

Tests
- Wrist synovitis or wrist pathology

Procedure
- Patient sitting in a chair. Patient holds on to both arms of the chair and pushes themselves up so they are suspended above the seat using only their arms for support

Positive Sign
- Inability to support their weight through their wrists

SWEATER FINGER SIGN

Tests
- Rupture of flexor digitorum profundus tendon

Procedure
- Patient makes a fist

Positive Sign
- Inability of one of the distal interphalangeal joints to flex

TINEL'S TEST (AT THE WRIST)

Tests
- Median nerve pathology
- Carpal tunnel syndrome

Procedure
- Patient sitting with the elbow supinated and hand resting on a table. Tap over the midpoint of the carpal tunnel with your fingers or a percussion hammer

Positive Sign
- Tingling or paraesthesia in the median distribution in the hand (palmar aspect of the thumb, index and middle fingers)

THUMB GRIND TEST

Tests
- Stability and/or degeneration of the first trapeziometacarpal joint

Procedure
- Stabilise the wrist and apply an axial compressive force to the first metacarpophalangeal joint and then medial and lateral rotation

Positive Sign
- Pain, crepitus

TRIANGULAR FIBROCARTILAGE COMPLEX (TFCC) LOAD TEST

Tests
- Triangular fibrocartilage complex integrity

Procedure
- Hold the patient's forearm. With the other hand, hold the wrist in ulnar deviation, then move it through supination and pronation while applying a compressive force

Positive Sign
- Pain, clicking, crepitus

WRIST FLEXION AND COMPRESSION TEST

Tests
- Aids diagnosis of carpal tunnel syndrome

Procedure
- Patient sitting with the elbow in extension and supination. Flex the wrist to 60°, place the thumb over the course of the median nerve, just distal to the wrist crease, and press firmly for up to 30 seconds

Positive Sign
- Reproduction of symptoms (paraesthesia and/or pain) within 30 seconds

Pelvis

COMPRESSION TEST

Tests
- Sprain of the posterior sacroiliac joint or ligaments

Procedure
- Patient supine or side-lying. Push the right and left anterior superior iliac spine (ASIS) toward each other

Positive Sign
- Reproduction of symptoms

GAENSLEN'S TEST

Tests
- Sacroiliac joint involvement

Procedure
- Patient lies supine near the edge of the plinth with their leg hanging over the side. Patient hugs both knees to their chest, and then lowers the test leg into extension. Place one hand above the knee of the extended leg and the other hand over the knee of the flexed leg. Apply an opposing force to each leg simultaneously

Positive Sign
- Reproduction of pain in the sacroiliac joints

ANTERIOR GAPPING TEST (DISTRACTION PROVOCATION TEST)

Tests
- Sacroiliac joint involvement

Procedure
- Patient supine. Push down and outward on the medial aspect of the right and left ASIS

Positive Sign
- Reproduction of symptoms around the sacroiliac joint

GILLET'S TEST (STORK TEST)

Tests
- Sacroiliac joint dysfunction

Procedure
- Patient standing. Palpate the posterior superior iliac spine (PSIS) with one thumb, and place the other thumb in line with the first thumb on the sacrum. Patient is asked to flex the hip to 90° on the side being palpated while standing on the opposite leg. Repeat the test on the other side and compare

Positive Sign
- If the PSIS on the side tested moves minimally or upward in relation to the sacrum, it indicates hypomobility on that side

PIEDALLU'S SIGN (SITTING FLEXION)

Tests
- Movement of the sacrum on ilia

Procedure
- Patient sitting. The left and right PSIS are palpated while the patient forward flexes

Positive Sign
- One side moves higher than the other, indicating hypomobility on that side

SHEAR TEST

Tests
- Sacroiliac joint involvement

Procedure
- Patient prone. Apply downward and superior pressure to the sacral base

Positive Sign
- Reproduction of pain

STANDING FLEXION TEST

Tests
- Movement of ilia on the sacrum

Procedure
- Patient standing. The left and right PSIS are palpated while the patient forward flexes

Positive Sign
- One side moves higher than the other, indicating hypomobility on that side

SUPINE TO SIT TEST

Tests
- Sacroiliac joint dysfunction caused by pelvic torsion or rotation

Procedure
- Patient supine. Note the level of the inferior borders of the medial malleoli. Patient sits up, and the relative position of the malleoli is noted

Positive Sign
- One leg moves up more than the other

THIGH THRUST TEST (FEMORAL SHEAR TEST)

Tests
- Sacroiliac joint

Procedure
- Patient supine. Place hip and knee in 90° flexion. Place one hand on top of the flexed knee and the other hand under the sacrum. Apply a longitudinal force down the femur

Positive Ssign
- Reproduction of pain

Hip

ANTERIOR LABRAL TEAR TEST

Tests
- Anterior superior impingement
- Anterior labral tear

Procedure
- Patient in a supine position. The hip is placed in full flexion, lateral rotation and full abduction. The hip is then extended while adding medial rotation and adduction

Positive Sign
- Reproduction of symptoms (with or without a click) or apprehension

FABER TEST (PATRICK'S TEST)

Tests
- Hip joint or sacroiliac joint dysfunction
- Spasm of the iliopsoas muscle

Procedure
- Patient supine. Place the foot of the test leg on the opposite knee. Patient gently lowers the knee of the test leg while the pelvis on the opposite side is stabilised

Positive Sign
- Knee remains above the opposite leg
- Reproduction of symptoms

LEG LENGTH TEST

Tests
- Leg length discrepancy

Procedure
- Patient supine. Measure between the anterior superior iliac spine and the medial or lateral malleolus. Repeat on the other side

Positive Sign
- A difference of more than 1.3 cm between the two sides is considered significant

NOBLE COMPRESSION TEST

Tests
- Integrity of iliotibial band

Procedure
- Patient supine. Place knee in 90° flexion accompanied by hip flexion. Apply pressure with your thumb to the lateral femoral epicondyle. Maintain pressure and slowly extend the knee

Positive Sign
- Pain over the lateral femoral condyle when the knee reaches approximately 30° flexion
- Reproduction of symptoms

OBER'S TEST

Tests
- Tensor fascia lata and iliotibial band contractures

Procedure
- Patient in a side-lying position with the hip and knee of the lower leg flexed. Stabilise the pelvis. Passively abduct and extend the upper leg with the knee extended or flexed to 90°, then lower it toward the plinth

Positive Sign
- Upper leg remains abducted and does not lower to the plinth

POSTERIOR LABRAL TEAR TEST

Tests
- Posterior-inferior impingement
- Labral tear

Procedure
- Patient in a supine position. The hip is placed in full flexion, adduction and lateral rotation. The hip is then extended while adding lateral rotation and abduction

Positive Sign
- Reproduction of symptoms (with or without a click), groin pain, or apprehension

SCOUR ADDUCTION TEST

Tests
- Intra-articular hip joint pathology

Procedure
- Patient supine. Place hip in 90° flexion and adduction. Apply a longitudinal compressive force through the femur while passively moving the hip into flexion and extension

Positive Sign
- Pain, locking, crepitus, clicking, apprehension

THOMAS TEST

Tests
- Hip flexion contracture

Procedure
- Patient supine. Patient hugs one knee to their chest

Positive Sign
- Opposite leg lifts off the plinth

MODIFIED THOMAS TEST

Tests
- Flexibility of the iliopsoas, rectus femoris and tensor fascia lata/iliotibial band

Procedure
- Patient lies supine toward the bottom edge of the plinth, allowing the lower leg to hang off the end. The patient hugs their knees to their chest, then lowers the contralateral leg as far as possible

Positive Sign
- Leg is unable to reach a neutral position (contact with plinth)

- Tightness of the iliopsoas or rectus femoris
- To differentiate between the cause of the tightness, passively flex the knee:
  - Increased hip flexion indicates tightness of the rectus femoris
  - Unchanged hip flexion indicates tightness of the iliopsoas
  - Increased hip abduction may indicate tightness of the tensor fascia lata/iliotibial band

TRENDELENBURG TEST

Tests
- Stability of the hip
- Strength of the hip abductors

Procedure
- Patient stands on one leg

Positive Sign
- Pelvis on the opposite side drops

WEBER-BARSTOW MANOEUVRE

Tests
- Leg length asymmetry

Procedure
- Patient supine with the hips and knees flexed. Hold the patient's feet while palpating medial malleoli with thumbs. Patient lifts their pelvis off the bed and then returns to the starting position. Passively extend their legs, and compare the relative position of medial malleoli

Positive Sign
- Leg length asymmetry

Knee

ABDUCTION (VALGUS) STRESS TEST

Tests
- Full knee extension: integrity of the medial collateral ligament, posterior oblique ligament, posteromedial capsule, cruciate ligaments, medial quadriceps expansion, semimembranosus muscle
- With 20-30° knee flexion: integrity of the medial collateral ligament, posterior oblique ligament, posterior cruciate ligament

Procedure
- Patient supine. Stabilise the ankle with one hand and, with the other hand, apply medial pressure (valgus stress) to the knee joint while in full extension and then again with slight knee flexion (20-30°)

Positive Sign
- Reproduction of medial knee pain
- Excessive movement (>15°) compared to the opposite knee

ADDUCTION (VARUS) STRESS TEST

Tests
- Full knee extension: integrity of the cruciate ligaments, lateral gastrocnemius muscle, lateral collateral ligament, arcuate-popliteus complex, posterolateral capsule, iliotibial band, biceps femoris tendon
- With 20-30° knee flexion: integrity of the lateral collateral ligaments, arcuate-popliteus complex, posterolateral capsule, iliotibial band, biceps femoris tendon

Procedure
- Patient supine. Stabilise the ankle. Apply lateral pressure (varus stress) to the knee joint at 0° and then at 20-30° flexion

Positive Sign
- Excessive movement compared to the opposite knee

ANTERIOR DRAWER TEST

Tests
- Integrity of the anterior cruciate ligament, posterior oblique ligament, arcuate-popliteus complex, posteromedial and posterolateral capsules, medial collateral ligament, and iliotibial band

Procedure
- Patient supine with the hips flexed to 45° and knee flexed to 90°. Stabilise foot. Apply posteroanterior force to the tibia

Positive Sign
- Tibia moves more than 6 mm on the femur

APLEY'S TEST

Tests
- Meniscal integrity

Procedure
- Patient prone with the knee flexed to 90°. Fix the lower thigh with your knee. Medially and laterally rotate the tibia – first with distraction and then compression

Positive Sign
- Pain and/or apprehension with compression
- Reduced pain and/or apprehension with distraction

BRUSH TEST

Tests
- Mild effusion

Procedure
- Patient in a supine position with the knee extended as much as possible. Stroke the medial side of the patella from just below the joint line up to the suprapatellar pouch two or three times. Use the opposite hand to stroke down the lateral side of the patella

Positive Sign
- Fluid travels to the medial side and appears as a bulge below the distal border of the patella

CLARKE'S TEST (PATELLOFEMORAL GRIND TEST)

Tests
- Whether the patellofemoral joint is the origin of pain

Procedure
- Patient in a supine or long sitting position with knees extended. Place the web of your hand over the superior pole of the patella. Apply downward and inferior pressure to the patella as the patient contracts their quadriceps muscles
- To test different parts of the patella, the test should be performed in 30°, 60°, and 90° flexion and full extension

Positive Sign
- Reproduction of symptoms
- Patient unable to hold the contraction

EXTERNAL ROTATION RECURVATUM TEST

Tests
- Posterolateral rotary stability in knee extension

Procedure
- Patient supine. Grip both big toes and lift both feet off the bed. Patient is instructed to keep the quadriceps relaxed. Observe the extension and rotational movement of the tibial tuberosity

Positive Sign
- Excessive hyperextension, genu varum and lateral rotation of the tibia and tibial tuberosity

HUGHSTON'S PLICA TEST

Tests
- Inflammation of the suprapatellar plica

Procedure
- Patient supine. Flex and medially rotate the knee while applying a medial glide to the patella and palpating the medial femoral condyle. Passively extend and flex the knee

Positive Sign
- Popping of the plica band over the femoral condyle

LACHMAN'S TEST

Tests
- Possible injury to any of the following structures: anterior cruciate ligament, posterior oblique ligament, arcuate-popliteus complex

Procedure
- Patient supine with the knee flexed 0-30°. Stabilise the femur with one hand, and apply a posteroanterior force to the tibia with the other

Positive Sign
- Soft end feel or excessive movement

MCCONNELL TEST FOR CHONDROMALACIA PATELLAE

Tests
- Chondromalacia patellae

Procedure
- Patient in a high sitting position with the femur laterally rotated. Isometric quad contractions are performed at 0°, 30°, 60°, 90° and 120° of knee flexion for 10 seconds. If pain is produced with any of these movements, repeat the test with the patella pushed medially

Positive Sign
- Decrease in the symptoms with medial glide

MCMURRAY'S TEST

Tests
- Medial meniscus and lateral meniscus injury

Procedure
- Patient supine with the test knee completely flexed. To test the medial meniscus, laterally rotate the knee, and passively extend it to 90° while palpating the joint line. To test the lateral meniscus, repeat the test with the knee in medial rotation

Positive Sign
- A snap or click
- Reproduction of symptoms

MEDIAL PATELLAR PLICA TEST (MITAL-HAYDEN TEST)

Tests
- Pain originating from the medial patellar plica

Procedure
- Patient supine with the knee in 30° flexion and supported on the examiner's knee. Apply a medial glide to the patella with your thumb

Positive Sign
- Pain or click

PASSIVE PATELLAR TILT TEST

Tests
- Patellofemoral syndrome

Procedure
- Patient supine. The knee is extended and the quads relaxed. Lift the lateral edge of the patella away from the lateral femoral condyle

Positive Sign
- Less than 15° tilt

PATELLA APPREHENSION TEST (FAIRBANK'S)

Tests
- Patellar subluxation or dislocation

Procedure
- Patient supine with the knee in 30° flexion and quads relaxed. Passively glide the patella laterally

Positive Sign
- Patient apprehension or excessive movement

PIVOT SHIFT TEST

Tests
- Integrity of the anterior cruciate ligament

Procedure
- Patient supine. Place the hip in 45° flexion and 30° abduction, and flex the knee to 45°. One hand supports the knee while applying a valgus force to the proximal fibula. The other hand cradles the foot while applying an internal rotation force to the tibia, using the foot as a lever. As both forces are applied, slowly extend the knee

Positive Sign
- A 'jerk' or 'clunk' as the tibia reduces backward at approximately 30° knee flexion

POSTERIOR DRAWER TEST

Tests
- Posterior cruciate ligament integrity

Procedure
- Patient supine with the hips flexed to 45° and knees flexed to 90°. Stabilise the foot. Apply an anteroposterior force to the tibia

Positive Sign
- Excessive movement compared to the unaffected knee

POSTERIOR SAG SIGN

Tests
- Posterior cruciate ligament integrity

Procedure
- Patient supine with the hips flexed to 45° and knee flexed to 90° with their feet on the plinth. The hamstrings and quadriceps are relaxed

Positive Sign
- Tibia drops posteriorly with visible posterior sag

SLOCUM TEST FOR ANTEROLATERAL ROTARY INSTABILITY

Tests
- Anterolateral rotary instability

Procedure
- Patient supine with the hips flexed to 45° and the knee flexed to 90°. Place foot in 30° medial rotation and stabilise. Apply a posteroanterior force to the tibia

Positive Sign
- Excessive movement on the lateral side when compared with other knee

SLOCUM TEST FOR ANTEROMEDIAL ROTARY INSTABILITY

Tests
- Anteromedial rotary instability

Procedure
- Patient supine with the hips flexed to 45° and knee flexed to 90°. Place the foot in a 15° lateral rotation and stabilise. Apply a posteroanterior force to the tibia

Positive Sign
- Excessive movement on the medial side when compared with the other knee

STEP UP TEST

Tests
- Patellofemoral pain
- Quadriceps weakness

Procedure
- Patient steps up sideways with their unaffected leg onto a stool that is 25 cm high. This is repeated with the affected leg

Positive Sign
- Inability to step up with the affected leg

THESSALY TEST

Tests
- Integrity of the menisci

Procedure
- Patient standing on the affected leg with slight knee flexion (20°). Hold the patient's hands for support. The patient rotates their body from left to right several times (rotating the femur on the tibia medially and laterally)

Positive Sign
- Pain, catching, locking, or apprehension

Ankle and Foot

ANTERIOR DRAWER TEST

Tests
- Medial and lateral ligament integrity

Procedure
- Patient supine with the hips flexed to 45° and knee flexed to 90° with feet on the plinth. Apply a posteroanterior force through the tibia and fibula

Positive Sign
- Excessive anterior glide of the talus

SYNDESMOSIS SQUEEZE TEST

Tests
- Integrity of the interosseous membrane/ligaments

Procedure
- Patient in a long sitting or supine position. Squeeze the fibula and tibia together proximal to the ankle joint

Positive Sign
- Reproduction of pain

TALAR TILT TEST

Tests
- Instability of the ankle joint

Procedure
- Patient prone with the legs over the end of the plinth. Fix the tibia and fibula with one hand, and tilt the talus medially with the other

Positive Sign
- Excessive movement on the affected side relative to the non-affected side

THOMPSON'S TEST

Tests
- Achilles tendon rupture

Procedure
- Patient prone with the feet over the edge of the plinth. Gradually squeeze the calf muscles

Positive Sign
- Absence of plantarflexion

Cervical Spine

SPURLING'S TEST

Tests
- Nerve root compression

Procedure
- Patient sitting. Bend or side flex the head to the affected side. Apply gentle downward pressure to the head

Positive Sign
- Radiating pain into the shoulder or arm on the affected side

2.18

Common Vascular Tests

Adson's Manoeuvre

Tests
- Thoracic outlet syndrome

Procedure
- Patient sitting. The patient turns their head toward the test arm and extends it. The examiner laterally rotates and extends their shoulder and arm while palpating the radial pulse. The patient takes a deep breath and holds it

Positive Sign
- Disappearance of the radial pulse

Costoclavicular Syndrome (Military Brace) Test

Tests
- Thoracic outlet syndrome

Procedure
- Patient sitting. Draw the patient's shoulder down and back while palpating their radial pulse

Positive Sign
- Loss of radial pulse

Halstead Manoeuvre

Tests
- Thoracic outlet syndrome

Procedure
- Patient sitting. Palpate the radial pulse while applying downward traction on the patient's arm while their head is rotated to the opposite side and hyperextended

Positive Sign
- Absence or loss of radial pulse

Homan's Test

Tests
- Deep vein thrombophlebitis

Procedure
- Patient supine. Apply passive dorsiflexion to the ankle with the knee extended

Positive Sign
- Pain in the calf
- Tenderness on palpation of the calf

Provocation Elevation Test

Tests
- Thoracic outlet syndrome

Procedure
- Patient standing with their arms above their head. The patient opens and closes their hands 15 times

Positive Sign
- Fatigue, cramp, tingling

Roos Test (Elevated Arm Stress Test)

Tests
- Thoracic outlet syndrome

Procedure
- Patient standing. Abduct the arm to 90°, laterally rotate the shoulder and flex the elbows to 90°. The patient opens and closes their hands slowly for 3 min

Positive Sign
- Unable to maintain starting position
- Pain, heaviness or weakness on the affected side

Wright Test (Modified)

Tests
- Thoracic outlet syndrome

Procedure
- Patient sitting. With the elbow in 90° flexion, place the shoulder in 90° abduction, lateral rotation and horizontal extension. Rotate the patient's head away from the test side while feeling their radial pulse

Positive Sign
- Pulse disappears with rotation of the head

2.19

Diagnostic Criteria and Clinical Scoring Systems

Budapest Criteria – Diagnosis of Complex Regional Pain Syndrome (CRPS) (Harden, 2007)

To make the clinical diagnosis, the following criteria must be met:
1. Continuing pain, which is disproportionate to any inciting event

2. Must report at least one symptom in all four of the following categories:
- **Sensory**
  - Reports of hyperaesthesia and/or allodynia
- **Vasomotor**
  - Reports of temperature asymmetry and/or skin colour changes and/or skin colour asymmetry
- **Sudomotor/oedema**
  - Reports of oedema and/or sweating changes and/or sweating asymmetry
- **Motor/trophic**
  - Reports of decreased range of motion and/or motor dysfunction (weakness, tremor, dystonia) and/or trophic changes (hair, nail, skin)

3. Must display at least one sign at the time of evaluation in two or more of the following categories:
- **Sensory**
  - Evidence of hyperalgesia (to pinprick) and/or allodynia (to light touch and/or temperature sensation and/or deep somatic pressure and/or joint movement)
- **Vasomotor**
  - Evidence of temperature asymmetry ($>1\,°C$) and/or skin colour changes and/or asymmetry
- **Sudomotor/oedema**
  - Evidence of oedema and/or sweating changes and/or sweating asymmetry
- **Motor/trophic**
  - Evidence of decreased range of motion and/or motor dysfunction (weakness, tremor, dystonia) and/or trophic changes (hair, nail, skin)

4. There is no other diagnosis that better explains the signs and symptoms

Beighton Hypermobility Score (Beighton, 1973)

Component	Score
1. Passive dorsiflexion and hyperextension of the fifth MCP joint beyond 90°	_/2
2. Passive apposition of the thumb to the flexor aspect of the forearm	_/2
3. Passive hyperextension of the elbow beyond 10°	_/2
4. Passive hyperextension of the knee beyond 10°	_/2
5. Active forward flexion of the trunk with the knees fully extended so that the palms of the hands rest flat on the floor	_/1
Total	_/9

A positive Beighton score for adults is five out of the nine possible points.
For children, a positive score is at least six out of the nine possible points.

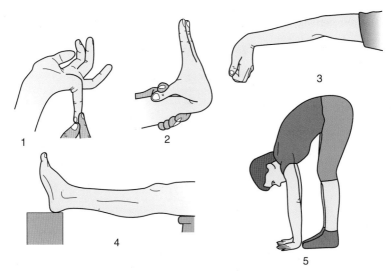

Fig 2.19.33 Beighton score for joint hypermobility

Ottowa Ankle Rules for Ankle Injury Radiography (Stiell, 1994)

An ankle X-ray series is only required if there is any pain in the malleolar zone and any of these findings:

- Bone tenderness over the distal 6 cm of the posterior edge or tip of the lateral malleolus (A on the illustration)

OR

- Bone tenderness at the base of the fifth metatarsal (B on the illustration)

OR

- Inability to bear weight immediately following trauma and/or an inability to walk four steps when examined

A foot X-ray series is only required if there is any pain in the midfoot zone and any of these findings:
- Bone tenderness at the posterior edge or tip of the medial malleolus (C on the illustration) OR
- Bone tenderness at the navicular (D on the illustration) OR
- Inability to bear weight immediately following trauma and/or an inability to walk four steps when examined

Recommendations on how to apply the Ottawa ankle rules accurately:
- Palpate the entire distal 6 cm of the fibula and tibia
- Do not neglect the importance of medial malleolar tenderness
- Do not use for patients under 18 years of age
- Clinical judgement should prevail over the rules if the patient:
  - Is intoxicated or uncooperative
  - Has other distracting painful injuries
  - Has diminished sensation in the legs
  - Has gross swelling which prevents palpation of malleolar bone tenderness

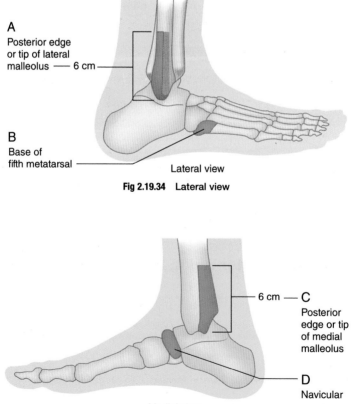

A
Posterior edge
or tip of lateral
malleolus —— 6 cm

B
Base of
fifth metatarsal

Lateral view

Fig 2.19.34   Lateral view

6 cm — C
Posterior
edge or tip
of medial
malleolus

D
Navicular

Medial view

Fig 2.19.35   Medial view

Diagnostic Criteria for Fibromyalgia (Wolfe et al, 2010)

Diagnostic Criteria

A patient may be diagnosed with fibromyalgia if the following three conditions are met:

1. Widespread pain index of **seven or more** and symptom severity score of **five or more OR** widespread pain index between three to six and symptom severity score of nine or more.
2. Symptoms have been present for at least three months.
3. The patient does not have a disorder that would otherwise explain the pain.

Widespread Pain Index

The widespread pain index quantifies the number of places that the patient has had pain or **tenderness over the past seven days.**

Region	Left	Right
Shoulder girdle		
Hip (buttock and/or greater trochanter)		
Jaw		
Arm (upper)		
Arm (lower)		
Leg (upper)		
Leg (lower)		
Abdomen		
Chest		
Neck		
Upper back		
Lower back		
Total	**/19**	

Symptom Severity Score

Part 2a

Symptom	No Problem (0)	Slight or Mild Problem (1)	Moderate Problem (2)	Severe Problem (3)
Fatigue				
Trouble thinking or remembering				
Waking up tired (unrefreshed)				
Total	**_ /9**			

Part 2b

Consider the Somatic Symptoms* in General, Does the Patient Have	No Symptoms (0)	Few Symptoms (1)	A Moderate Number of Symptoms (2)	A Great Deal of Symptoms (3)
Score	**/3**			

Continued on following page

Diagnostic Criteria
Total (part 2a+2b)   /12

Total (2a+2b)

*Somatic symptoms include: muscle pain, irritable bowel syndrome, fatigue, insomnia, cognitive problems (memory, thinking), muscle weakness, headache, pains and cramps in the abdomen, numbness and tingling, dizziness, insomnia, depression, constipation, pain in the upper abdomen, nausea, nervousness, chest pain, blurred vision, fever, diarrhoea, dry mouth, itching, wheezing, Raynaud's, phenomenon, hives, welts, ringing in ears, vomiting, heartburn, oral ulcers loss/change in taste, seizures, dry eyes, shortness of breath, loss of appetite, rash, sun sensitivity, hearing difficulties, easy bruising, hair loss, frequent urination, painful urination and bladder spasms.
From the American College of Rheumatology 2010 revised criteria.

Diagnostic Criteria for Hypermobile Ehlers-Danlos Syndrome (hEDS) (Tinkle et al, 2017)

Criteria	Generalised joint hypermobility with a Beighton score of: 1. ≥6 for pre-pubertal children and adolescents 2. ≥5 for pubertal men and women up to the age of 50 3. ≥4 for those >50 years of age for hEDS
Criteria 2	A: Five or more out of 12 extra-articular symptoms B: Positive family history (one or more first-degree relatives with confirmed hEDS) C: One or more out of three musculoskeletal features
Criteria 3	Exclusion of other conditions, including: 1. Other types of EDS, Marfan's syndrome 2. Other heritable/acquired connective tissue disorder (e.g. SLE) 3. Autoimmune conditions (e.g. rheumatoid arthritis) 4. Neuromuscular disorders (e.g. myopathy) 5. Skeletal disorders (e.g. osteogenesis imperfecta)
Requires three criteria to be met:	

The key 12 extra-articular features are:
1. Skin hyperextensibility – defined as stretching over 1.5 cm at distal forearms and the dorsum of the hands; 3 cm at neck, elbow and knees and 1 cm on the volar surface of the hand (palm)
2. Smooth/velvety skin that bruises easily
3. Atrophic (wide or flat) scars (in at least two sites)
4. Unexplained stretch marks (striae)
5. Soft, skin-coloured papules found on the heels (piezogenic papules)
6. Recurrent abdominal hernias
7. Prolapse of the pelvic floor, rectum or uterus
8. Dental crowding and high/narrow palate
9. Arachnodactyly
10. Arm span to height ≥1.05
11. Mitral valve prolapse
12. Aortic root dilatation

The key three musculoskeletal features are
1. Pain > three months affecting two or more limbs
2. Chronic widespread pain > three months
3. Recurrent dislocations or instability of joints (without trauma)

References

Harden, R. N., Bruehl, S., Stanton-Hicks, M., Wilson, P. R. (2007). Proposed new diagnostic criteria for complex regional pain syndrome. *Pain Medicine (Malden, Mass.), 8*(4), 326-331.

Beighton, P. H., Solomon, L., Soskolne, C. L. (1973). Articular mobility in an African population. *Annals of the Rheumatic Disease, 32*(5), 413-418.

Stiell, I. G., et al. (1994). Implementation of the Ottawa ankle rules. *JAMA, 271,* 827–832.

Wolfe, F., et al. (2010). The American College of Rheumatology preliminary diagnostic criteria for fibromyalgia and measurement of symptom severity. *Arthritis Care & Research, 62*(5), 600–610.

Tinkle, B., et al. (2017). Hypermobile Ehlers-Danlos syndrome (a.k.a. Ehlers-Danlos syndrome Type III and Ehlers-Danlos syndrome hypermobility type): Clinical description and natural history. *Am J Med Genet C Semin Med Genet, 175*(1), 48–69.

Fractures – An Overview

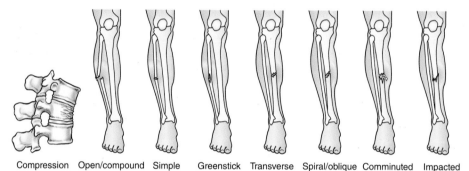

Compression Open/compound Simple   Greenstick Transverse Spiral/oblique Comminuted Impacted

Fig 2.20.36   Common classifications of fractures. From Rollins, J. H., Long, B. W., Curtis, T. (2023). *Merrill's atlas of radiographic positioning & procedures* (15th ed.). St. Louis, MO: Elsevier.

A fracture describes either a partial or complete break in a bone.
   Fractures can be classified according to their characteristics:
- **Location**
  - Proximal, middle or distal
  - Any involvement of a nearby joint surface
- **Closed**
  - No overlying soft tissue injury
- **Open**
  - Where there is direct communication between the fracture site and the external environment through an open wound or break in the skin. This is important in terms of infection risk and delayed healing
- **Complete**
Where the fracture runs all the way through the bone
  - Transverse
    - The fracture line runs at a right angle to the body of the bone
  - Spiral
    - Runs around the bone and is usually the result of a twisting injury
  - Oblique
    - Running at an angle to the body of the bone
  - Comminuted
    - Means the bone has broken into two or more pieces
  - Impacted
    - The fracture has collapsed into itself, sometimes seen in a fractured neck of the femur
- **Incomplete**

The fracture only goes part way through the bone, more commonly seen in children

- **Greenstick**
  - Seen with bending of the shaft or body of the bone with a fracture only affecting the convex surface of the bone
- **Salter-Harris**
  - A partial fracture of the growth plate
- **Buckle or torus**
  - With an identifiable bulge in the bony cortex
  - Normally due to the loading of a bone along its axis
- **Bowing**
  - With an identifiable bend in the shaft of the bone causing deformation and angulation without a clear fracture line
  - Normally seen in long bones in children (radius and ulna most commonly):
- **Pathological fracture**
  - A fracture in an abnormal or diseased bone where a relatively minor load can cause a fracture that would not normally affect healthy bone
  - Used to describe fractures related to bone tumours (both benign and malignant)
  - Can also describe fractures relating to metabolic conditions such as Paget's disease
  - They are most commonly seen in the femur, humerus or vertebral body
- **Insufficiency fractures**
  - Although technically a form of pathological fracture, this describes a type of stress fracture that is the result of (often multiple) normal loading events on a thinning, osteoporotic bone
  - More commonly seen in athletes and may be a sign of reduced quality of bone (e.g. in older patients or athletes with a nutritional deficiency)
- **Fragility fracture**
  - Is similar to an insufficiency fracture but describes an acute, symptomatic or asymptomatic fracture from a low level event or trauma (e.g. vertebral fracture in osteoporosis on stepping off a pavement)
- **Stress fracture**
  - Generally seen with repeated loading or mechanical stress of a bone
  - Most commonly seen in athletes or the military (e.g. march fractures)
  - Can be thought of as an overuse injury and may overlap with insufficiency fractures

Subjective Assessment

Body Chart

- Location of current symptoms
- Type of pain
- Depth, quality, and intensity of symptoms
- Intermittent or constant
- Abnormal sensation (e.g. pins and needles, numbness)
- Relationship of symptoms
- Check other relevant regions

Behaviour of Symptoms

- Aggravating factors
- Easing factors
- Severity
- Irritability
- Daily activities/functional limitations
- 24 h behaviour (night pain)
- Stage of the condition

History of the Present Condition

- Mechanism of injury
- History of each symptomatic area
- Relationship of onset of each symptomatic area
- Change of each symptom since the onset
- Previous episodes of the present complaint
- Previous treatment and outcome
- Recent X-rays or investigations

Special Questions

- Red flags
- Dizziness or other symptoms of vertebrobasilar insufficiency (diplopia, drop attacks, dysarthria, dysphagia, nausea)

Past Medical History

- **THREAD** (**T**hyroid disorders, **H**eart problems, **R**heumatoid arthritis, **E**pilepsy, **A**sthma or other respiratory problems, **D**iabetes)
- Osteoporosis
- Past surgery
- Previous episodes of the same problem, their impact, and management

Family History

- Heritable conditions (e.g. spondyloarthropathy, thyroid disease), particularly in first - degree relatives

Drug History

- Current medication
- Previous medications tried for the current problem
- Medication that may influence treatment (e.g. steroids, anticoagulants)
- Allergies

Social History

- Home circumstances (e.g. flat or house, stairs, upstairs bedrooms or bathrooms or adapted bathrooms)
- Finances
- Support network - partner, family, friends
- Work history - full - or part - time, nature of work, support from colleagues and supervisors, occupational hazards
- Dependants
- Leisure activities and hobbies
- Exercise

Personal History

- Alcohol history
- Substance use/misuse
- Smoking history

Physical Assessment

Observation

- Posture
- Function
- Gait
  - Pattern
  - Distance
  - Velocity
  - Use of walking aids
  - Orthoses
  - Assistance from others
- Structural abnormalities
- Muscle bulk and tone
- Soft tissues

Palpation

- Skin and superficial soft tissue
- Muscle and tendon
- Nerve
- Ligament
- Joint
- Bone
- Pulses

Palpation Active Joint Movements

- Repeated movements
- Sustained movements
- Fatiguability
- Functional range
- End feel

Passive Joint Movement

- Repeated movements
- Sustained movements
- End feel
- Passive accessory movements

Joint Integrity Tests (i.e. Valgus and Varus Stress Test)

Muscle Tests

- Muscle strength
- Muscle control and stability
- Muscle length
- Isometric muscle testing

Neurological Tests

Integrity of the Nervous System

- Dermatomes
- Reflexes
  - Biceps (C5/6)
  - Triceps (C7/8)
  - Knee (L3/4)
  - Ankle (S1/2)
- Plantar reflex (Babinski's sign)
- Hoffman's reflex
- Myotomes
- Sensation
  - Light touch
  - Pinprick
  - Two-point discrimination
  - Vibration sense
  - Joint position sense
  - Temperature
  - Vision and hearing
- Tone
  - Decreased/flaccid
  - Increased
    - Spasticity (clasp-knife or clonus)
    - Rigidity (cogwheel or lead pipe)

Sensitivity of the Nervous System

- Straight leg raise
- Slump test
- Slump knee bend
- Passive neck flexion
- Upper limb neurodynamic tests

Other Tests (i.e. Vascular, Cranial)

Musculoskeletal Regional Conditions

Spine

3.1.1 Cervical Sponydylotic Myelopathy

Cervical spondylotic myelopathy (CSM) is a disorder involving progressive compression of the spinal cord and surrounding structures due to degenerative changes in the cervical spine leading to spinal stenosis (e.g. disc herniation, facet joint and ligamentum flavum hypertrophy). CSM is the most common form of spinal cord dysfunction (myelopathy) and mainly affects adults over 50 years old. Clinical symptoms can vary, but the condition is associated with progressive loss of motor and sensory function.

History

Risk factors include:
- Increasing age
- Congenitally narrowed spinal canal (and rare disorders of the bony architecture of the neck, e.g. Klippel-Feil syndrome)
- Inflammatory diseases (e.g. rheumatoid arthritis)
- Smoking
- History of trauma or surgery to the cervical spine

Symptoms

- Neck pain - may refer to occipital region and be associated with headaches
- May be worse with movement (extension and/or flexion) and prolonged standing
- Neck stiffness

- Radicular arm or leg pain (i.e. sharp, shooting or lancinating pain which may be worse with activity, e.g. pseudo claudication)
- Arm weakness and parasthesia - related to cervical radiculopathy
- Clumsiness and problems with fine motor skills
- Gait instability and falls
- Bladder, bowel or sexual dysfunction
- Paraesthesia in limbs

Examination

- Kyphosis and/or scoliosis may be apparent
- Loss of spinal range of movement
- Hyperreflexia on testing
- Increased tone
- Loss of balance and/or coordination
- Sensory loss and spasticity (trunk and legs)
- Muscle weakness and wasting (chronic feature)

Special Tests

- Hoffman's sign
- Babinski test
- Clonus of the ankle
- Deep tendon reflexes (biceps, brachioradialis, triceps and knee jerk)

Investigations

- X-ray
  - May be used to identify bony pathologies (e.g. spondylosis, spondylolisthesis and fracture)
- MRI
  - Shows a detailed view of the soft tissue structures and spinal cord – usually with gadolinium enhancement to improve sensitivity
- Myelography
  - X-rays taken after injection of contrast into the spinal canal to evaluate the spinal canal (rarely used)
- Electromyography (EMG)
  - May be normal and can be used to rule out alternate diagnoses (e.g. multiple sclerosis)

Management

Surgical intervention is considered first line treatment in those with acute, moderate or severe symptoms with the aim of preventing further deterioration. Conservative approaches may be used for milder symptoms or poor surgical candidates.

CONSERVATIVE

- Use of a hard cervical collar may be used for people who are unable to have surgery
- Education and advice on managing the condition
- Postural advice - advise patient to avoid maintaining static neck positions (reading, writing, working at a computer, telephone etc) or prolonged sitting or standing

- Home exercise programme - aimed at maintaining strength and flexibility in the neck, increasing or maintaining range of movement and improving mobility and proprioception

MEDICATION

- Non-steroidal anti-inflammatories (NSAIDs) where safe and tolerated
- Weak opiates with or without paracetamol if NSAIDs contraindicated, not tolerated or ineffective
- Avoid strong opiates, gabapentinoids or antidepressants

INJECTIONS

- Facet joint injection/denervation – for focal pain where relevant
- Epidural corticosteroid injection or nerve root block – may be used for associated radicular pain

SURGERY

- Surgical decompression of the spinal cord and/or nerve roots (e.g. laminectomy, anterior cervical discectomy) is indicated for significant pain or progressive neurological symptoms. Fusion or immobilisation of spinal segments may be used in cases with severe underlying degenerative joint disease
- Outcomes are better for younger people with shorter duration of symptoms and those with well defined, localised areas of pathological changes in the spine

3.1.2 Acute Mechanical Neck Pain

Acute neck pain describes non-traumatic pain that can be located anywhere between the occipital condyle and the vertebra prominens (spinous process of C7), lasting less than four weeks, though the majority usually resolve before then. Identifying a specific structure responsible for mechanical neck pain remains controversial and elusive.

History

Risk factors for developing mechanical neck pain include:
- Previous episode of neck pain
- Prolonged static postures
- Twisting or bending of the trunk
- Pain secondary to traffic collision or related to occupation (higher likelihood of chronicity)
- Obesity
- Women are affected more than men

Symptoms

- Pain may be unilateral, bilateral or central
- Pain is generally worse with movement
- It may radiate to the head, chest, shoulders and thoracic spine
- Can be described as gnawing, aching or burning pain
- Stiffness may be associated with stiffness lasting <30 min
- May be associated with acute and/or episodic muscle spasms

Examination

- Reduced range of movement
- Tenderness around the extensor muscles of the neck
- Pain more commonly on extension +/- rotation
- Absence of central bony tenderness

Differential Diagnosis

- Gastric and diaphragmatic disorders (e.g. reflux)
- Cardiac ischaemia (e.g. angina)
- Carotid or vertebral artery dissection
- Thyroid disorders (e.g. thyroiditis)
- Inflammatory conditions (e.g. axial spondyloarthropathy, rheumatoid arthritis)
- Infection (e.g. shingles [herpes zoster], epidural abscess, meningitis, vertebral osteomyelitis)
- Malignancy (e.g. myeloma or secondary [metastatic] disease)
- Osteomalacia
- Cervical myelopathy
- Cervical radiculopathy

Investigation

- Acute, mechanical neck pain is primarily a clinical diagnosis that only requires further investigations if there is clinical uncertainty or other pathologies are suspected

Management

CONSERVATIVE

- Reassurance regarding prognosis – the majority settle within a few weeks
- Advise to stay active and avoid bed rest
- Signpost to self-management resources
- Develop a home exercise plan
- Activity modification in the short term (e.g. adopt the position of most comfort and reduce provocative activities)
- Remain in or return to work as soon as possible

MEDICATION

- Non-steroidal anti-inflammatories (NSAIDs) where safe and tolerated
- Weak opiates with or without paracetamol if NSAIDs contraindicated, not tolerated or ineffective
- Avoid strong opiates, gabapentinoids or antidepressants

3.1.3   Acute Lower Back Pain

Acute lower back pain is also known as acute, non-specific, mechanical or simple back pain. It describes pain between the posterior ribs and above the lower margins of the buttocks lasting less than four weeks. Exact causes are difficult to pinpoint in many cases with uncertain involvement of localised structures (e.g. muscles, joints, ligaments).

History

Risk factors for mechanical lower back pain include:
- Obesity
- Sedentary lifestyle
- Previous back pain
- Family history of low back pain
- Poor flexibility
- Stress and psychiatric comorbidities
- Psychosocial factors:
  - Depression
  - Stress
  - Dissatisfaction in the workplace
  - Perceived lack of control over workload
- Less reliable risk factors include:
  - Heavy physical and work-related activities
  - Smoking
  - Prolonged sitting, standing or walking
  - Increasing age

Symptoms

- Pain may be described as dull, tearing or burning
- Pain is usually located in the lower lumbar area
- May be unilateral, bilateral or central
- Generally sudden onset
- Pain tends to build over a period of hours and may be associated with muscle spasms and stiffness lasting <30 mins
- Pain does not normally radiate below the knee

Examination

- Restricted range of movement in the lumbar spine
- Localised muscle tenderness and/or increased tonicity
- Absence of marked localised bony tenderness
- Neurological examination of lower limbs (tone, power, sensation, reflexes) is normal
- Normal straight leg test and slump test

Differential Diagnosis

- Radiculopathy/sciatica
- Spinal stenosis

- Ankylosis spondylitis
- Spinal tumour
- Spinal infection (osteomyelitis, discitis, abscess)
- Spinal compression fracture
- Abdominal aortic aneurysm
- Kidney stone or infection (pyelonephritis)

Investigations

- Mechanical back pain is primarily a clinical diagnosis that only requires further investigations if there is clinical uncertainty or other pathologies are suspected

Management

CONSERVATIVE

- Assurance regarding prognosis – the majority settle within a few weeks
- Advise to stay active and avoid bed rest
- Signpost to self-management resources
- Develop a home exercise plan
- Activity modification in the short term (e.g. adopt the position of most comfort and reduce provocative activities)
- Remain in or return to work as soon as possible

MEDICATION

- Non-steroidal anti-inflammatories (NSAIDs) where safe and tolerated
- Weak opiates with or without paracetamol if NSAIDs contraindicated, not tolerated or ineffective
- Avoid strong opiates, gabapentinoids or antidepressants

3.1.4   Cauda Equina Syndrome

Cauda equina syndrome (CES) is a rare condition caused by compression of the bundle of nerves originating from the bottom of the spinal cord that are involved in bladder, bowel, sexual and lower limb function. These include all spinal nerves below the level of L2 (including sacral and coccygeal nerves). Compression or damage to these nerves due to disc herniation, narrowing of the spinal canal, infection, inflammation, haematoma, fracture or malignant tumour can cause significant, lifelong disability, so early diagnosis and management are vital.

History

Risk factors include:
- Previous diagnosis of disc pathology or spinal stenosis
- History of cancer
- Recent spinal operation
- Spinal epidural abscess (consider if there are risk factors for infection e.g. diabetes, recent surgery, intravenous drug use or other causes of immunosuppression)
- Recent trauma
- Congenital malformations of the spine (e.g. spina bifida, congenital spinal stenosis or kyphoscoliosis)

Symptoms

- Saddle anaesthesia
  - Loss or altered sensation in the perineal and/or perianal region
- Bladder disturbance
  - Difficulty initiating urination
  - Loss of sensation when passing urine
  - Loss of full bladder sensation
  - Inability to pass urine
  - Incontinence of urination
- Bowel disturbance
  - Constipation
  - Loss of sensation when passing a motion
  - Incontinence
- Back and/or nerve root pain
  - Lower back pain
  - Radicular nerve pain (especially if progressing from unilateral to bilateral or alternating lower limb radicular pain) and associated myotomal or dermatomal deficit may precede the symptoms of CES
- Loss of sexual function
  - Unable to achieve an erection
  - Unable to ejaculate and or orgasm
  - Loss of sensation during intercourse

These features can present in different stages of progression, as defined below (Todd 2016). The rate of progression is not fixed, and features can vary and intermingle between the stages.

- CES suspected
  - Bilateral radicular pain
  - No frank signs of CES but at risk of progression
- CES incomplete
  - Urinary difficulties of neurogenic origin
  - Loss of desire to void
  - Poor stream
  - Needing to strain to empty their bladder
  - Loss of urinary sensation
- CES retention
  - Painless urinary retention
  - Overflow incontinence
- CES complete
  - Objective loss of the cauda equina function
  - Absent perineal sensation and reflex
  - Loss of anal tone
  - Paralysed bladder and bowel

Examination

The following features may be found:
- Reduced range of lumbar spine movement
- Difficulty walking due to leg weakness
- Myotomal deficit (e.g. loss of dorsiflexion of the foot [L4] and toes [L4,5], and of eversion and plantarflexion [S1])
- Altered sensation in a dermatomal distribution
- Loss or diminished tendon reflexes (e.g. loss of ankle jerk)
- Digital rectal examination may show altered perianal sensation and/or anal tone. Note that a rectal examination is not always required to make a diagnosis of CES
- Positive straight leg raise or slump test

Differential Diagnosis

- Conus medullaris syndrome – damage to the tip of the spinal cord (note that this presents with upper and lower motor neurone signs)
- Mechanical back pain +/- sciatica
- Multiple sclerosis
- Motor neurone disease
- Carcinomatous meningitis – late-stage symptom of cancer with a spread of cancerous cells to the meninges giving symptoms that can mimic CES
- Vasculitis of the spinal cord
- Spinal artery thrombosis or aneurysm
- Guillain-Barre syndrome
- Medication effects
  - Cholinergic drugs (e.g. acetylcholine and pilocarpine) may cause unexpected voiding of urine
  - Anticholinergic drugs (e.g. oxybutynin or amitriptyline) can cause urinary retention
  - Opioids (e.g. tramadol, codeine) may cause constipation and reduced bladder sensation

Investigation

- MRI
  - The gold standard investigation should be undertaken urgently for suspected CES to confirm the diagnosis, identify the level of compression and underlying cause and inform surgical planning
  - The most common findings (in descending order) are:
    - Disc herniation – most commonly at L4–5 and L5–S1 levels
    - Tumour (e.g. metastases, lymphoma, meningioma)
    - Infection (e.g. tuberculosis, abscess)
    - Lumbar spinal stenosis
    - Haematoma (epidural, subdural)
    - Inflammatory (e.g. rheumatoid arthritis, ankylosing spondylitis)
    - Vascular (e.g. arteriovenous malformations)
- Ultrasound
  - To visualise the bladder contents and assess for a significant retained volume of urine after urinating

Management

- The diagnosis is a clinical one in primary care. If CES is suspected, then immediate referral to accident and emergency (A&E) department or spinal orthopedics/neurosurgery is advised for definitive imaging and treatment
- Time is of the essence, and there should be no delay to onward assessment in secondary care
- The aim is to prevent progressive, irreversible damage to the nerves and save or restore function

SURGERY

- Emergency surgical decompression of the spine (e.g. decompressive laminectomy)
  - Ideally within 48 h (or within 24 h if no bladder symptoms have yet emerged to reduce the chance of them having post-operative problems)
  - Poor prognostic indicators include bilateral sciatica and complete perineal anaesthesia
  - Longer-term multidisciplinary support may be required for any residual bladder and sexual dysfunction
  - Incomplete CES has a better prognosis than complete CES

Reference

Todd, N. V., Dickson, R. A. (2016). Standards of care in CES. *British Journal of Neurosurgery*, 30(5), 518–522.

3.1.5   Cervical Radiculopathy

Cervical radiculopathy describes the cluster of clinical symptoms caused by the irritation or compression of one or more cervical nerve roots. The majority of patients with cervical radiculopathy will improve with non-operative management.

History

- Cervical radiculopathy may be caused by:
  - Herniated intervertebral discs (in up to a quarter of cases)
  - Cervical spondylosis
  - Cervical instability
  - Trauma
  - Cancer (e.g. metastatic deposits)
  - Infection (e.g. epidural abscess)
- This is more commonly seen in:
  - Middle-aged patients
  - Smokers
  - Prior history of radiculopathy
  - Occupational factors
    - Lifting heavy objects
    - Driving heavy equipment (vibration and shaking)

Symptoms

- Radicular pain may be described as sharp, lancinating or burning in nature
- Often severe
- Pain radiates in the dermatomal distribution of the affected nerve root – most commonly C7
- May include radiation to the posterior aspect of the shoulder
- Can occur with or without neck pain
- Often worse with movement (e.g. bending), prolonged sitting and can be eased with lying down
- May involve 'impulse pain' (i.e. provoked or worsened by cough or sneeze)
- Can present with neurological symptoms and no pain
- Upper limb weakness causing difficulty with grip strength, carrying and lifting objects
- Paraesthesia – pins and needles, numbness in the upper limb or hand
- Secondary headaches
- Stiffness and pain in shoulders and muscles of the upper back
- Symptoms are usually unilateral
- Bilateral symptoms may suggest widespread degenerative changes or a very large, herniated disc with a risk of central stenosis and cervical myelopathy

Examination

- Structural abnormalities may be apparent (e.g. kyphosis, scoliosis, loss of lordosis)
- Asymmetry – atrophy, postural asymmetry (head tilted away from the affected side)

- Reduced range of movement of the cervical spine may be found, especially cervical extension
- Altered or reduced sensation in a dermatomal pattern
  - Thumb (C6)
  - Index, middle and ring fingers (C7)
  - Little finger (C8)
- Formal myotome testing may show a reduction of the following:
  - Shoulder elevation (shrug) (C4)
  - Shoulder abduction (C5)
  - Wrist extension (C6)
  - Elbow extension and wrist flexion (C7)
  - Thumb extension and finger flexion (C8)
  - Finger abduction (T1)
- Altered reflexes:
  - Diminished biceps reflex (C5)
  - Diminished brachioradialis reflex (C6)
  - Diminished triceps reflex (C7)

Tests

- Spurling test
- Lhermitte's sign – a sudden electric shock sensation that passes down the neck and into the spine when the neck is flexed

Differential Diagnosis

- Peripheral nerve entrapment
- Brachial plexus pathology
- Shoulder pathology
  - Rotator cuff dysfunction
  - Acromioclavicular joint pathology
  - Adhesive capsulitis
  - Bicipital disease
  - Osteoarthritis of the glenohumeral joint
- Spinal tumour
- Cervical myelopathy
- Polyneuropathy
- Cervical arterial dysfunction
- Thoracic outlet syndrome
- Cardiovascular disease
  - Angina
  - Myocardial infarction
  - Beurger's disease (non-atherosclerotic vasculitis most commonly seen in smokers)
- Pancoast tumour (apical lung tumour causing Horner's syndrome, shoulder pain and lower brachial plexus dysfunction)
- Shingles
- Parsonage Turner syndrome (acute brachial neuritis)

Investigations

Cervical radiculopathy is primarily a clinical diagnosis. It only requires further investigations if there is diagnostic uncertainty or there is progressive neurology, failure to respond to conservative therapy or as part of planning interventions (injection therapies or surgery).

- MRI
  - Gold standard to identify structural pathologies (e.g. spondylosis, osteophytes, disc herniations and nerve root impingement)
- X-ray
  - Of limited value but may show a prevalence of degenerative changes
- CT
  - Considered when MRI is contraindicated (e.g. pacemakers, spinal implants) or when more detail of bony structures is required
- Nerve conduction studies/EMG
  - May be helpful to distinguish between cervical radiculopathy and peripheral nerve entrapment

Management

CONSERVATIVE

- Careful explanation of diagnosis and natural history, as the majority of cases resolve within four weeks without the need for intervention
- Signposting information and self-management resources
- Stretching and strengthening exercises
- Joint and soft tissue mobilisations
- Exercise to improve cervical range of movement
- Neurodynamic exercises to reduce nerve sensitivity (e.g. gliding, sliding techniques)
- Postural re-education

MEDICATION

- Oral analgesia may be considered
  - Paracetamol, NSAIDs and codeine may be used, taking into account risks and side effects
  - The use of neuropathic painkillers for radicular pain (e.g amitriptyline, gabapentin, pregabalin) continues to debated and needs to be informed by local guidelines

INJECTION

- Epidural corticosteroid +/- local anaesthetic injection may be considered for acute, severe pain or pain persisting despite conservative measures

SURGERY

- Urgent referral to intermediate or secondary care should be considered if:
  - Major myotomal weakness – a drop to grade 3/5 or below
  - Significant functional impairment
  - Severe, unremitting/uncontrolled pain
- Routine referral to intermediate or secondary care should be considered if:
  - Persistent pain that is not resolving with conservative measures
  - Progressive neurological deficit (may require urgent referral)
  - Complex presentation and/or diagnostic uncertainty
- Surgery usually involves spinal decompression (e.g. anterior cervical decompression)

3.1.6 Chronic Lower Back Pain

Chronic lower back pain, also known as chronic or persistent mechanical or non-specific back pain, describes pain between the posterior ribs and above the lower margins of the buttocks lasting more than 12 weeks.

It includes pain that may arise from facet joints, intervertebral discs, muscles, ligaments and fascia. However, accurate identification of the sub-types of mechanical back pain remains elusive and controversial.

History

Many factors have been identified as influencing the likelihood of developing chronic lower back pain, including:

- Biomechanical
  - Muscle strain or sprain or other soft tissue changes secondary to a traumatic incident or repetitive overuse
  - Anatomical or functional abnormalities in the spine
    - Degenerative changes in the spine (e.g. facet joints, discs)
    - Congenital deformities (e.g. scoliosis, kyphosis)
- Social
  - Influence of friends and family, beliefs about symptoms, illness and treatment
  - Past (personal and family) experiences of healthcare services
  - Overprotective spouse or family
  - Lack of support
  - Occupational
    - Manual roles and injuries
    - Poor job satisfaction or support at work
    - Legal cases, compensation or ongoing claims
- Psychological
  - Thoughts: negative health beliefs, hypervigilance, catastrophising
  - Feelings: stress, fear, anxiety, depression
  - Behaviours: fear avoidance, poor coping strategies, pain behaviour

Symptoms

- Pain can be described as throbbing, aching or dull in nature but also stabbing and sharp with the potential for 'flares-ups' or spasms
- It can radiate into the buttocks and posterior thighs
- Follows a 'mechanical' pattern of pain
  - Worse with movement and/or activity
  - Varies over time
  - Generally eased with rest or lying down
- Can report pain on coughing, sneezing
- May be more pronounced on prolonged standing or walking uphill, lying on their front and eased by sitting or bending forwards
- May co-exist with radicular pain and radiculopathy

Examination

- Spinal asymmetry
  - May be able to observe abnormal curvature of the spine (functional or structural scoliosis, kyphosis)
- Restricted lumbar range of movement, especially in flexion and extension – more so with added side bending or rotation
- Palpation of the paraspinal musculature may reveal tenderness and hypertonicity or spasm
- Abnormal movements
  - Pain going into flexion that may ease towards the end of range and return on movement back toward neutral
  - Walking hands up thighs to return to neutral from flexion (Gower sign)
- Normal gait and neurological examination

Differential Diagnosis

- Disc herniation
- Vertebral fracture – traumatic, fragility
- Spondylolisthesis
- Spinal stenosis
- Congenital disease – kyphosis, scoliosis, transitional vertebrae
- Inflammatory disease (e.g. ankylosing spondylitis)
- Infection – osteomyelitis, discitis or abscess
- Metabolic disease (e.g. Paget's disease)
- Malignancy
- Referred visceral pain
- Chronic primary pain and other persistent pain syndromes (e.g. fibromyalgia)

Investigations

- Diagnosis of mechanical back pain is based primarily on history and examination. Investigations have a limited role and are predominantly used to exclude rarer causes of back pain, including sinister or serious pathologies
- X-ray
  - Are of limited value as they do not identify soft tissue structures but can be used to exclude fracture or structural abnormality (e.g. spondylolisthesis, scoliosis)
- MRI
  - Consider if persistent or progressive symptoms and, as part of the workup, identify a target for potential intervention
  - Gold standard for identifying cauda equina syndrome, cancers, herniated discs and spinal stenosis
  - MRI findings need to be discussed in relation to the incidence of radiographic findings in people who do not have back pain (see table below)

Age-Specific Prevalence Estimates of Degenerative Spine Imaging Findings in Asymptomatic Patients

Imaging Finding	Age (years)						
	20	30	40	50	60	70	80
Disc degeneration	37%	52%	68%	80%	88%	93%	96%
Disc signal loss	17%	33%	54%	73%	86%	94%	97%
Disc bulge	24%	34%	45%	56%	67%	76%	84%
Disc protrusion	30%	40%	50%	60%	69%	77%	84%
Annular fissure	19%	20%	22%	23%	25%	27%	29%
Facet degeneration	4%	9%	18%	32%	50%	69%	83%
Spondylolisthesis	3%	5%	8%	14%	23%	35%	50%

Source: Brinkji, W, et al. (2015). Systemic literature review of imaging features of spinal degeneration in asymptomatic populations. *American Journal of Neuroradiology, 36*(4), 811–816.

- CT
  - If MRI is contraindicated. It may have a role in further detailing bone pathologies
- Diagnostic injections
  - Anaesthetic injections to a joint (facet or sacroiliac joints) or the nerves that supply a joint (e.g. the medial branch(es) of the dorsal ramus of the spinal nerve in the case of facet joints)
  - Significant improvement in reported pain (ideally 80% or more) is used to identify the target for further interventions (facet joint or sacroiliac joint denervation)

Management

No single intervention or treatment is likely to be highly effective when used in isolation in patients with chronic low back pain, especially those with a longer duration and substantial disability.

CONSERVATIVE

- Pain education to all patients to help them understand their pain and functional restrictions
- Reassure and encourage patients to remain as active as possible to avoid further physical or psychological disability
- Avoid bed rest
- Signpost to self-management resources
- Develop a home exercise plan
- Stay in or return to work as soon as possible
- Consider referral to a pain management service to consider multidisciplinary care and access to a pain management programme

MEDICATION

- Non-steroidal anti-inflammatories (NSAIDs) where safe and tolerated
- Weak opiates with or without paracetamol if NSAIDs contraindicated, not tolerated or ineffective
- Avoid strong opiates, gabapentinoids or antidepressants

INJECTIONS

- Therapeutic injections of steroids with local anaesthetic either to joints, muscles (including trigger point injections) or connective tissue give limited, short-term benefits
- Spinal epidural injections have been used historically for short-term relief of spinal stenosis but have been shown to be of limited value

RADIOFREQUENCY DENERVATION

- Consider referral for assessment for radiofrequency denervation for people with chronic low back pain when:
  - Non-surgical treatment has not worked
  - The main source of pain is thought to come from structures supplied by the medial branch nerve
  - They have moderate or severe levels of localised back pain
  - Radiofrequency denervation should only be performed in people with chronic low back pain after a positive response to a diagnostic medial branch block

SURGERY

- Spinal fusion and disc replacement are no longer widely recommended for isolated back pain

3.1.7   Lumbar Radiculopathy

Lumbar radiculopathy, also known as sciatica, describes the cluster of clinical symptoms caused by the irritation or compression of one or more lumbar nerve roots. Most patients who present with acute sciatica have a good prognosis, with pain and disability usually improving within two to four weeks with or without treatment

History

- May be caused by:
  - Herniated intervertebral disc in around 90% of cases
    - Most commonly at L4–5 or L5–S1 level
  - Spondylolisthesis
  - Lateral recess or foraminal stenosis
  - Infection (e.g. epidural abscess, discitis, osteomyelitis)
  - Cancer (e.g. metastatic deposits)
- This is more commonly seen in:
  - Middle-aged patients
  - Smokers
  - Those with a prior history of radiculopathy
  - Occupational factors or leisure activities (use of vibrating equipment and driving)
  - Family history of disc degeneration
  - There is weak evidence for associations with:
    - Obesity
    - Diabetes
    - Atherosclerosis

Symptoms

- Leg pain that can exist in isolation or be accompanied by back and/or buttock pain
- Described as sharp or burning pain most commonly radiating down the posterior or lateral aspect of the leg to the foot
- Usually relatively acute in onset and can be severe and disabling in nature
- May involve 'impulse pain' (i.e. provoked or worsened by cough or sneeze)
- May worsen on bending or sitting and ease with standing
- May be associated with numbness or paraesthesia of the leg and/or foot
- May be associated with motor weakness
  - Patient may report foot 'slapping' the ground as walking (sign of foot drop in L4/L5 nerve root compromise)

Note: pathologies that cause radiculopathy may progress to cause cauda equina compression. Features that should raise suspicion include:
- Bilateral sciatica
- Severe or bilateral progressive neurological deficit
- Urinary disturbance – initially, difficulty initiating micturition or impaired sense of flow can lead to urinary retention with overflow incontinence
- Bowel disturbance – loss of sense of bowel fullness, which can progress to faecal incontinence
- Perineal, perianal or genital paraesthesia or numbness

Examination

- Muscle weakness
  - L4 reduced foot dorsiflexion (e.g. inability to heel walk)
  - L5 reduced great toe dorsiflexion
  - S1 reduced foot plantar flexion (e.g. inability to toe walk)
- Reflexes altered.
  - Diminished patella reflex (L5)
  - Diminished ankle reflex (S1)
- Dermatomal sensory change
  - Asymmetrical reduced fine touch or pinprick sensation
- Important to elicit an absence of upper motor neurone signs (routinely screen for hyper-reflexia, clonus, +ve Hoffman's and Babinski)
- May co-exist with features of chronic or acute lower back pain
  - Restricted range of movement in the lumbar spine
  - Localised muscle tenderness or increased tonicity

Special Tests

- Straight leg raise
- Slump test

Differential Diagnosis

- Hip osteoarthritis
- Sacroiliitis
- Facet joint pain
- Greater trochanteric pain syndrome
- Peroneal palsy or other neuropathies
- Spinal stenosis (spinal claudication)
- Myelopathy or a higher cord lesion
- Malignancy – metastatic disease including spinal cord compression, neuromas or other pelvic mass with associated nerve compression

Investigations

Lumbar radiculopathy is primarily a clinical diagnosis that only requires further investigations if there is diagnostic uncertainty or if there is progressive neurology, failure to respond to conservative therapy or as part of surgical planning.

- MRI
  - To identify structural pathologies (e.g. spondylosis, osteophytes, disc herniations and nerve root impingement)
- X-ray
  - Of limited value but may show relevant structural or degenerative changes (e.g. spondylolisthesis)
- CT
  - Considered when MRI is contraindicated (e.g. in the presence of pacemakers or spinal implants) or when more detail of bony structures is required
- Nerve conduction studies/electromyography (EMG)
  - May be helpful to distinguish between lumbar radiculopathy and peripheral nerve entrapment

Management

CONSERVATIVE

- Explanation of diagnosis and natural history as the majority of cases resolve within four to six weeks without the need for intervention
- Signposting to information and self-management resources
- Stretching and strengthening exercises
- Joint and soft tissue mobilisations
- Range of movement exercises
- Neurodynamic exercises to reduce nerve sensitivity (e.g. gliding, sliding techniques)
- Postural re-education

MEDICATION

- Oral analgesia may be considered
  - Paracetamol, NSAIDs and codeine may be used, taking into account risks and side effects
  - The use of neuropathic painkillers for radicular pain (e.g amitriptyline, gabapentin, pregabalin) continues to be debated and needs to be informed by local guideline

INJECTIONS

- Epidural corticosteroid +/- local anaesthetic injection may be considered for acute, severe pain or pain persisting despite conservative measures

SURGERY

- Urgent referral should be considered if:
  - Major myotomal weakness – a drop to grade 3/5 or below
  - Within 48 h of developing foot drop
  - Significant functional impairment
  - Severe, unremitting or uncontrolled pain
- Routine referral should be considered if:
  - Persistent pain that is not resolving with conservative measures
  - Progressive neurological deficit (may require urgent referral)
  - Complex presentation/diagnostic uncertainty
- Surgical options include:
  - Discectomy – removal of the herniated disc that is compressing the nerve root or spinal cord
  - Laminectomy – part of the lamina is removed to create space for the spinal canal

3.1.8 Metastatic Spinal Cord Compression

Metastatic spinal cord compression (MSCC) involves an acute compression of the spinal cord or cauda equina due to direct pressure from a tumour or vertebral collapse due to metastases in the spine. Whilst rare, it is important to be aware of those at risk of MSCC and to take swift action if suspicious of it being present to prevent significant disability.

History

- A history of cancer, especially those that metastasise to bone (e.g. breast, lung, bowel, kidney, prostate and thyroid)
- A history of multiple myeloma
- Although rare, it may be caused by primary bone cancers, spinal cord tumours and leukaemia
- MSCC may be the first sign of a previously undiagnosed primary cancer

Symptoms

- Progressive, severe or unremitting pain
- Significant localised back pain, which may be described as 'band-like'
- More commonly found in the thoracic spine (followed by the lumbar and then cervical spine)
- Aggravated by cough, sneeze or straining to pass a stool
- Night pain that prevents sleep
- Radicular pain in limb(s)
- Limb weakness or difficulty in walking
- Bladder and/or bowel dysfunction
- Sexual dysfunction (e.g. erectile dysfunction)
- Saddle region paraesthesia
- Symptoms relating to the primary malignancy (e.g. cough, shortness of breath, breast lump, change in bowel habit)

Examination

- Marked focal tenderness of the spine
- Compression of spinal nerve roots may produce lower motor neurone (LMN) signs, including:
  - Radicular pain
  - Diminished reflexes
  - Myotomal weakness
  - Dermatomal sensory changes
- Compression of the spinal cord itself shows sensory impairment and upper motor neurone (UMN) signs below the level of the lesion
- Spinal 'shock' is characterised by UMN features but with flaccid paralysis and loss of distal reflexes and is the result of an acute spinal cord insult

Investigation

Investigation and onward management of MSCC are usually undertaken as an emergency in secondary care.

- MRI
  - A whole spine MRI is necessary to localise the lesion and aid surgical planning
- CT
  - May provide additional information on spinal stability and further support surgical planning
- Myelography
  - Can be used if other techniques are inadequate or contraindicated
- X-ray
  - Not advised to diagnose or exclude spinal metastases

Management

- Suspected MSCC is to be treated as a surgical emergency with immediate referral into secondary care
- Patient should be kept flat with neutral spinal alignment until stabilised for transfer into hospital
- Options for further management depend on individual circumstances and may include corticosteroids, radiotherapy, surgical decompression and stabilisation
- In some cases, investigation and admission may be avoided where there is well established paralysis (more than one week), the expected lifespan is very limited due to underlying illness or in keeping with patient preference

3.1.9   Spinal Infections

Spinal infections are rare conditions that can be localised or more widespread and arise either from the outside the body (e.g. during surgery or following injections) or spread to bone via the bloodstream from another existing infection (most commonly urinary tract infection). Spinal infections can occur in the vertebral column (vertebral osteomyelitis), intervertebral disc (discitis), spinal canal (epidural abscess) or in the adjacent soft tissues (paravertebral or psoas abscess).

They have potentially severe consequences and are often difficult to diagnose as they can present both acutely or as a more chronic condition.

History

- There may be a history of predisposing factors, including:
  - Diabetes mellitus
  - HIV infection
  - Long-term steroid use
  - Use of disease modifying anti-rheumatic drugs (DMARDs)
  - Chronic alcoholism
  - History of recent spinal intervention, surgery or trauma
  - Intravenous drug use
  - Local or systemic infection, including endocarditis, tuberculosis or urinary tract infection
  - Rheumatoid arthritis
  - Chronic kidney disease
  - Cancer

Symptoms

- Malaise and fatigue
- Fever (though may be absent)
- Severe, unremitting back pain
- Pain worse at night, not relieved by rest
- Neurological deficit
- Focal bony tenderness
- Weight loss in late stage
- Radicular limb pain
- Paraspinal abscess may cause flank pain or abdominal pain
- Psoas abscess may radiate to hip or thigh regions

Examination

- Localised tenderness on palpation and percussion
- Neck stiffness or torticollis in patients with an epidural abscess at the cervical level
- Restricted range of movement
- Paravertebral muscle spasm
- Erythema, warmth and pus from any surgical site, lumbar puncture or injection site
- Neurological deficit distal to the level of the lesion, including:
  - Limb weakness
  - Sensory disturbance
  - Loss of tendon reflexes

- Upper motor neurone signs may be found if there is spinal cord compression
  - Cauda equina features if compression below L2

Investigations

- MRI
  - Are often undertaken using gadolinium-enhanced views to identify and locate the spread of inflammation and infection
- CT
  - Used if MRI is contraindicated and/or to identify bony damage
- Blood tests
  - May be normal despite active infection
  - Blood cultures
  - Full blood count – raised white cell count (WCC)
  - Raised ESR/CRP– CRP rises earlier than ESR
- Biopsy and polymerase chain reaction of aspirate to identify the infective organism

Management

Is usually initiated in secondary care with a focus on identifying and treating the underlying organism, managing sepsis (if present) and managing the increased risk of thromboembolism.

MEDICATION

- Antimicrobial therapy (antibiotics or antifungals)
  - Generally administered as an inpatient (intravenous administration) and usually required for a minimum of six weeks

SURGERY

- Indicated if there is progressive neurological compromise or failure of antibiotic therapy
- May involve surgical drainage and debridement of infection
- Aim to eliminate infection and provide segmental stabilisation if there is spinal column involvement or destruction

3.1.10 Spinal Stenosis

Spinal stenosis is a narrowing of the spinal canal and its lateral recesses, including the neural foramina, that can cause compression of spinal nerve roots, giving a characteristic back, buttock and leg pain with exercise (also called neurogenic claudication).

Spinal stenosis is usually associated with age-related changes of the spine, including intervertebral disc degeneration and herniation, facet joint hypertrophy, spinal ligament hypertrophy and spondylolisthesis combining to reduce the diameter of the spinal canal and neuroforamina.

History

- Predominantly seen in an older age group (>40 years of age)
- Associated with:
  - Previous back surgery
  - Prior back injury
  - Acromegaly
  - Achondroplasia
  - Congenitally narrowed spinal canal

Symptoms

- Insidious onset
- Steady progression of symptoms
- Lower back and buttock pain
- Neurogenic claudication – classically described as bilateral leg pain that can be relieved with rest or eased with leaning forwards (e.g. easier to walk using a trolley)
- Development of a stooped posture when walking – especially in the later stages
- Leg pain may be accompanied by paraesthesia and weakness
Note: Spinal stenosis can be an asymptomatic finding on imaging

Examination

- Reduced lumbar range of movement, especially in extension and side bending
- Diminished knee or ankle jerk reflexes
- Straight leg raise may be negative
- Pedal pulses should be checked to exclude vascular claudication
Note: Examination may be relatively normal, and neurological deficits may be absent

Tests

- Bicycle stress test - involves the patient pedaling on a static bike while sitting upright with the lumbar spine in neutral lordosis for a set time and distance. The test is repeated with the patient in a slumped position (reduced lumbar extension and increased lordosis) for the same length of time. If they are able to pedal further the second time, then lumbar spinal stenosis may be suspected
- Two-stage treadmill test - in the first stage the patient walks on a level treadmill for a set period of time and the distance walked is noted. The test is repeated with the treadmill on an incline (10-15 degrees) for the same length of time. If the patient can walk further during the second stage, then lumbar spinal stenosis may be suspected

Differential Diagnosis

- Mechanical lower back pain
- Peripheral vascular disease
- Spinal tumour (primary or secondary)
- Spinal infection (abscess/osteomyelitis)
- Lumbar radiculopathy
- Trochanteric bursitis
- Hip osteoarthritis
- Diabetic neuropathy
- Spinal compression fracture

Investigation

- MRI
  - Is not routinely required to confirm the diagnosis but may be used as part of surgical planning
  - Usually shows a combination of lumbar degenerative changes, including intervertebral disc degeneration and herniation, facet joint hypertrophy, spinal ligament hypertrophy and spondylolisthesis
- CT
  - Useful when MRI contraindicated (e.g. pacemakers, spinal implants)
  - Some bony changes may be better visualised using CT to inform surgical planning (e.g. spondylosis)

Management

Focusses on reducing leg and/or back pain, improving function and preventing progression.

CONSERVATIVE

- Prolonged rest should be avoided
- Activity modification with limitation of provocative movements
- Lumbar flexion exercises for symptomatic relief
- Aerobic and strengthening exercises to improve mobility and walking tolerance
- Improve stability and strength to help decrease the risk of falls

MEDICATION

- Limited efficacy with any medication, including neuropathic medication (e.g. amitriptyline, gabapentin or pregabalin)

INJECTIONS

- Epidural injections have been shown to be of limited value

SURGERY

- Considered in cases where there is severe pain or significant or progressive motor weakness or when conservative measures have not improved pain or function after three to six months
- Options include spinal decompression (e.g. laminectomy, bilateral laminotomies or partial facetectomy)
- Surgery is more effective in reducing leg symptoms rather than back pain

3.1.11   Thoracic Back Pain

Thoracic spinal pain is less common than neck or lower back pain. This is primarily due to the fact that the thoracic spine is attached to the rib cage and is therefore more stable and has less movement than the cervical or lumbar spine.

Thoracic back pain can be due to a range of factors including trauma or injury, poor posture, repetitive activities, muscle or soft tissues lesions, nerve irritation, disc herniations etc.

However, pain in the thoracic spine is also associated with a number of serious or sinister pathologies which need to be taken into consideration when patients present with pain in the mid-spinal area.

- Features that may indicate serious pathology include:
  - Unremitting pain that is not related to movement or eased with rest
  - Pain that is worsening, or failing to improve, despite treatment
  - Recent trauma (e.g. road traffic accident, fall from height) with increased risk of fracture
  - History of cancer that metastasis to bone (breast, bowel, prostate, lung, thyroid, kidney)
  - Systemically unwell with fever, weight loss, sweats, malaise, loss of appetite (malignancy, infection)
  - Severe or progressive neurological deficit in lower limbs (spinal cord compression)
  - History of immunosuppression, prolonged steroids, intravenous drug use (increased risk of infection)
  - Low-impact injury in someone with osteoporosis (fragility fractures)
  - Prolonged morning stiffness, enthesopathies (axial spondyloarthropathy)
  - Sudden onset chest pain radiating to back and not eased with lying down – associated with nausea, palpitation, sweating, dizziness (aortic aneurysm/cardiac pain)
  - Epigastric pain radiating to the thoracic area that may be associated with reflux and nausea and is changed on eating or drinking (peptic ulcer). Be aware that these can overlap with cardiac symptoms

History

- Risk factors for mechanical thoracic pain include:
  - Repetitive bending movements
  - Occupational factors
    - Job where there is a perception of a high workload or lack of breaks
    - Frequent or sustained neck flexion +/- repetitive tasks
    - Driving vehicles for prolonged periods

Symptoms

- Thoracic back pain may co-exist with cervical or lumbar pain
- Pain may be described as dull, tearing, or burning
- May be unilateral, bilateral or central
- May be associated with a movement
- May be associated with muscle spasms and/or stiffness

Examination

- Mechanical thoracic back pain may include:
  - Restricted range of movement
  - Localised muscle tenderness and/or increased tonicity

- Focal bony tenderness would raise suspicion of serious or sinister pathologies
- Tenderness to percussion
- Demonstrable pain-provoking movement or activity
- Postural dysfunction (lordosis, kyphosis, flat or sway back)

Differential Diagnosis

- Malignancy – primary or secondary
- Fracture – vertebral includes fragility and pathological
- Cardiac – angina, myocardial infarction
- Dissecting thoracic aortic aneurysm
- Peptic ulcer
- Cholecystitis
- Kidney infection or kidney stones
- Axial spondyloarthropathy
- Infection – osteomyelitis, discitis, epidural abscess
- Shingles
- Scheurman's disease
- Thoracic disc prolapse/herniation

Investigation

Mechanical or non-specific thoracic back pain is primarily a clinical diagnosis that only requires further investigations if there is clinical uncertainty or other pathologies are suspected.

- MRI
  - May be used to aid diagnosis and exclude sinister or serious pathologies
- CT
  - May be used where MRI contraindicated

Management

CONSERVATIVE

- Pain education to help the individual understand their pain/restriction
- Stretching and strengthening to increase range of motion and function
- Encourage patients to remain as active as possible
- Stretching and strengthening exercises
- Exercise to improve thoracic range of movement
- Joint and soft tissue mobilisations - should be delivered alongside exercise therapies

MEDICATION

- Non-steroidal anti-inflammatory drugs (NSAIDs) where safe and tolerated
- Weak opiates with or without paracetamol if NSAIDs contraindicated, not tolerated or ineffective
- Avoid strong opiates, gabapentinoids or antidepressants

INJECTIONS

- Therapeutic injections of steroids with local anaesthetic either to joints, muscles (including trigger point injections) or connective tissue give limited, short-term benefits

RADIOFREQUENCY DENERVATION

- Consider referral for assessment for radiofrequency denervation for people with chronic thoracic pain when:
  - Non-surgical treatment has not worked
  - The main source of pain is thought to come from structures supplied by the medial branch of the dorsal spinal ramus
  - They have moderate or severe levels of localised back pain
  - Radiofrequency denervation should only be done after a positive response to a diagnostic medial branch block

SURGERY

- Is generally not indicated for thoracic pain

3.1.12   Thoracic Outlet Syndrome

Thoracic outlet syndrome (TOS) describes compression, elongation or angulation of one or more of the neurovascular structures that traverse through the narrow space between the clavicle and first rib towards the axilla.

The most common type is neurogenic TOS, affecting the lower elements of the brachial plexus (C8 and T1 nerves). Vascular TOS is a lot less common and is caused by compression of the subclavian artery or vein. It can also present as a mixture of both neurogenic and vascular types (neurovascular TOS).

History

- More common in women
- Usually in the 30–40 year age group

Risk factors include:

- Local structural variance causing narrowing in the inter-scalene triangle including:
  - Presence of a cervical rib
  - Enlargement of the transverse process of the seventh rib
  - Fibrous bands in the inter-scalene triangle
  - Abnormal or additional muscles
- Secondary causes include:
  - Trauma (rib or clavicle fractures and hyperextension injuries)
  - Surgery (thoracic, cardiovascular, breast implants)
  - Postural changes (i.e. dropped shoulder)
  - Repetitive occupational or leisure activities
    - Repeated overhead activities
    - Prolonged time spent at a keyboard
    - Overhead racquet sports (e.g. tennis)

Symptoms

NEUROLOGICAL TOS

- Dull ache in the head, neck, shoulder, upper back or anterior chest with radiation to forearm and/or hand
- Increased pain with movements that cause compression or obstruction of the thoracic outlet (e.g. overhead activities or those involving head forward and/or shoulder protraction)
- Paraesthesia in hands and fingers (unilateral or bilateral)
  - Occurs more often at night as a 'release' phenomenon with the cessation of compressive activities or postures increasing blood flow to the nerve
- Weakness in the shoulder girdle and hand that worsens with sustained activity
- Numbness along the medial aspect of the forearm and hand
- Sympathetic nerve involvement
  - Cold, warm or sweaty arm(s)
  - Raynaud's phenomenon

VASCULAR TOS

- Pain that worsens with exertion or activity (claudication)
- Paraesthesia in hand and fingers
- Weakness in the shoulder girdle and hand that worsens with sustained activity
- Colour changes in hand or fingers (i.e. going blue or white)
- Additional features depending on the vessels involved:
  - Arterial (caused by emboli from the subclavian artery)
    - Thrombosis (pain and swelling in the arm)
    - Ischaemia
    - Aneurysm
  - Venous (caused by subclavian vein obstruction and/or thrombosis)
    - Venous distention
    - Oedema
    - Effort thrombosis (onset of swelling and pain in the arm after an increase in provocative activity)

Examination

- Hand muscle wasting with neurological TOS (thenar eminence and interossei)
- Tender points in shoulder girdle (including scalene, supraclavicular region, trapezius and chest wall)
- Sweaty hands (sympathetic feature)
- Weakness (especially in hand and thumb muscles)
- Difference in blood pressure between arms (arterial TOS)
- Pale, cold or cyanotic upper limb
- Cervical rib may be visible or palpable
- Systolic bruit (audibly turbulent blood flow in the systolic phase of the cardiac cycle) in the supraclavicular region when auscultated with the shoulder abducted

Tests

- Adson's manoeuvre
- Roos test (elevated arm stress test)
- Halstead manoeuvre
- Costoclavicular syndrome (military brace)
- Provocation elevation test
- Wright test (modified)
- Upper limb tension tests

Differential Diagnosis

- Angina or myocardial infarction
- Beurger's disease (non-atherosclerotic vasculitis most commonly seen in smokers)
- Polymyalgia rheumatica
- Carpal tunnel syndrome
- Cubital tunnel syndrome
- Parsonage Turner syndrome (acute brachial neuritis)
- Cervical radiculopathy
- Multiple sclerosis
- Rotator cuff dysfunction

- Acromioclavicular joint pathology
- Adhesive capsulitis
- Bicipital disease
- Osteoarthritis of the glenohumeral joint
- Complex regional pain syndrome (CRPS)
- Pancoast tumour

Investigations

- Nerve conduction studies/electromyography (EMG)
  - May help exclude an alternative diagnosis in suspected neurological TOS (e.g. cervical radiculopathy, cubital/carpal tunnel syndrome)
- X-ray
  - May identify cervical rib, abnormal transverse processes or apical lung tumour (Pancoast's syndrome)
- MRI
  - May identify soft tissue abnormalities (e.g. fibrous bands)
- Doppler ultrasound
  - If venous TOS is suspected, this can be used to reveal thrombus, stenosis or compression of the subclavian or axillary vein
- Arteriography or contrast venography
  - May show thrombus, stenosis or compression of the subclavian or axillary vein or artery
- Blood tests
  - Full blood count and clotting tests to exclude a hypercoagulable state as a cause for focal thrombosis

Management

CONSERVATIVE

- Physical therapy approaches may include:
  - Strengthening of the shoulder girdle muscles to open the thoracic outlet
  - Exercises to improve range of movement
  - Manual therapy to mobilise the first rib
- Ergonomics – adaptations to work environment and activities where relevant

MEDICATION

- Short-term use of non-steroidal anti-inflammatory drugs (NSAIDs) where tolerated and safe

INJECTION

- Botox injections to scalene muscles may help reduce pain and muscle spasm

SURGERY

- Is indicated if there is evidence of a significant motor deficit (e.g. muscle atrophy or objective weakness)
- Surgery involves decompression of the thoracic outlet by targeting relevant structures causing compression of the nerves and/or vessels

Arterial

- Urgent surgical intervention is indicated if there is suspicion of ischaemia (e.g. acute onset pain, pallor, reduced pulses, reduced capillary refill time)
- Involves thrombolysis of any embolus or bypass surgery, arterial repair and surgical decompression where relevant

Venous

- Intervention is often required for thrombus, stenosis or compression of the subclavian or axillary vein
- May involve thrombolysis of any thrombus and surgical decompression where relevant

3.1.13   Differential Diagnosis of Neck Pain

Diagnosis	History	Examination	Investigations
Simple, mechanical or non-specific neck pain	• Unilateral, bilateral or central neck pain • May be described as gnawing, aching or burning pain • Absence of red flags • Absence of upper limb neurology	• Reduced range of movement • Paravertebral tenderness • Pain more commonly on extension +/- rotation • Absence of central bony tenderness	• Not routinely recommended
Cervical radiculopathy	• Pain in the neck (may be central/unilateral/bilateral) radiating to arm in a dermatomal distribution • May be described as shooting or electric pain • Associated with stiffness, weakness and/or sensory disturbance	• Altered sensation in the dermatomal distribution • Weakness in myotomal pattern • +ve Spurling test	• MRI is imaging modality of choice to identify the target for intervention • CT scan if MRI contraindicated – findings may include herniated cervical intervertebral disc, spinal stenosis or spondylolisthesis
Rheumatoid arthritis	• History of rheumatoid arthritis • Typically radiates to the head • May be associated with sensory loss in the hands and feet	• Tenderness of the cervical spine • Cervical subluxation • Limb weakness/spasticity/hyperreflexia • Evidence of synovitis in the peripheral joints (hands, wrists, elbows) • Rheumatoid nodules (extensor surfaces of tendons)	• Imaging • MRI • X-ray • Blood tests (including inflammatory markers/rheumatoid factor/anti-cyclic citrullinated peptide) may be normal in up to 30% of people
Acute torticollis	• There may be a history of minor injury/accident • Pain – localised to neck	• Unilateral contraction of neck muscles (causing asymmetry) • Increased tone and tenderness on palpation • Absence of neurological signs	• Not routinely recommended

Continued on following page

Diagnosis	History	Examination	Investigations
Cervical myelopathy	• Is usually a slow, progressive disorder • Long history of neck pain • New onset of sensory changes in the upper and lower limbs • Clumsiness (hands/feet) • Gait changes – patients report loss of balance/confidence in walking • Disturbances in sexual, bladder and bowel function	• Subtle gait changes (slower, wider based, shorter steps) • Limb weakness • Increased muscle tone • Hyperreflexia of lower limbs • Conus • +ve Babinski test • +ve heel toe walk	• MRI reveals multiple degenerative changes (spondylosis), including cervical intervertebral disc herniation, facet joint hypertrophy causing central canal narrowing and spinal cord compression • Oedema/inflammation seen on T2 weighted images, enhancement with gadolinium
Spinal tumour – primary/ secondary	• History of cancer that metastasises to the bone (e.g. breast, prostate, lung, bowel, thyroid) • Localised neck pain • Weight loss, fatigue • Acute metastatic spinal cord compression	• Localised tenderness (significant focal central/bony tenderness) • Metastatic spinal cord compression – may present acutely with upper motor neurone signs in the lower limbs (upper going plantars, hyperreflexia, spasticity and clonus) and lower motor neurone signs in the upper limbs (atrophy and hyporeflexia) • Lymphadenopathy – supraclavicular lymph nodes may be present in cancer or infection	• MRI – may reveal localised erosions and tumour • Blood tests • Full blood count (FBC) (anaemia), raised C-reactive protein and erythrocyte sedimentation rate (but may be normal)
Cervical osteomyelitis or abscess	• Insidious onset over weeks/months • Pain worse at night • Low-grade fever	• Fever • Focal/point tenderness • Neurological symptoms (myotomal/dermatomal deficit/myelopathy) present if advanced	• MRI – increased signal intensity lesions on T2 weighted images • Blood tests • Biopsy

Diagnosis	History	Examination	Investigations
Meningitis	• Stiff neck • Headache • Photophobia • Fever • Confusion • Rapid onset	• Fever • Non-blanching pete-chial rash is a late sign • Altered mental status • Kernig's sign: patient supine with hips flexed to 90° – test is posi-tive if there is pain on passive extension of the knee • Brudzinski's sign: patient supine and passively flex their neck – test positive if this causes reflex flexion of the hip and knee	• Blood tests – FBC, inflammatory markers, blood cultures (all are done as inpatient procedures) • Cerebrospinal fluid culture
Cervical fracture	• Trauma (e.g. diving, RTA or fall from height ([less than one m]) • Neurological deficit – numbness, weakness or paralysis (upper and/or lower limbs) • Age 18–25 or >65 years	• Weakness in limbs – pyramidal pattern: flexors stronger than extensors, upper limbs and extensors stronger than flexors in lower limb • Altered sensation in limbs • Urine/faecal retention/incontinence • Priapism (prolonged erection) in men • Hoffman/Babinski's sign may be +ve	• High-resolution CT is the gold standard in emergency care and may reveal fracture, misalignment and oedema of soft tissues
Shingles	• Itch • Pain – burning or tingling • Abnormal sensation (in dermatomal distribution) • Above may precede developing a rash (prodromal phase one to five days) • Fever • Malaise • Headache	• Rash – characteristically a blistering rash in a dermatomal pattern that becomes crusted over after five to seven days • Fever • Lymphadenopathy • Allodynia/hyperaes-thesia in affected area	• Swab may be taken for polymerase chain reaction testing to de-tect viral DNA, or viral culture may be used

Continued on following page

Diagnosis	History	Examination	Investigations

Cardiac: angina/ myocardial infarction	• Pain – Tight/dull or heavy pain in the chest, which can radiate to the jaw/neck or to one or both arms, generally the axilla, inside of the arm – Worsened with activity and eased with rest but may occur at rest (unstable angina/ myocardial infarction)
	• NB atypical presentation (in women/elderly) including radiation to the back, right arm, abdomen, burping, sense of impending doom)
	• May be associated with
	  • Palpitations
	  • Breathlessness
	  • Sweats
	  • Nausea
	  • Fatigue
		• Examination may be normal (more so in chronic angina), but the following may be found:
		  • Tachycardia (fast heartbeat)
		  • Abnormal heart sounds (murmur on auscultation)
		  • Carotid bruit
		  • Reduced peripheral pulses
			• Requires medical assessment – urgent/ same day if symptomatic at rest
			• Typical initial workup includes:
			  • ECG
			  • Blood tests (haemoglobin, lipid profile, HbA1c, thyroid function test)
			• Further lab/hospital-based tests may include
			• Coronary angiography
			• Exercise ECG
			• Chest X-ray

Carotid/vertebral artery dissection)	• Unilateral neck pain, headache (may have facial pain • Weakness • Sensory loss • Transient loss of vision in one or both eyes (amaurosis fugax – transient unilateral or bilateral loss of vision)	• Pulsatile mass may indicate carotid artery aneurysm • Hemiplegia – weakness, stiffness (spasticity) and lack of control in one side of the body • Hemisensory loss – altered/absent sensation on one side of the body • Visual field defect (homonymous hemianopia)	• CT or MR angiography may reveal asymmetrical vessels, decreased/ asymmetrical blood flow, blood clot or damage within the vessel wall

Shoulder

3.2.1 Subacromial Shoulder Pain

Subacromial shoulder pain (SSP) is the most common cause of shoulder pain. It arises from the subacromial space and is associated with loss of movement and impaired function, especially in relation to overhead activities. Pain in this region is largely due to impingement between the rotator cuff tendons and the underside of the acromion due to rotator cuff pathology. A number of other terms are used to describe the condition, including subacromial impingement syndrome, shoulder impingement, rotator cuff tendinopathy and cuff-related shoulder pain.

There is no single cause of SSP; rather, it is a consequence of multiple factors, including altered shoulder biomechanics, structural abnormalities, rotator cuff and scapular dysfunction, shoulder instability, capsular tightness or laxity, calcific tendinosis, bursitis and overuse.

History

- Involvement in sporting or occupational activities that involve repetitive, sustained or forced overhead movements (i.e. tennis, volleyball, swimming, painters, carpenters)
- In non-traumatic cases, onset is often gradual or insidious
- Increased risk of rotator cuff tears due to tendon degeneration and poor vascularity in older adults (>40 years old)
- Trauma – falling onto an outstretched arm or a sudden, wrenching movement (dog pulling on lead or grabbing a rail to prevent a fall), especially when the tendon is already weakened

Symptoms

- Lateral arm pain localised over the deltoid region
- Pain when lifting and lowering the arm
- Difficulty with overhead or repetitive activities
- Pain with specific movements (e.g. reaching behind the back or head)
- Difficulty lying or sleeping on the affected side

- Pain is worse at night
- Improves with rest
- Pain may radiate to the lateral mid-humerus

Examination

- Asymmetry in muscle bulk around the shoulder and scapular with atrophy on the affected side
- Tenderness on palpation over the subacromial space
- Painful arc with active movement between approximately 70–120°
- Passive range of movement is generally unaffected
- Weakness with resisted testing – though it can be difficult to determine whether the weakness is due to pain inhibition or tendon rupture
- Possible scapular dyskinesia with forward elevation of the arm
- Positive findings with impingement tests

Special Tests

- Hawkins-Kennedy impingement test
- Neer's sign
- Painful arc test
- Internal rotation resistance strength test
- Yokum's test

Differential Diagnosis

- Rotator cuff tear
- Adhesive capsulitis
- Bicipital tendinitis
- Acromioclavicular injury
- Acromioclavicular osteoarthritis
- Glenohumeral osteoarthritis
- Subscapularis bursitis
- Avascular necrosis
- Labrum tear
- Joint infection
- Shoulder dislocation
- Fracture

Investigations

- X-ray
  - An X-ray, preferably with an outlet view to demonstrate the coracoacromial arch, can be used to assess the shape of the acromion (structural abnormalities may narrow the subacromial space) and rule out other pathologies such as glenohumeral or acromioclavicular arthritis
- MRI
  - MRI is the primary imaging modality used to assess SSP and differentiate it from other shoulder conditions
  - It can identify changes that narrow the subacromial space or change shoulder dynamics, such as subacromial osteophytes and sclerosis, rotator cuff tears, subacromial bursitis, labral tears, bony oedema and joint effusion

- Ultrasound
  - Ultrasound can be used diagnostically to detect superficial tendon damage and cuff rupture

Management

CONSERVATIVE

- Relative rest
- Activity modification – avoiding activities that exacerbate symptoms (i.e. overhead movements, pushing or pulling, throwing, lifting heavy objects) but maintaining usual activities within the limits of pain
- Rotator cuff strengthening
- Exercises to improve flexibility and range of movement
- Postural correction (i.e. excessive thoracic kyphosis)
- Restore scapular control and scapulohumeral function
- Graded return to activity or sport

MEDICATION

- In the initial stages, non-steroidal anti-inflammatory drugs (NSAIDs) where safe and tolerated
- Weak opiates with or without paracetamol if NSAIDs contraindicated, not tolerated or ineffective

INJECTION

- A subacromial corticosteroid injection may be considered to reduce inflammation and pain
- The use of repeated corticosteroid injections as a single therapy is not recommended as there is an association with poor long term outcomes (including tendon weakening and rupture)

SURGERY

- Surgery may be appropriate if symptoms have not responded to exhaustive conservative treatment
- Surgical management includes:
  - Arthroscopic subacromial decompression
  - Bursectomy
  - Rotator cuff repair – if rotator cuff tears co-exist

3.2.2   Rotator Cuff Tears

Rotator cuff tears are a common source of shoulder pain and disability. In older adults, degenerative cuff tears are a normal part of ageing and are often asymptomatic. However, a low impact fall or wrenching injury can rupture or tear a degenerative tendon.

In younger adults, rotator cuff tears usually result from acute trauma. Tears resulting from significant trauma are often accompanied by other traumatic injuries to the shoulder, such as dislocation/subluxation, labral tears, fractures and soft tissue injury. Most rotator cuff tears occur in the supraspinatus tendon.

History

- Direct trauma or an abrupt or forceful movement of the shoulder
- Repetitive lifting or overhead movements (throwing sports, swimming, house painting)
- History of previous shoulder trauma or instability
- Risk factors include:
  - Age (>40 years)
  - Obesity (BMI >25)
  - Smoking
  - Diabetes mellitus
  - Poor blood supply
  - Genetics

Symptoms

- Immediate onset of intense pain with an acute tear
- Characterised by severe pain for the first six weeks
- Insidious onset with degenerative cuff tears
- Pain with lifting and lower arm and with certain movements
- Pain over the lateral deltoid
- Loss of shoulder movement
- Difficulty sleeping on the affected side
- Pain worse at night
- Weakness – though in some cases, patients can have a full-thickness tear without any noticeable weakness on assessment
- Difficulty reaching behind the back
- Pain at rest

Examination

- Loss of active range of movement
- Painful active range of movement
- Greater or full passive range of movement
- Tenderness over greater tuberosity
- Painful arc with active movement
- Supraspinatus and infraspinatus atrophy can be seen in large rotator cuff tears
- Tendon defects may be palpable

Special Tests

- Supraspinatus (empty can or Jobe) test
- External rotation lag sign
- Lift off test
- Hornblower's test
- Neer's test
- Hawkins-Kennedy test
- Drop arm test

Differential Diagnosis

- Adhesive capsulitis
- Acromioclavicular osteoarthritis
- Glenohumeral osteoarthritis
- Cervical radiculopathy
- Labral tears
- Glenohumeral ligament injury
- Coracoacromial and acromioclavicular ligament tears

Investigations

- X-ray
  - Although X-rays cannot identify a rotator cuff tear, they are helpful in excluding other causes of shoulder pain, such as calcification of the coracohumeral ligament, osteoarthritis and fracture and can identify bony spurs and cystic and sclerotic changes
  - A high-riding humeral head seen on X-ray may indicate a large rotator cuff tear
- MRI/MR arthrogram (MRA)
  - An MRI scan, but ideally an MRA if due to traumatic injury, is effective in determining the size, shape and thickness of full or partial tears, the degree of tendon retraction, the presence of muscle atrophy and fatty infiltration
  - It is also used to rule out other shoulder pathology
- Ultrasound
  - Ultrasound is a cost-effective way of evaluating rotator cuff tendon pathology. They are accurate in detecting full-thickness tears but are less so in diagnosing partial tears

Management

CONSERVATIVE

- Activity modification – avoid aggravating factors (overhead movements, repetitive activities)
- Rotator cuff strengthening exercises
- Restore range of movement
- Improve strength and flexibility deficits or imbalances
- Review scapular stability and mobility
- Address postural issues

- Treatment should take into consideration:
  - Age of the patient
  - Activity levels
  - Mechanism of the tear (degenerative or traumatic)
  - Extent of the tear (partial or complete rupture)

INJECTION

- A corticosteroid injection may be considered for short-term pain relief, but there are concerns that the use of steroids may impact long-term recovery

MEDICATION

- Non-steroidal anti-inflammatory medications or paracetamol +/- weak opiates may be used where safe and tolerated to reduce pain and inflammation

SURGERY

- Full-thickness tears and rotator cuff injuries that have not responded to conservative management may require surgery
- If indicated, surgery should not be delayed as it can lead to rotator cuff tendon retraction, muscle atrophy and fatty infiltration
- In the active elderly, the decision to proceed with surgery will depend on the level of pain and discomfort felt during activity as well as the patient's expectations

3.2.3 Adhesive Capsulitis (Frozen Shoulder)

Adhesive capsulitis is a condition characterised in its initial stages by severe shoulder pain and an insidious onset of shoulder stiffness. It can occur in isolation or alongside other shoulder conditions, such as rotator cuff tendinopathy or bursitis. Although adhesive capsulitis is often self-limiting and generally resolves in approximately one to three years, a proportion of patients develop long-term symptoms.

The condition progresses through three overlapping clinical phases:
- **Freezing (pain) phase**
  - Insidious onset of shoulder pain
- **Frozen (stiff) phase**
  - Pain begins to subside
  - Decrease in glenohumeral movement in all planes
- **Thawing (resolution) phase**
  - Progressive improvement in range of movement

History

Shoulder stiffness can be classified as primary or secondary
- Primary frozen shoulder
  - Primary frozen shoulder develops without trauma or specific trigger, and there is no identifiable underlying cause
  - Commonly affects 40–60 years olds
  - More prevalent among women
  - Often associated with conditions such as:
    - Diabetes
    - Dupuytren's contracture
    - Hypothyroidism
    - Hyperthyroidism
    - Cerebrovascular disease
    - Autoimmune disease
    - Parkinson's disease
- Secondary stiff shoulder
  - Develops from a known cause
    - Shoulder trauma
    - Shoulder surgery
    - Immobilisation of shoulder due to another shoulder condition such as subacromial impingement, rotator cuff tear, biceps tendinopathy

Symptoms

- **Freezing phase** – typically lasting two to nine months
  - Insidious and progressively worsening shoulder pain
  - Pain around lateral deltoid
  - Pain worse with movement
  - Gradual loss of shoulder movement – impaired forward flexion, abduction and external and internal rotation (external rotation is often affected first)

- Severe pain at the end of range
- Diffuse pain at rest
- Pain worse at night
- **Frozen phase (stiff phase)** – lasting four to 12 months
  - Pain levels diminishing
  - Severely limited active and passive movement
  - Difficulties with activities of daily living
- **Thawing phase** (resolution or thawing phase) – lasting 12–42 months
  - Pain has resolved
  - Progressive increase in shoulder movement
  - Increased function

Examination

- Loss of active and passive range of movement in all planes as the condition progresses to the frozen phase
- Loss of passive external rotation
- Increasing pain towards the end of range
- Firm block at the end of range
- In pain-free ranges, shoulder strength is not affected
- Frozen shoulder is characterised by a loss of both active and passive movement, as opposed to some shoulder conditions where passive range of movement is often preserved

Tests

There are no specific tests for adhesive capsulitis, but the principal diagnostic indicator is a loss of passive external rotation

Differential Diagnosis

- Glenohumeral joint arthritis
- Rotator cuff disorders
- Calcific tendinitis

Investigations

- There are no reliable imaging modalities for diagnosing frozen shoulder. However, imaging may be used to rule out other causes of pain and stiffness, such as glenohumeral arthritis, pathological fracture or rotator cuff tendinopathy

Management

The aims of treatment are to reduce pain, improve shoulder range of movement, reduce symptoms and encourage a return to normal function

CONSERVATIVE

- Education and advice – inform the patient about the condition, its progression and that it is usually self-limiting
- Activity modification – in the initial stages, advise the patient to avoid movements that increase pain but to continue to move arm within tolerated ranges to maintain joint mobility and function
- Range of movement exercises – maintain available range of movement with active, active-assist and passive exercises and stretches
- Increase exercise intensity and stretching as the condition progresses toward the thawing phase
- Consider hot and cold packs and transcutaneous electrical nerve stimulation (TENS) pain relief

MEDICATION

- Consider paracetamol or non-steroidal anti-inflammatory drugs (NSAIDs) where safe and tolerated
- Weak opiates with or without paracetamol if NSAIDs are contraindicated, not tolerated or ineffective
- If no early benefit, discontinue

INJECTION

- Consider intra-articular corticosteroid injection if the patient does not respond to conservative treatment or they cannot tolerate attempts at conservative management due to high pain levels
- Corticosteroid injections should be combined with physiotherapy to improve patient outcomes

SURGERY

- Arthrographic joint distention
  - A large volume of fluid is injected into the joint space to distend the capsule and increase the intracapsular volume. The aim is to provide pain relief, improve the range of movement and increase function
- Manipulation under anaesthesia
  - Involves mobilising the shoulder while the patient is under general anaesthesia. The aim is to rupture and stretch the joint capsule and break down adhesions to improve shoulder movement
- Arthroscopic capsular release
  - A radiofrequency thermal probe is inserted arthroscopically to incise and remove sections of the thickened joint capsule. This releases the tightened structures, restoring movement in the shoulder
- Open capsulotomy
  - Similar to an arthroscopic capsular release but the capsule is accessed by an open incision in the shoulder

3.2.4 Shoulder Instability (Atraumatic and Traumatic Dislocations)

The glenohumeral joint provides a large range of motion in all planes but is inherently unstable due to a shallow glenoid that only articulates with a small portion of the humeral head. It, therefore, relies heavily on a range of dynamic (rotator cuff and scapulothoracic muscles and sensorimotor control systems) and static (glenoid labrum, glenohumeral ligaments, joint capsule, intraarticular pressure, osteoarticular surface) stabilisers to maintain the humeral head in the glenoid fossa during movement. Any disruption to these stabilisers can lead to shoulder instability.

Classification of Shoulder Instability

Shoulder instability can be classified according to a range of factors.

This may include their cause (traumatic, atraumatic), direction (anterior, posterior, inferior), frequency (acute, recurrent, chronic) or type (dislocation, subluxation, labral tear, laxity). A number of classification systems have been developed to help guide management by identifying the underlying cause of the instability (i.e. structural changes due to significant trauma or changes in muscle patterning).

The Stanmore classification system (Lewis et al., 2004) identifies three polar types of shoulder instability:

- Type I traumatic structural
  - Significant trauma
  - Unilateral instability
  - Usually, Bankart lesion
- Type II atraumatic structural
  - No trauma
  - Structural damage
- Type III muscle patterning, non-structural
  - No trauma
  - No structural damage
  - Abnormal muscle patterning

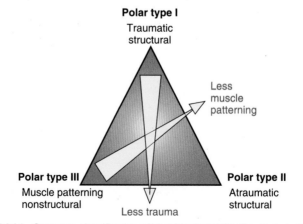

Fig 3.2.4.1   Stanmore classification of shoulder instability (Lewis et al., 2004)

Because patients may display a spectrum of pathologies that do not always fit neatly into specific types, they are arranged in a triangle, with each polar group occupying its own corner. The triangular relationship recognises a continuum between pathologies and that some patients may lie between two polar types. For instance, a patient with a traumatic dislocation or a structural lesion may later develop abnormal muscle patterning.

ATRAUMATIC SHOULDER INSTABILITY

History

- A number of mechanisms can lead to the development of symptomatic atraumatic instability:
  - Increasing joint laxity due to microtrauma to the joint capsule caused by repetitive movements (i.e. throwing and overhead activities)
  - Forceful external rotation with the humerus abducted and extended (i.e. baseball pitching), placing stress on the joint capsule
  - Weakening of the anterior and inferior static stabilisers through repetitive, mainly overhead, activity
  - Rotator cuff weakness resulting in a loss of dynamic stabilisation and reduced compression of the humeral head against the glenoid
  - Loss of muscle control and altered movement patterns in the shoulder girdle
  - Tight posterior capsule pushing the humeral head forward
  - Lack of neuromuscular control (i.e. injury to the axillary nerve)
  - Habitual, voluntary dislocation due to muscle patterning instability – may provide psychological gratification or be done as a 'party trick'
  - History of involuntary subluxations and dislocations and functional deficits
  - Increased glenoid retroversion
- Atraumatic shoulder instability predominantly affects adolescents and young adults

Symptoms

- Apprehension and pain when doing specific activities, especially overhead activities
- Recurrent shoulder dislocations/subluxations
- Patients report that the shoulder feels 'loose' or that it wants to come out of the socket when in a provocative position or during certain movements
- Diffuse pain around the shoulder area
- Numbness and/or pins and needles down the arm

Examination

- Assess shoulder symmetry and muscle wasting
- Check for generalised laxity – use Beighton Scale and specific laxity tests
- Active range of movement – look at the quality of movement, motor control, signs of apprehension and onset of pain
- Review scapular position and control
- Passive range of movement
- Palpation of tissue and structures around the shoulder girdle
- Neurological examination
- Review posture

Special Tests

- Load and shift test
- Apprehension and relocation test
- Apprehension test anterior release method
- Apprehension test fulcrum method
- Anterior drawer test
- Posterior drawer test
- Norwood stress test
- Sulcus sign

Investigations

- Imaging is generally limited for investigating atraumatic shoulder instability as capsule stretch and laxity are difficult to assess. However, scans and X-rays may be requested to exclude other shoulder pathology, review rotator cuff integrity, identify labral lesions and reveal possible anatomical and structural abnormalities

Management

CONSERVATIVE

- Treatment is aimed at addressing factors that may be contributing to instability, including:
  - Muscle imbalances and neuromuscular control around the shoulder and scapular
  - Rotator cuff weakness
  - Scapular dyskinesia
  - Proprioception
  - Soft tissue tightness – especially posterior capsule
  - Posture

SURGERY

- Surgery is rarely indicated in the management of atraumatic shoulder instability but may be considered when conservative treatment fails to prevent recurrent dislocations and sub-luxations or to meet the specific needs of the patient
- Surgery aims to improve stability by reducing or shrinking the capsule using procedures such as arthroscopic capsular plication, thermal capsulorrhaphy or open capsular shift

TRAUMATIC SHOULDER INSTABILITY – DISLOCATION

History

ANTERIOR DISLOCATIONS:

- Occurs mainly in young athletes involved in contact sports (football, rugby, wrestling, judo) but can be due to other trauma pushing the humeral head out of the glenoid fossa (falls, motor vehicle accidents)
- Mechanism of injury is usually hyperabduction and external rotation
- Direction of force is posterior to anterior
- Sudden onset of pain with decreased range of motion

- Report of popping sensation or feeling of the shoulder 'slipping out' as humorous translates anteriorly out of the glenoid

POSTERIOR DISLOCATIONS:

- Mechanism of injury is often due to a fall onto an internally rotated outstretched arm, which forces the head of the humerus posteriorly out of the glenoid cavity
- Seizure or electrocution causing a sudden and extreme contraction of the internal rotator cuff, which pulls the head of the humerus posteriorly
- Report of popping sensation as humorous translates posteriorly out of the glenoid fossa
- Sudden onset of pain with decreased range of motion

INFERIOR DISLOCATIONS:

- The least common form of dislocation
- Caused by sudden, forceful hyperabduction of the arm (i.e. falling off a motorbike), which pushes the humeral neck up against the acromion, usually with resultant inferior glenohumeral capsule tear and rotator cuff disruption
- Although less common, it can also be the result of direct trauma to a straight, fully abducted and internally rotated arm

Symptoms

- Visible deformity around the shoulder
- Severe pain localised to the shoulder region
- Loss of passive and active movement
- Apprehension with certain movements or activities
- Swelling
- Bruising
- Numbness and/or pins and needles in arm and hand
- Muscles spasm around the shoulder

Examination

- Visible or palpable bulge
- Muscle spasm around the shoulder
- All shoulder movements limited by pain and apprehension
- Possible areas of numbness around the lateral deltoid due to nerve damage
- Asymmetric radial pulses may indicate reduced patency of the axillary artery
- The arm is presented in a characteristic position:
  - *Anterior dislocation:* the arm is held away from the body in slight abduction and external rotation, and the weight of the injured arm is supported by the other hand to reduce pain
  - *Posterior dislocation:* the arm is adducted and internally rotated with the arm held against the abdomen
  - *Inferior dislocation:* the arm is maintained in a fully abducted position with the forearm resting on the head. It is often referred to as *Luxatio Erecta* (erect dislocation)

Associated Injuries

ANTERIOR DISLOCATION

- Bankart lesion (avulsion of the anterior inferior aspect of the glenoid labrum and capsular attachments at the glenoid rim)
- Hill-Sachs lesion (a cortical depression in the posterolateral head of the humerus caused by the posterior humerus forcefully impacting the anterior glenoid rim)
- Nerve damage
- Fractures

POSTERIOR DISLOCATION

- Fractures of surgical neck or tuberosity
- Reverse Hill-Sachs lesion (a cortical depression on the anterior head of the humerus caused by the anterior humerus impacting the posterior glenoid rim)
- Reverse Bankart lesion (detachment of posteroinferior labrum with avulsion of posterior capsular periosteum)
- Rotator cuff tears

INFERIOR DISLOCATION

- Neurovascular injury
- Axillary nerve damage
- Internal capsule tears
- Rotator cuff injury

Differential Diagnosis

- Humeral fracture
- Clavicle fracture
- Scapula fracture
- Acromioclavicular joint injury
- Rotator cuff injury
- Bicipital tendinitis
- Rheumatoid arthritis
- Shoulder subluxation
- Biceps or triceps tendon rupture

Investigations

- X-ray
  - Usually, a shoulder X-ray will be sufficient to make a diagnosis. It will show the direction of the dislocation and rule out any associated fractures
- MRI
  - An MRI, but ideally an MR arthrogram, should be ordered if there is suspected cuff damage or labral lesions. It can also rule out any soft tissue pathologies
- CT
  - Used to assess traumatic fractures around the glenoid, Bankart lesions, labral tears, tendon and ligament damage

Management

CONSERVATIVE

- Prompt reduction of the glenohumeral joint – with either intraarticular injection or under conscious sedation. In some instances, it may need to be done under general anaesthetic
- Immobilisation in a sling – usually with the shoulder in a small degree of external rotation
- Maintain active range of movement of elbow, wrist and fingers while in the sling
- Begin active and passive shoulder movements when appropriate and the patient is out of the sling
- Gradually restore range of movement
- Provide rotator cuff strengthening exercises

SURGERY

Arthroscopic or, occasionally, open surgery to repair and tighten damaged tissue may be recommended for:

- Recurrent shoulder dislocations
- Young, active patients where there is a high rate of recurrence
- If non-surgical and conservative management has not helped

Reference

Lewis, A., Kitamura, T., Bayley, J. I. L. (2004). Mini symposium: shoulder instability (ii) the classification of shoulder instability: new light through old windows! *Current Orthopaedics, 18*, 97–108.

3.2.5 Acromioclavicular Joint Injury

Acromioclavicular (AC) injuries are common in athletes, especially those involved in contact sports (hockey, rugby and football). They usually result from falling directly onto the top of the shoulder while the arm is at the side in an adducted position but may also result from falling onto an outstretched hand.

Traumatic AC joint injuries can range from mild to severe and can be classified from low-grade joint sprains to higher-grade AC and coracoclavicular ligament ruptures and joint displacement.

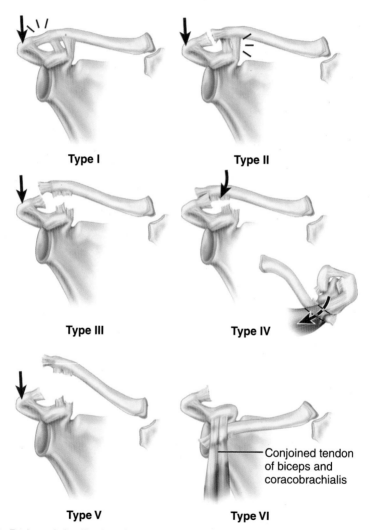

Fig 3.2.5.2 Rockwood classification of acromioclavicular separations. From Azar, F., Canale, F., Beaty, J. (2020). *Campbell's operative orthopaedics.* (14th Ed) Elsevier.

Rockwood Classification of Acromioclavicular Separation

Type	Description
I	Acromioclavicular (AC) joint sprain; ligaments intact
II	AC ligaments torn, coracoclavicular (CC) ligament intact. Lateral end of the clavicle may be mildly elevated
III	AC and CC ligaments torn, resulting in complete dislocation of the joint; more than five mm elevation of the clavicle
IV	Complete dislocation of the joint with the distal clavicle displaced posteriorly into or through the trapezius muscle
V	Complete dislocation with superior elevation of the clavicle one to three mm above its normal position. Complete disruption of deltoid and trapezius attachments from the distal clavicle
VI	Complete dislocation with the clavicle displaced inferior to the acromion and coracoid process

Adapted from: Rockwood, C.A., Jr. (1984). Fractures and dislocations of the shoulder. In: Rockwood, C.A., Jr, Green. D.P., editors. *Fractures in adults*. Philadelphia, PA: Lippincott; 860–910.

History

- Direct or indirect trauma to the AC joint
- Usually sports related
- Occurs mainly in people younger than 35 years old
- Men are far more likely to be affected than women
- Although uncommon, the patient may describe popping or catching around the AC joint

Symptoms

- Localised pain and swelling around the AC joint
- Painful and reduced shoulder movements
- Difficulty with overhead movements
- Difficulty with reaching across the body
- Pain when lying on the affected side
- Shoulder may catch with movement
- Increased pain when carrying heavy objects by the side of the body

Examination

- Focal tenderness on palpation of the AC joint
- Distal clavicle may be more prominent with a visible step or bump
- Loss of active and passive shoulder range of movement
- Muscle weakness

Tests

- Active compression test (O'Brien)
- Scarf test (Crossed-arm adduction test)
- Shear test

Differential Diagnosis

- Clavicle fracture
- Acromioclavicular osteoarthritis
- Distal clavicle osteolysis
- Shoulder dislocation
- Rotator cuff injury
- Labral tear
- Pectoralis major tendinosis/tear
- Biceps tenosynovitis
- Adhesive capsulitis

Investigations

- X-ray
  - An X-ray can be used to make a diagnosis of AC joint injury and can also identify other causes of traumatic shoulder pain
- MRI
  - An MRI scan may be ordered if there is any uncertainty in diagnosis and to rule out any additional intra-articular and/or extra-articular glenohumeral joint pathology

Management

CONSERVATIVE

- Mild cases can be treated conservatively, while more severe cases may require surgery and postoperative rehabilitation.

Type I–II Injuries

Initial treatment consists of:
- RICE protocol (Rest, Ice, Compression, Elevation)
- Immobilise arm in a sling
- Relative rest
- Activity modification – avoid overhead reaching, reaching across the body, heavy lifting or sleeping on the affected side
- When appropriate, commence muscle strengthening and range of movement exercises

Type III

- Initial management is the same as that for Type I and II, but the arm may be immobilised for longer
- Although conservative treatment is the main option for Type III injuries, surgery may be considered for younger, more active patients. The decision to proceed will reflect the individual's demands and may allow a high-level athlete or manual worker a quicker return to activity

Type IV–VI

- Surgery is often indicated for Type IV–VI patients, but this will depend on various factors, including the patient's activity levels, whether there is associated muscle or nerve damage, other existing health conditions and the expectations of the patient

MEDICATION

- Non-steroidal anti-inflammatory drugs (NSAIDs) where safe and tolerated
- Weak opiates with or without paracetamol if NSAIDs contraindicated, not tolerated or ineffective

INJECTION

- A steroid injection into the AC joint may be considered to help to reduce inflammation and pain

SURGERY

- Type IV–VI injuries usually require surgery. This is aimed at correcting the displacement of the clavicle and easing pressure on the nearby trapezius muscles, and/or repairing or reconstructing injured ligaments

3.2.6 Glenohumeral Arthritis

Glenohumeral arthritis (GA) is a progressive joint disease characterised by degeneration of the articular cartilage and subchondral bone with narrowing of the glenohumeral joint space. It is described as either primary (no history of injury, disease or illness) or secondary (due to trauma, injury or infection). The progression of primary GA is difficult to predict as the changes to the articular surface and subchondral bone occur over months to years, and there is often little correlation between the changes observed on imaging and the patient's symptoms.

History

- Gradual onset of pain deep in the shoulder joint
- Often asymmetric
- Pain worse with prolonged activity or after periods of inactivity
- Progressive loss of range of movement
- Pain and disability worsen over time
- Poor sleep – unable to sleep on the affected side and waking with night pain
- Incidence increases with age – >50–55 years old – although symptoms may appear earlier

Symptoms

- Joint pain and stiffness
- Morning stiffness – improves with gentle movement and lasts less than 30 min
- Increased pain with shoulder movements
- Reduced shoulder range of movement
- Crepitus with movement

Examination

- Loss of passive and active glenohumeral range of movement, especially external rotation, forward flexion and internal rotation
- Crepitus in the shoulder
- Joint tenderness
- Muscle wasting and a feeling of weakness
- Joint effusion

Differential Diagnosis

- Rotator cuff dysfunction
- Shoulder impingement
- Adhesive capsulitis
- Rheumatoid arthritis
- Biceps tendinitis
- Calcific tendinitis
- Bursitis
- Labral tear
- Cervical radiculopathy

Investigations

There is often little correlation between the changes seen on X-ray and MRI and the level of pain and distress described by the patient. Many patients with significant changes remain asymptomatic and vice versa.

- X-ray
  - An X-ray will be able to identify some of the principal signs of GA, such as subchondral sclerosis, osteophyte formation, bony erosion and subchondral cyst formation, joint space narrowing and posterior glenoid wear
- Ultrasound
  - Ultrasound can be used to assess bony changes associated with GA and the presence of joint effusion and synovial swelling, inflammation and thickening
- MRI
  - GA can be diagnosed without an MRI scan but is often used to assess for cartilage and labral pathology, bone marrow oedema, joint effusion, synovitis and the rotator cuff muscles. This information is often an integral part of surgical planning

Management

CONSERVATIVE

- The aim of treatment is to manage pain, improve the range of movement and restore function
- Education and advice on managing the condition
- Activity modification – avoid aggravating activities and prolonged inactivity
- Home exercise programme – aimed at strengthening and stretching exercises for the upper limb, increasing or maintaining range of movement and improving proprioception and function

MEDICATION

- Non-steroidal anti-inflammatory drugs (NSAIDs) where safe and tolerated
- Weak opiates with or without paracetamol if NSAIDs contraindicated, not tolerated or ineffective

INJECTIONS

- A corticosteroid injection may help to manage an exacerbation of shoulder pain or when severe symptoms are limiting movement and function and preventing the patient from engaging with conservative treatment

SURGERY

- Surgery may be considered if conservative measures have not helped. Ideally, patients are referred for surgical consideration before significant functional limitations develop or pain becomes severe. Although function can be affected by GA, the primary aim of surgery is to reduce pain
- Surgical interventions include:
  - Arthroscopic debridement or osteotomy
  - Shoulder resurfacing
  - Hemiarthroplasty
  - Total shoulder replacement
  - Reverse shoulder replacement
  - Autologous cartilage implantation and autograft

3.2.7   Long Head of Biceps Tendinopathy

Biceps tendinopathy refers to pain and dysfunction of the long head of the biceps (LHB) tendon resulting from degeneration, inflammation, overuse or trauma. It is often associated with other shoulder conditions, such as rotator cuff disorders, superior labrum anterior-posterior (SLAP) lesions, shoulder instability, acromioclavicular joint disorders and subacromial impingement.

History

- Gradual, progressive onset of anterior shoulder pain
- Declining function over time
- Aggravated by repetitive overhead activities, lifting or pulling
- Worse at night
- Difficulty sleeping on the affected shoulder

Symptoms

- Pain localised to the area of the bicipital groove
- Shoulder weakness
- Pain may radiate to the biceps muscle belly and, sometimes, down to the elbow and hand
- Patients may report clicking or popping with rotational movements

Examination

- It is often difficult to differentiate LHB tendinopathy as findings are similar to other conditions that affect the glenohumeral joint
- The most common finding is focal tenderness over the bicipital groove while palpating an area about three to six cm below the anterior margin of the acromion with the arm in 10° of internal rotation

Tests

- Speed's test
- Yergason's test

Differential Diagnosis

- Rotator cuff dysfunction
- Subacromial impingement
- Glenohumeral instability
- Adhesive capsulitis
- Glenohumeral osteoarthritis
- Acromioclavicular joint pathology
- Subacromial bursitis
- SLAP lesions
- Cervical spine pathology

Investigations

- X-ray
  - Does not diagnose LHB tendinopathy but may be ordered to exclude bony abnormalities and glenohumeral osteoarthritis
- MRI/MR arthrography (MRA)
  - An MRI, but ideally an MRA, allows visualisation of the bicipital groove and biceps and is able to detect other associated pathology and rule out other possible causes
- Ultrasound
  - Cost-effective and accurate method of visualising thickened and degenerative tendons and ruling out other possible pathologies

Management

CONSERVATIVE

- Relative rest
- Activity modification – avoiding repetitive overhead activities, lifting and pulling
- Exercises that progressively load the tendon (initially isometric and then progressing to eccentric and then concentric movements)
- Stretching exercises
- Graded strengthening of the rotator cuff muscles, scapular stabilisers and biceps
- Postural advice and correction

MEDICATION

- Non-steroidal anti-inflammatory drugs (NSAIDs) where safe and tolerated
- Weak opiates with or without paracetamol if NSAIDs contraindicated, not tolerated or ineffective

INJECTION

- A corticosteroid injection may be helpful in managing pain and inflammation, especially in patients who have not responded to NSAIDs and other pain management strategies

SURGERY

- Surgery may be appropriate if symptoms have not responded to conservative treatment
- Surgical techniques include:
  - Arthroscopic or open tenotomy
    - The LHB tendon is released from its attachment to the glenoid
  - Arthroscopic or open tenodesis
    - The LHB tendon is detached from the glenoid and reattached to the humerus

3.2.8   Glenoid Labrum Tear

The glenoid labrum is a fibrocartilaginous ring that encircles and deepens the glenoid cavity, increasing the stability of the shoulder joint. Repetitive shoulder movements or a traumatic event can lead to a labral tear, causing pain and instability of the shoulder. Tears can be located in the upper or lower part of the glenoid socket.

A superior labrum, lateral, anterior to posterior (SLAP) lesion is a tear of the upper glenoid rim that may also involve the biceps tendon, while a Bankart lesion is a tear below the middle of the socket that involves the inferior glenohumeral ligament.

History

- Risk factors for a SLAP lesion include:
    - Being involved in overhead sports (tennis, baseball pitching, volleyball)
    - Falling on an outstretched arm
    - Lifting a heavy load (weightlifting)
    - Direct shoulder trauma
- A Bankart lesion typically occurs as a result of an anterior shoulder dislocation
- Increasing age is also a risk factor due to age-related changes weakening the attachment of the labrum to the glenoid

Symptoms

- Pain with overhead movement
- A feeling of instability in the shoulder
- Catching, clicking, grinding or popping sensation with shoulder movement
- Decreased range of movement
- Muscle weakness
- Shoulder subluxation/dislocation

Examination

It is difficult to differentiate between labral tears, rotator cuff dysfunction and shoulder instability during an examination. Diagnosis is therefore reliant on the patient's history, special tests and/or diagnostic imaging or arthroscopy

Special Tests

- Clunk test (Bankart)
- Anterior slide test (Bankart/SLAP)
- Active compression of O'Brien (SLAP)
- Biceps tension test (SLAP)
- Biceps load test (SLAP)
- SLAP prehension test (SLAP)
- Labral Crank test (Bankart/SLAP)

Differential Diagnosis

- Rotator cuff injury
- Cervical radiculopathy
- Shoulder impingement
- Supraspinatus tendonitis
- Shoulder dislocation
- Clavicle fracture
- Acromioclavicular joint injury

Investigations

- X-ray
  - A glenoid labrum tear will not show up on X-ray but may be ordered to rule out other shoulder pathologies such as osteoarthritis and fractures
- MRI/ MR arthrogram (MRA)
  - If a labral tear is suspected, an MRA should be ordered to diagnose the tear and rule out other potential causes of injury
  - An MRI can often miss a labral tear and produce a negative result, which may lead to the patient needing to have further investigations (i.e. MRA)
  - Smaller tears may be difficult to identify, and arthroscopy may be needed to make a clear diagnosis

Management
CONSERVATIVE

- Relative rest
- Activity modification
- Strengthening exercises – rotator cuff, shoulder and scapular muscles
- Increasing shoulder range of movement
- Improving dynamic shoulder stability
- Posterior capsule stretching, if appropriate

MEDICATION

- Non-steroidal anti-inflammatory drugs (NSAIDs), where safe and tolerated
- Weak opiates with or without paracetamol if NSAIDs are contraindicated, not tolerated or ineffective

SURGERY

- Surgery may be considered when conservative management has failed to reduce symptoms or to facilitate a return to activity

- Surgery is primarily via arthroscopy and includes:
  - Debridement of the glenoid labrum (trimming or removing the damaged part of the labrum)
  - Reattachment of the superior labrum to the glenoid and anchoring of the biceps tendon
  - Biceps tenodesis (the long head of the biceps is detached from the glenoid and reattached to the upper part of the humerus)

Elbow

3.3.1 Lateral Epicondylitis (Tennis Elbow)

Lateral epicondylitis is a common overuse disorder affecting the extensor tendons (particularly those of extensor carpi brevis and extensor carpi ulnaris) and is usually driven by repetitive wrist dorsiflexion with supination and pronation. It has historically been called tennis elbow; although it is commonly seen in non-athletes.

History

May include the following risk factors:
- Prior history of epicondylitis
- Occupations with repetitive actions (e.g. bricklayer, gardener)
- Sports (e.g. racquet sports, golf)
    - Using heavier or wet balls, overhitting, using a new racquet that is a different size or requires a changed grip
    - Poor mechanics (e.g. overhitting or backhand with an extended elbow or flexed wrist)
- Leisure activities
    - Knitting, DIY with prolonged, repeated use of hand tools (e.g. screwdriver) or playing a musical instrument
- Smoking
- Fluoroquinolone antibiotics (e.g. ciprofloxacin), especially in the first month of use

Symptoms

- Pain is located around the lateral epicondyle
- May radiate to the lateral forearm
- Worsens during or after elbow flexion or extension
- Exacerbated by holding or gripping objects while holding the wrist in neutral or extension

- Pain may increase with repetition of activity
- Acute onset or can be delayed up to 24–72 h after a recent change in activity or overloading event (e.g. trimming the garden hedges)
- Loss of grip strength

Examination

- Tenderness over the lateral epicondyle and common extensor tendon
- Pain on resisted wrist or middle finger extension
  - This is more provocative with the elbow in extension and the wrist pronated
- Reduction in grip strength
- Pain reproduced on lifting in overhand grip
- Positive extensor carpi radials brevis stretch
- Range of movement should be preserved in all but very late stage
- Loss of range of movement, especially with clicking, may suggest loose bodies
- Swelling and warmth may be found

Differential Diagnosis

- Cervical radiculopathy
- Synovitis of radio-humeral joint
- Radio-humeral bursitis
- Osteochondritis dissecans of capitellum or radius
- Osteoarthritis of radio-humeral joint
- Posterior interosseous nerve entrapment (radial tunnel syndrome)
- Lateral collateral ligament complex injury
- Radial head fracture
- Intra-articular loose bodies – may be associated with trauma
- Enthesopathy associated with systemic inflammatory disorder

Investigations

Lateral epicondylitis is primarily a clinical diagnosis that only requires further investigations if there is clinical uncertainty or other pathologies are suspected

- Ultrasound
  - May identify areas of hypoechogenicity and partial tears
- MRI
  - May show increased signal intensity and oedema around the tendon as well as excluding complete rupture of the extensor origin

Management

CONSERVATIVE

- Education and information – inform patients that the condition can be self-limiting, but recovery can take between six and twelve months
- PRICE (Protection, Relative rest, Ice, Compression, Elevation)
- Activity modification – to reduce the load on the tendon

- Graduated loading programme
- Eccentric exercise programme
- Elbow brace

MEDICATION

- Non-steroidal anti-inflammatory drugs (NSAIDs) where safe and tolerated
- Weak opiates with or without paracetamol if NSAIDs contraindicated, not tolerated or ineffective.

INJECTION

- Corticosteroid injection may be considered to reduce inflammation and pain if symptoms are not resolved with conservative measures but are associated with poorer long term outcomes (including tendon damage and rupture)

SURGERY

- Its use is limited to cases where there are signs of elbow instability or when extensive conservative measures have failed
- May include excision of the degenerative section of the tendon in addition to localised debridement

3.3.2   Medial Epicondylitis (Golfer's Elbow)

Medial epicondylitis is an overuse disorder that affects the flexor tendons of the wrist (particularly those of flexor carpi radialis and pronator teres). It is less common than tennis elbow and is usually driven by repeated loading of the forearm muscles.

History

May include the following risk factors:
- Prior history of epicondylitis
- Occupational risk factors
  - Manual handling of heavy loads, use of hand tools (e.g. repeated use of hammer)
- Throwing activities that place valgus stress on the elbow (e.g. baseball pitch, javelin throwing)
- Sports with repeated wrist flexion and forearm pronation (e.g. golf and tennis) or excessive use of wrist flexors (e.g. tennis players who put a lot of topspin on the forehand)
- Smoking
- Fluoroquinolone antibiotics (e.g. ciprofloxacin), especially in the first month of use

Symptoms

- Medial elbow pain that is often described as sharp and persistent
- May radiate along the medial side of the elbow to the forearm
- Worsens on activities, including opening doors or shaking hands
- Can be acute or, more usually, insidious in onset
- May occur alongside other upper limb disorders (e.g. carpal tunnel syndrome, ulnar neuritis, lateral epicondylitis or rotator cuff disorders)

Examination

- Localised tenderness at or below the medial epicondyle and over pronator teres and flexor carpi radialis
- Pain on resisted wrist flexion and forearm pronation (starting with elbow fully extended and forearm supinated)
- Range of movement should be preserved in all but very late or advanced stage
- Negative Tinel's sign over cubital tunnel
- Normal neurology in the upper limb is expected
- Instability on valgus stress suggests medial collateral ligament sprain
- May be associated with:
  - Ulnar neuritis with Tinel's sign over the cubital tunnel, paraesthesia in the ring and little finger and weakness in the hand (Froment's sign)
  - Ulnar collateral ligament injury

Differential Diagnosis

- Medial collateral ligament sprain
- Ulnar neuritis
- Avulsion fracture of the medial epicondyle
- Apophysitis
- Referred pain – C6/7 radiculopathy

- Ulnar or median nerve neuropathy (including cubital tunnel syndrome)
- Osteoarthritis

Investigation

Not usually required as medial epicondylitis is primarily a clinical diagnosis
- Ultrasound
  - May help in complex cases with areas of hypoechogenicity and partial tears the most common finding
- MRI
  - May show increased signal intensity and oedema around the tendon

Management

CONSERVATIVE

- Education and information – inform patients that the condition can be self-limiting, but recovery can take between six and twelve months
- PRICE (Protection, Relative rest, Ice, Compression, Elevation)
- Activity modification – to reduce the load on the tendon
- Graduated loading programme
- Eccentric exercise programme
- Elbow brace

MEDICATION

- Non-steroidal anti-inflammatory drugs (NSAIDs) where safe and tolerated
- Weak opiates with or without paracetamol if NSAIDs contraindicated, not tolerated or ineffective

INJECTION

- Corticosteroid injection may be considered to reduce inflammation and pain if symptoms are not resolving with conservative measures but are associated with poorer long term outcomes (including tendon damage and rupture)

SURGERY

- Limited to use in cases where there are signs of elbow instability or when extensive conservative measures have failed
- May include excision of the degenerative section of the tendon and tends to be an open approach to avoid damage to the ulnar nerve and ulnar collateral ligament

3.3.3 Osteoarthritis of the Elbow

Osteoarthrtitis of the elbow describes degenerative changes usually involving the articular surfaces of the olecranon and the coronoid processes of the humerus with associated osteophyte formation limiting the range of movement. Primary osteoarthritis of the elbow is very rare and it is more usually secondary to previous trauma to the elbow creating disruption to the articular surface, ligament instability or malunion of a fracture or related to overhead sports or activities.

History

- Primary osteoarthritis
  - More common in men
  - Usually in the dominant arm
  - Associated with heavy manual work
  - May be found in sports that place repeated, heavy burden on the affected limb
- Secondary osteoarthritis
  - Usually follows trauma to the elbow (e.g. fracture causing altered biomechanics and changes to the articular surfaces)

Symptoms

- Joint pain – usually in the lateral aspect of the joint
- Patient may describe pain at the end range of movement in the early stages, but this may develop into pain throughout the range of movement as the condition progresses
- Loss of range of movement may precede the onset of pain
  - Extension tends to be lost first (especially for secondary osteoarthritis)
- Mechanical symptoms, including clicking, catching and blocks to movement – suggestive of intra-articular loose bodies
- Ulnar neuropathy may accompany elbow osteoarthritis with features of hand weakness and paraesthesia

Examination

- Deformity and muscle atrophy may be observed in comparison to the other arm
- Reduced range of movement
- May have features of ulnar neuropathy, including a positive elbow flexion test and Tinel's signs over the cubital tunnel

Differential Diagnosis

- Cervical radiculopathy or referred pain
- Ligament sprain or tear
- Medial or lateral epicondyle tendinopathy
- Ulnar neuropathy
- Fracture

Investigation

- X-ray
  - May identify osteophytes on the coronoid process and olecranon. Joint space narrowing and loose bodies may be seen (but not always)
- CT
  - May identify loose bodies, deformity or mal-alignment of prior fractures

Management

CONSERVATIVE

- Education and information
- Splinting
- Ice or heat
- Exercise therapy – including range of movement and strengthening exercises

MEDICATION

- Topical non-steroidal anti-inflammatory gel or cream
- Oral paracetamol and non-steroidal anti-inflammatory drugs (NSAIDs) where safe and tolerated

INJECTION

- Intra-articular corticosteroid injection for pain and inflammation if symptoms are not resolving with conservative measures

SURGERY

- Techniques include debridement or arthroplasty (total or radio-capitellar)
- With more focal lateral compartment pain, resection of the radial head may be indicated

3.3.4   Olecranon Bursitis

Olecranon bursitis describes pain and swelling over the elbow representing thickening and inflammation of the olecranon bursa, a small synovial fluid-containing sac that lies on the bony tip of the olecranon. This is usually caused by localised pressure, friction, infection, inflammation or trauma.

History

There is an increased risk with:
- Occupational factors
  - Repeated prolonged pressure, irritation or friction over the elbow (e.g. mechanics, gardeners)
- History of inflammatory arthritis, including gout and rheumatoid arthritis
- Previous history of olecranon bursitis
- Immunosuppression (e.g. cancer, diabetes, steroids) increases the risk of infection
- History of localised trauma or damage to superficial skin with a laceration or puncture wound that may lead to infection (usually with *Staphylococcus aureus*)

Symptoms

- Acute onset associated with trauma or infection
- Chronic, insidious onset if driven by prolonged or repeated irritation or friction
- Systemic features, including fever, malaise and rigours, suggest infection or sepsis
- An acute crystal bursitis can present with similar features

Examination

- Tender swelling over olecranon with the appearance of an egg or golf ball
- Decreased range of movement, especially flexion, which stretches the inflamed bursa
- Severe tenderness, swelling or erythema with fever may suggest infection, especially in those with risk factors
- The presence of nodules may indicate gout or rheumatoid arthritis
- There may be evidence of an abrasion, puncture wound or contusion
- Peri-bursal cellulitis with erythema spreading beyond the localised swelling may be found
- Presence of focal inflammation may be found in gout and rheumatoid arthritis

Differential Diagnosis

- Rheumatoid arthritis
- Gout or pseudogout
- Triceps tendinopathy
- Posterior impingement
- Olecranon fracture

Investigation

- Blood tests
  - Are of limited use but may show an elevated erythrocyte sedimentation rate, C-reactive protein level and uraemia. However, urate may be normal in acute gout or a positive rheumatoid factor or anti-cyclic citrullinated peptide. A raised white cell count would suggest infection
- Aspiration of the bursa
  - Gram stain and culture to identify organisms in septic bursitis
  - Microscopy looking for crystals to identify gout or pseudogout
- X-ray
  - May reveal evidence of olecranon spurs in chronic or recurrent bursitis

Management

CONSERVATIVE

- PRICE (Protection, Relative rest, Ice, Compression, Elevation)
- Support – elbow pad to cushion and prevent direct contact
- Treatment of underlying gout, if present
- Referral to rheumatology if features suggestive of rheumatoid arthritis

MEDICATION

- Non-steroidal anti-inflammatory drugs, where safe and tolerated
- Antibiotic treatment if signs of infection – be aware of spreading infection and sepsis (signs include spreading erythema, fever, increased pulse rate and low blood pressure). This may necessitate urgent admission for intravenous antibiotics, fluids and close monitoring

INJECTION

- Aspiration may be both diagnostic and therapeutic
- Corticosteroid injection may be considered to reduce inflammation and pain if symptoms are not resolving with conservative measures in the absence of any infection

SURGERY

- Surgery may be considered in case of failure to respond to conservative therapies
- May include open or arthroscopic bursectomy

3.4

Hand and Wrist

3.4.1 Carpal Tunnel Syndrome

Carpal tunnel syndrome (CTS) is the most common entrapment neuropathy encountered in practice. It is caused by compression and ischaemia of the median nerve in the carpal tunnel of the wrist (the space between the carpal bones and the flexor retinaculum) resulting in symptoms of numbness, pins and needles and pain in the hand, wrist and forearm.

History

- Tends to affect females more than males
- More common in people >30 years old
- There is an increased risk with:
  - Obesity
  - Rheumatoid disease
  - Diabetes mellitus (carpal tunnel may also precede the development of diabetes)
  - Acromegaly
  - Hypothyroidism
  - Pregnancy
  - Previous wrist fracture (e.g. Colle's fracture)
  - Occupational factors (e.g. computer use, use of hand-held vibrating instruments, repetitive flexion or twisting of the wrist)
  - Tumours or space-occupying lesions (e.g. lipomas, ganglion)
  - Congenital carpal tunnel stenosis

Symptoms

- Pain and paraesthesia, usually in median nerve distribution (thumb, second, third and radial side of the fourth finger)
- May also describe a burning sensation in the hand
- Pain may radiate to the wrist and forearm
- Intermittent and gradual onset of symptoms that can become more constant in severe cases
- Pain worse at night

- Pain is eased with movement (e.g. by flicking or shaking the wrist)
- Decreased grip strength (e.g. difficulty opening jars) and clumsiness in more severe cases
- Sensation of swelling or tightness in hand or wrist
- May be unilateral (commonly in the dominant hand) or bilateral

Examination

- Weakness and wasting of the opponens policis and abductor pollicis brevis
- Atrophy of thenar eminence (indicator of severe CTS)
- Normal reflexes (useful to distinguish between CTS and radiculopathy)
- Examination may reveal no findings

Tests

- Phalen's test
- Hand elevation test
- Tinel's sign
- Durkan's test

Differential Diagnosis

- Cervical radiculopathy (C6/7)
- Multiple sclerosis
- Osteoarthritis (base of the thumb)
- Median nerve entrapment at another point (e.g. pronator teres syndrome)
- Diabetic neuropathy
- Inflammatory arthritis (small joints of hand)
- De Quervain's tenosynovitis

Investigation

CTS is primarily a clinical diagnosis that only requires further investigations if there is clinical uncertainty.

- Ultrasound/MRI
  - Is rarely used but may help diagnose and grade CTS by assessing the cross-sectional area of the median nerve and changes in the flexor retinaculum
- Electromyelography (EMG) and nerve conduction studies (NCS)
  - Not routinely required but may help identify and locate lesions if the diagnosis is uncertain
  - May show slowing of median nerve conduction velocity and reduced or absent motor responses if severe
  - Can also assess the severity of damage to the median nerve as part of surgical planning

Management

CONSERVATIVE

- Activity modification – adapt provocative movements or activities that place the wrist into flexion for prolonged periods (e.g. holding a phone, driving)
- Wrist splints – worn principally at night

INJECTIONS

- Corticosteroid injection may be considered to reduce inflammation and pain if symptoms are not resolving with conservative measures

SURGERY

- Surgery may be considered if there is a failure to respond to conservative therapies and/or significant symptoms, including:
  - Constant numbness and tingling during day and night
  - Symptoms significantly disturbing function (e.g. sleep or driving)
  - Thenar muscle atrophy
- Surgical release involves division of the flexor retinaculum and decompression of the carpal tunnel

3.4.2 De Quervain's Tenosynovitis

De Quervain's tenosynovitis is a chronic overuse condition affecting the abductor pollicis longus and extensor pollicis brevis tendons and tendon sheath of the thumb, causing pain and inflammation around the radial styloid and base of the thumb.

History

- Unusual, repeated or excessive loading of the thumb
  - Sporting activity (e.g. racquet sports, rowers)
  - Occupational roles (e.g. carpenters, gardeners)
  - Mothers repeatedly lifting or carrying their newborn babies
  - Affects females more than males
  - More prevalent in 30- to 50-year-old people
  - Associated with rheumatoid arthritis, insulin-dependent diabetics, menopause and pregnancy

Symptoms

- Pain over the radial styloid radiating proximally or distally
- Pain that is worse with gripping
- Pain with activities involving ulnar deviation with a clenched fist (e.g. gripping, lifting, hammering)
- Symptoms are initially activity related but may progress to become constant
- May disturb sleep

Examination

- Swelling of the tendon sheath at the distal radial styloid process
- Localised tenderness along the tendon sheath
- Pain is worse with resisted thumb abduction
- Palpable crepitus on thumb movements – particularly resisted extension and abduction
- Numbness of the dorsum of the thumb is a rare but occasional finding

Tests

- Finklestein's test

Differential Diagnosis

- Osteoarthritis (base of the thumb)
- Rheumatoid arthritis
- Fracture
- Septic arthritis
- Septic tenosynovitis
- Gout

Investigations

De Quervain's tenosynovitis is primarily a clinical diagnosis that only requires further investigations if there is clinical uncertainty

- Ultrasound
  - Ultrasound may identify tendon thickening, effusion and hyperaemia
- MRI
  - May show evidence of oedema in the tendon sheath and surrounding tissues with enlargement of the tendon in more advanced cases

Management

CONSERVATIVE

- Activity modification (e.g. lifting with an underhand grip, not an overhand grip)
- Thumb splint or spica
- Graded return to hand function

MEDICATION

- Non-steroidal anti-inflammatory drugs (NSAIDs) where safe and tolerated
- Weak opiates with or without paracetamol if NSAIDs contraindicated, not tolerated or ineffective

INJECTION

- Corticosteroid injection may be considered to reduce inflammation and pain if symptoms are not resolving with conservative measures
- May be used independently or alongside splinting

SURGERY

- Surgery may be considered in case of failure to respond to conservative therapies and/or in case of significant symptoms
- Options include the release of the extensor compartment and other compartment releases and may involve excision of the stenosed sheath

3.4.3 Trigger Finger

Trigger finger is a condition characterised by a restriction in finger extension due to inflammation of the flexor tendon as it penetrates its sheath at the metacarpophalangeal joint (MCPJ) level. The name is derived from a nodule in the tendon causing a restriction in extension at a certain point and a 'snap' as the obstruction is passed

The precise cause is uncertain in many cases, and along with de Quervain's disease, they form the most common types of tenosynovitis of the wrist.

History

- Affects females more than males
- Generally in people >40 years old
- Can affect any finger, but it most commonly occurs at the middle and ring fingers
- There is an increased risk with:
  - Diabetes
  - Rheumatoid arthritis
- May relate to trauma, inflammation and overuse during work activities, sports or leisure
- Congenital trigger finger presents in young children with the finger locked in flexion or extension

Symptoms

- Clicking with flexion or extension of the affected digit
- Pain may be present in the region of the thickened tendon
- Locking of the finger in flexion – patient may wake with the affected finger stuck in the flexed position
- May need to use the other hand to straighten out a locked finger

Examination

- Tenderness over the palmar aspect of the MCPJ
- Thickening may be palpable as a tender nodule along the line of the flexor tendon at the level of the A1 or, less commonly, A3 pulley
- Restriction in extension beyond a certain point and a 'snap' as the obstruction is passed
- The patient can often demonstrate the triggering action
- A fixed flexion deformity is unlikely. If present, it may suggest a Dupuytren's contracture

Differential Diagnosis

- Dupuytren's contracture
- Flexor tendon or sheath tumour
- Dislocation
- Infection of the flexor tendon or sheath
- Ulnar collateral ligament injury
- Extensor tendon rupture
- Metacarpophalangeal joint arthritis

Investigations

Trigger finger is primarily a clinical diagnosis that only requires further investigations if there is clinical uncertainty or other pathologies suspected

Management

CONSERVATIVE

- Splinting
  - Using a tongue depressor running from the proximal interphalangeal joint to the palm
  - Used mainly at night
- Buddy taping
  - Strapping the affected finger to an adjacent finger

MEDICATION

- Non-steroidal anti-inflammatory drugs are of limited use

INJECTION

- Corticosteroid injection may be considered to reduce inflammation and pain if symptoms are not resolved with conservative measures
  - Following injection, the pain usually resolves within a couple of days, but the locking and triggering may take a couple of weeks to resolve

SURGERY

- Surgery may be considered in case of failure to respond to conservative therapies and/or in case of significant symptoms
  - Consider urgent referral to the hand surgeons for release if the finger is stuck in flexion
  - May involve a pulley release or synovectomy

Hip

3.5.1   Hip Osteoarthritis

The hip is a major weight-bearing joint subjected to large static and dynamic forces that predispose the articular surfaces of the femur and acetabulum to osteoarthritis (OA). Although the articular cartilage is mainly affected, there are also changes in the subchondral bone, joint margins and surrounding tissue. This leads to the characteristic symptoms of pain, stiffness and reduced mobility and function.

History

- Insidious onset of pain that is poorly localised (though it is possible to have a sudden onset)
- Pain eased with gentle movement and activity
- Aggravated by more vigorous activity
- Difficulty with walking, bending down and getting up from a chair
- Pain and disability worsen over time
- Incidence increases with age

Symptoms

- Dull, aching pain in the groin area
- May radiate into the thigh, buttocks and down to the knee
- Morning stiffness – improves with movement and lasts less than 30 min
- Pain and stiffness after sitting and resting
- Difficulty weight-bearing on the affected side – affects gait pattern and mobility
- Can be worse at night

Examination

- Muscle weakness and tightness, especially gluteals and quadriceps
- Decreased range of movement in the hip, especially hip internal rotation

- Altered gait pattern
- Joint crepitus may be present with hip movement

Tests

- Hip quadrant test

Differential diagnosis

- Hip fractures – femoral neck, acetabulum, pubic ramus
- Referred lumbar spine pain
- Lumbar radiculopathy
- Trochanteric bursitis
- Acetabular labral tear
- Transient synovitis
- Meralgia parasthetica
- Rheumatoid arthritis
- Septic arthritis
- Avascular necrosis
- Polymyalgia rheumatica
- Prostate cancer
- Intrapelvic pathology

Investigations

- X-ray
  - Radiography is the main investigation for diagnosing hip OA. It allows visualisation of joint space narrowing, osteophytes at the joint margins, joint space narrowing, subchondral cysts and remodelling of the femoral head in chronic cases
  - It is worth noting that there is often a mismatch between X-ray findings and the severity of the patient's symptoms. Patients with severe OA findings on X-ray may be asymptomatic and vice versa
- MRI
  - Not normally required for a diagnosis of hip OA but may be ordered to review secondary causes or abnormalities arising from the bone marrow, ligaments and synovium
  - An MRI may also be used to inform surgical planning
- CT (computed tomography) examination
  - Can be used to identify OA changes, including subchondral cysts, bone sclerosis and osteophytes and their adjacent soft tissue
  - May also be used for surgical planning to review acetabular and femoral head anatomy
- Ultrasound
  - Ultrasound can detect and evaluate joint effusions, synovitis, cartilage abnormalities and osteophytes

Management
CONSERVATIVE

- Education and advice

- Activity modification – avoiding aggravating activities and prolonged inactivity
- Weight management
- Exercise programme – aimed at strengthening and stretching exercises for the muscles around the hip, increasing or maintaining range of movement and improving muscle control and function
- Hydrotherapy – if indicated and available
- Walking aids, if appropriate, to decrease joint loading

MEDICATION

- Non-steroidal anti-inflammatory drugs (NSAIDs) where safe and tolerated
- Weak opiates with or without paracetamol if NSAIDs contraindicated, not tolerated or ineffective

INJECTIONS

- Intra-articular corticosteroid injections offer short-term pain relief and should be used in conjunction with other treatments to reduce pain and swelling and provide an opportunity to engage in rehabilitation

SURGERY

- Surgery may be indicated when:
  - Severe pain limits daily activity
  - There is ongoing pain, inflammation and swelling that does not respond to rest or medication
  - The hip has not improved with conservative treatment
- Surgery is aimed at significantly decreasing pain and improving function. Surgical options include:
  - Total hip arthroplasty (also called total hip arthroplasty) – the arthritic cartilage and bone of the femoral head and acetabulum are removed and replaced with prosthetic components
  - Hip resurfacing – the surface of the femoral head is trimmed and replaced with a smooth metal cap. In addition, the damaged bone and cartilage within the acetabulum are also removed, and a metal cup is inserted in its place. Hip resurfacing is generally offered to younger (>60 years old), active patients with good bone health and those with larger frames. The benefits of hip resurfacing are that they may be easier to revise, and there is a decreased risk of dislocation.

3.5.2 Greater Trochanteric Pain Syndrome

Greater trochanteric pain syndrome (GTPS) is a common cause of lateral hip pain. It was previously referred to as trochanteric bursitis, as it was attributed to inflamed bursae. However, its symptoms are now attributed to tendinopathy of the gluteus medius and/or gluteus minimus, and bursal pathology or inflammation is not always present.

History

- Gradual onset of lateral hip pain that can radiate down the thigh and into the buttock
- Linked to inflammation or trauma affecting muscles, tendons, fascia or bursae
- Triggered by a number of factors, including falls, prolonged weight-bearing, excessive or repetitive loading, an altered gait or a sudden change in activity
- Patient may have associated conditions such as low back pain, knee osteoarthritis, rheumatoid arthritis or fibromyalgia
- Can progressively worsen over time

Symptoms

- Pain in the lateral hip localised to the greater trochanter
- Symptoms aggravated with physical activity, overuse, prolonged weight-bearing or sitting or lying on the affected side

Examination

- Tenderness with palpation around the greater trochanter
- Replication of pain with passive hip adduction
- Pain with resisted active abduction, resisted internal rotation and/or resisted external rotation of the affected hip
- Weak hip abductors
- Lateral hip pain within 30 s of maintaining a single leg stance on the affected side

Tests

- Trendelenburg test

Differential Diagnosis

- Hip osteoarthritis
- Avascular necrosis of the femoral head
- Labral tear
- Hip impingement
- Hip fracture (stress or neck of femur)
- Meralgia paraesthetica
- Inflammatory joint disease
- Lumbar radiculopathy

Investigations

GTPS is primarily a clinical diagnosis so imaging studies are not usually required. It may, however, be indicated when treatment is not working or if there is a more complex picture and other pathologies need to be identified or excluded

- X-ray
    - Will often come back as normal. May be ordered to exclude other possible causes of symptoms such as hip osteoarthritis, calcific tendinopathy and fractures
- MRI
    - MRIs may be ordered if an alternative pathology is suspected
- Ultrasound
    - Can confirm the diagnosis of GTPS. Ultrasound can visualise thickened and fluid-filled trochanteric bursa or muscle tears and rule out other pathology

Management

CONSERVATIVE

- Relative rest
- Ice
- Activity modification - avoid activities that place load on the muscle/tendon (climbing stairs, walking uphill or standing on one leg)
- Gluteal and hip abductor strengthening exercises with gradual, increasing load
- Advise not to sit cross-legged or lie on the affected side
- Sleep with a pillow between legs and ankles to reduce load
- Avoid stretching the iliotibial band and other lateral structures
- Promote weight loss if necessary

MEDICATION

- Non-steroidal anti-inflammatory drugs (NSAIDs) where safe and tolerated
- Weak opiates with or without paracetamol if NSAIDs contraindicated, not tolerated or ineffective

INJECTIONS

- A corticosteroid injection may be offered for short-term analgesia
- This may also provide an analgesic window in which patients can engage in rehabilitation

SURGERY

- May be indicated in cases where optimal conservative management has failed to manage severe pain that limits activity
- Surgery may involve:
    - Lengthening or releasing the iliotibial band (ITB) and fascia lata
    - Gluteal tendon tear repair
    - Endoscopic bursectomy

3.5.3   Groin Pain in Athletes

Groin pain is a common condition in athletes involved in sports that require repetitive hip movements, such as kicking (football, rugby) and dynamic direction changes (hockey, skating). Historically, groin pain has been difficult to diagnose and manage as it relates to a number of separate pathologies and structures. In addition, there has been some confusion around the terminology and definitions used to describe the condition.

To address this, the Doha agreement in 2014 identified and classified groin pain in athletes and defined the following clinical entities (Weir et al., 2015).

Possible Causes of Groin Pain in Athletes

- **Defined entities**
  - Adductor-related groin pain
  - Iliopsoas-related groin pain
  - Inguinal-related groin pain
  - Pubic-related groin pain
  - Hip-related groin pain
- **Other musculoskeletal causes**
  - Inguinal or femoral hernia
  - Posthernioplasty pain
    - Nerve entrapment
    - Obturator
    - Ilioinguinal
    - Genitofemoral
    - Iliohypogastric
  - Referred pain
    - Lumbar spine
    - Sacroiliac joint
  - Apophysitis or avulsion fracture
    - Anterior superior iliac spine
    - Anterior inferior iliac spine
    - Pubic bone
- **Not to be missed**
  - Stress fracture
  - Neck of femur
  - Pubic ramus
  - Acetabulum
  - Hip joint
    - Slipped capital femoral epiphysis (adolescents)
    - Perthes' disease (children and adolescents)
    - Avascular necrosis/transient osteoporosis of the head of the femur
    - Arthritis of the hip joint (reactive or infectious)
  - Inguinal lymphadenopathy

- Intra-abdominal abnormality
  - Prostatitis
  - Urinary tract infections
  - Kidney stone
  - Appendicitis
  - Diverticulitis
- Gynaecological conditions
- Spondyloarthropathies
  - Ankylosing spondylitis
- Tumours
  - Testicular tumours
  - Bone tumours
  - Prostate cancer
  - Urinary tract cancer
  - Digestive tract cancer
  - Soft tissue tumours

Symptoms

- General symptoms:
  - Pain in the groin or lower abdomen
  - Onset is usually insidious but can be acute with a sensation of pulling or popping in the groin area
  - Pain can be aggravated with return to sporting activity (twisting, kicking, changing direction), increases in intra-abdominal pressure (sit-ups, sneezing, coughing) and dynamic or resisted adduction (getting into a car or out of bed)
  - Relieved with rest
- Specific symptoms (Weir et al., 2015)
  - *Adductor-related groin pain*

Pain around the insertion of the adductor longus tendon at the pubic bone. Pain may radiate distally along the medial thigh
  - *Iliopsoas-related groin pain*

Pain in the anterior part of the proximal thigh more laterally located than adductor-related groin pain
  - *Inguinal-related groin pain*

Pain in the inguinal region that worsens with activity. If pain is severe, often inguinal pain occurs when coughing or sneezing or sitting up in bed
  - *Pubic-related groin pain*

Pain in the region of the symphysis joint and the immediately adjacent bone

Examination Findings (from Thorborg et al., 2018)

- *Adductor-related groin pain*
  - Adductor tenderness and pain on resisted adduction testing
- *Iliopsoas-related groin pain*
  - Iliopsoas tenderness

- Iliopsoas-related groin pain is more likely if there is pain on resisted hip flexion and/ or pain on stretching the hip flexors
- *Inguinal-related groin pain*
  - Pain located in the inguinal canal region and tenderness on palpation of the inguinal canal
  - No palatable inguinal hernia is present
  - Inguinal-related groin pain is more likely if the pain is aggravated with resistance testing of the abdominal muscles or on Valsalva/cough/sneeze
- *Pubic-related groin pain*
  - Local tenderness on palpation of the pubic symphysis and the immediately adjacent bone
- *Hip-related groin pain*
  - If there is a clinical suspicion of hip-related pain, either through history or clinical examination, this should be investigated and treated appropriately

Differential Diagnosis

- Hip dysplasia
- Ankylosing spondylitis
- Osteoarthritis
- Rheumatoid arthritis
- Osteonecrosis
- Lumbar disc pathology
- Septic arthritis
- Osteomyelitis
- Bone malignancy or metastases

Investigations

Diagnosis is primarily based on history and clinical examination, as abnormal imaging findings are common in asymptomatic individuals

- X-ray
  - X-rays are generally normal in isolated cases of groin pain. However, they may pick up an avulsion injury, osteitis pubis, pelvic or hip stress fractures, bony impingement and other sources of groin pain
- MRI
  - MRI is the primary imaging modality for assessing groin pain as it can visualise soft tissue and osseous structures and diagnose bone marrow oedema around the pubic symphysis, stress fractures, avascular necrosis and osteitis pubis
  - It is also useful for assessing intraarticular hip pathologies such as articular cartilage defects and labral tears
- Ultrasound
  - Can be used to identify the area and extent of the injury and clarify the initial diagnosis and rule out other possible causes of groin pain

Management

CONSERVATIVE

- Treatment will depend on the related area of groin pain but will primarily be aimed at:
  - Improving range of movement
  - Increasing muscle strength – specifically hip adductors, hip abductors and abdominals
  - Correcting muscle imbalance
  - Improving coordination
  - Addressing functional deficits
  - Graduated rehabilitation programme aimed at restoring full range of movement, muscle strength, endurance, and ultimately, facilitating a return to sport

SURGERY

- If conservative measures fail to resolve symptoms adequately enough to enable a return to sport or activity, surgery may be considered
- Procedures include adductor tenotomy, adductor longus repair, open and laparoscopic mesh repairs and laparoscopic hernia repair

References

Weir, A., et al. (2015). Doha agreement meeting on terminology and definitions in groin pain in athletes. *British Journal of Sports Medicine*, *49*, 768–774.

Thorborg, K., et al. (2018). Clinical examination, diagnostic imaging, and testing of athletes with groin pain: an evidence-based approach to effective management. *Journal of Orthopaedic and Sports Physical Therapy*, 48, 239–249.

3.5.4　Piriformis Syndrome

Piriformis syndrome (PS) is an entrapment neuropathy where the sciatic nerve is irritated or compressed as it passes underneath the piriformis muscle, causing buttock, hip and lower limb pain. PS remains a controversial diagnosis for sciatic pain as no widely accepted tests are available for diagnosing the condition. Diagnosing PS is primarily based on ruling out other possible causes for a patient's symptoms.

History

Factors that predispose people to PS include:
- Hypertrophy, spasm, tightness or inflammation of the piriformis muscle caused by repetitive movements or overuse
- Hip or buttock trauma causing swelling or tissue scarring that may impinge or compress the sciatic nerve
- Occupations or activities requiring prolonged or excessive sitting
- Anatomical variants within the sciatic nerve and piriformis muscle – in some individuals, the sciatic nerve runs close to or even through the piriformis muscle

Symptoms

- Pain and tenderness in the buttocks and/or hip
- Burning, shooting pain radiating down the lower limb
- Paraesthesia and numbness down the posterior aspect of the leg
- Increased pain with sitting
- Pain worse with hip movements – especially hip adduction and internal rotation
- Pain when climbing stairs or walking up inclines

Examination

- Pain and tenderness with deep palpation around the gluteal and retro-trochanteric area
- Pain with passive internal rotation of the extended hip while the patient is supine (Freiberg's test)
- Pain and weakness with resisted abduction and external rotation of the hip while in a flexed or sitting position (Pace's sign)
- Pain on active hip abduction of the flexed leg while the patient is side lying on the unaffected side (Beatty manoeuvre)
- Pain in the gluteal area with passive hip flexion, adduction and internal rotation while the patient is side lying on the unaffected side (FAIR test)
- Neurological examination is usually unremarkable

Differential Diagnosis

- Facet arthropathy
- Sacroiliac joint dysfunction
- Spinal stenosis
- Trochanteric bursitis

- Pelvic tumour
- Lumbosacral disc
- Lumbosacral radiculopathy
- Inferior gluteal artery aneurysm

Investigations

- Imaging has a limited role in diagnosing PS
- Its main benefit is in ruling out other possible causes of symptoms and excluding the involvement of the spine or hip joint

Management

CONSERVATIVE

- Relative rest
- Activity modification – avoid prolonged sitting; especially on hard surfaces
- Stretching and strengthening exercises – especially gluteals and hamstring
- Soft tissue mobilisation
- Ice and heat packs
- Movement re-education

MEDICATION

- Non-steroidal anti-inflammatory drugs (NSAIDs) where safe and tolerated
- Weak opiates with or without paracetamol if NSAIDs contraindicated, not tolerated or ineffective

INJECTIONS

- A corticosteroid and local anaesthetic is sometimes injected into the piriformis to reduce pain and muscle spasm. This may be considered if the pain is preventing the individual from engaging in rehabilitation
- In some instances, a botox injection may be considered to reduce muscle spasms and relieve pressure on the sciatic nerve
- Injections can also be used diagnostically

SURGERY

- Surgery is rarely indicated and is usually only considered once all possible non-operative options have been attempted
- Surgery (open or endoscopic) involves decompressing the sciatic nerve by releasing the overlying piriformis muscle

3.5.5　Iliotibial Band Syndrome

Iliotibial band syndrome (ITBS) is a common overuse injury in athletes (especially runners) and presents as lateral knee pain caused by repetitive rubbing of the iliotibial band (ITB) over the lateral femoral condyle as the knee flexes and extends. This leads to inflammation and pain at the distal end of the ITB.

History

Often caused by a variety of factors, including:
- Repetitive and/or excessive training
- Altered biomechanics
- Muscle tightness
- Loss of flexibility
- Increased hip adduction, knee internal rotation or weakness of the external hip rotators place an increased strain on the ITB
- Knee varus

Symptoms

- Pain about two cm above the lateral joint line of the knee
- Pain may radiate up towards the hip or into the lower leg
- Worsens with activity
- Subsides with rest in less severe cases
- May describe a popping sensation around the lateral knee with activity

Examination

- Tenderness on palpation of the lateral knee just proximal to the lateral femoral epicondyle

Tests

- Noble compression test
- Ober's test
- Modified Thomas's test

Differential Diagnosis

- Lateral collateral ligament sprain
- Lateral meniscal tear
- Knee osteoarthritis
- Knee synovial cyst
- Lumbar spine radiculopathy
- Superior tibiofibular joint sprain
- Biceps femoris tendinopathy
- Patellofemoral stress syndrome
- Popliteal tendinopathy
- Myofascial pain

Investigations

- Diagnosis is based on clinical assessment and examination and does not usually require further investigation
- However, MRI or ultrasonography may be ordered if there is doubt about the diagnosis, the condition is not responding to treatment or there is a need to rule out other knee pathologies

Management

CONSERVATIVE

Acute phase (three to seven days)
- Non-steroidal anti-inflammatory drugs (NSAIDs)
- Ice
- Soft tissue therapy
- Activity modification

Subacute (three to 14 days)
- ITB stretches
- Start addressing altered biomechanics

Recovery and strengthening phase
- Strengthening exercises – gluteus medius and hip abductors
- Graded return to sport/activity

MEDICATION

- NSAIDs where safe and tolerated
- Weak opiates with or without paracetamol if NSAIDs contraindicated, not tolerated or ineffective

INJECTIONS

- Corticosteroid injections may be offered if the pain is still not responding to treatment or prevents the patient from engaging in rehabilitation

SURGERY

- Rarely indicated but may be considered if symptoms have not improved with at least six months of conservative treatment
- Surgery involves releasing or lengthening the ITB to reduce pain and restore function

3.5.6   Acetabular Labral Tear

Acetabular labral tears (ALTs) are a common cause of groin or anterior hip pain amongst athletes and can be caused by trauma, degenerative changes or microtrauma. Labral tears are often difficult to diagnose as they share features of other pelvic pathologies and are associated with hip conditions such as capsule laxity, hip hypermobility, degeneration, osteoarthritis, femoroacetabular impingement and hip dysplasia. It is worth noting that not all labral tears identified on imaging are symptomatic.

History

- Labral tears can occur as a result of the following:
  - A single traumatic event (e.g. motor accident, direct impact on the hip while playing sport, a fall, dislocation, a sudden block of hip flexion)
  - Degenerative tears due to sports or activities involving repetitive rotational movements (e.g. golf, ballet, hockey), repetitive movement into end-of-range hip flexion (e.g. running, tennis, football) or pivoting and twisting movements (e.g. football, rugby)
  - A sudden block of hip flexion (e.g. being tackled while about to kick a ball)
- With non-traumatic ALT, onset is often gradual and increases over time

Symptoms

- Patients complain of a dull, constant pain in the anterior hip or groin and, occasionally, the buttock
- Patients may describe hip clicking or, less frequently, locking or catching
- Pain is aggravated with certain movements, including walking, squatting, stepping up and prolonged sitting

Examination

- Pain and discomfort with hip flexion and adduction

Tests

- Anterior labral tear test (FADDIR test)
- Posterior labral tear test

Differential Diagnosis

- Groin pain
- Snapping hip
- Piriformis syndrome
- Osteitis pubis
- Avascular necrosis of the hip
- Trochanteric bursitis
- Legg-Calve-Perthes disease
- Slipped capital femoral epiphysis
- Lumbar radiculopathy

Investigations

- X-ray
  - X-rays cannot visualise a labral tear, but they may pick up conditions associated with ALT, such as femoroacetabular impingement or developmental dysplasia of the hip
- MRI
  - Is the main imaging modality for diagnosing labral tears and is also used to exclude other hip pathologies such as hip dysplasia, arthritis, acetabular cysts and bony abnormalities (coxa valga, acetabular retroversion) as a source of symptoms

Management

CONSERVATIVE

- Relative rest
- Activity modification (to limit pivotal movements and reduce load through the hip)
- Strengthening exercises
- Gait re-education
- Proprioception and balance training

MEDICATION

- Non-steroidal anti-inflammatory drugs (NSAIDs) where safe and tolerated
- Weak opiates with or without paracetamol if NSAIDs contraindicated, not tolerated or ineffective

SURGERY

- If conservative measures do not result in pain relief and a return to activity, surgical intervention may be considered
- Surgical options include:
  - Arthroscopic labral debridement
  - Labral repair
  - Labral reconstruction

3.5.7 Avascular Necrosis of the Femoral Head (Hip Osteonecrosis)

Avascular necrosis (AVN) of the femoral head occurs when there is a significant reduction in blood flow to the subchondral bone of the proximal femur. This results in bone cell death, progressive collapse of the articular surface and degenerative arthritis of the hip joint. It mainly affects people aged 25–50 years old, with males developing hip AVN more often than females do. Although the hip joint is most commonly affected, it can also occur in other joints, such as the shoulder, knee and ankle.

History

There are a large number of causes of AVN of the hip. It can be caused by trauma (i.e. hip dislocation or neck of femur fractures) or non-traumatic causes such as excessive alcohol use, chronic steroid use, congenital conditions, coagulopathy, haematologic and metabolic disorders, malignancy, pregnancy, and it is associated with conditions such as systemic lupus erythematosus, sickle cell anaemia, HIV and Gaucher disease.

Although a thorough history may reveal possible risk factors, there are many cases where a cause may not be clearly identified.

Symptoms

- In the early stages, there may be no pain or symptoms
- As the condition progresses, there is an insidious onset of pain and tenderness around the hip, groin or buttock, that worsens over time
- Active and passive range of movement may be restricted
- Pain with weight-bearing and sitting
- Pain relieved when lying down
- Development of a limp on the affected side

Examination

- In the early stages, a physical examination may not reveal much, and the condition is sometimes discovered incidentally when the patient undergoes a hip X-ray
- AVN can mimic a number of other hip conditions, so is often difficult to differentiate
- If a patient presents with signs of early-onset hip arthritis and has risk factors that may suggest possible AVN, then imaging may be indicated to rule out AVN

Differential Diagnosis

- Osteoarthritis
- Osteoporosis
- Labral tear
- Inflammatory synovitis
- Neoplastic bone conditions
- Osteomyelitis

Investigations

- X-ray
  - X-rays are usually the first investigation ordered when patients at risk of AVN present with hip pain. If the X-ray is normal or early signs of AVN are detected, then an MRI scan should be requested to confirm the diagnosis and evaluate the extent of the condition
- MRI
  - MRI is the gold standard for diagnosing AVN as it is able to detect early changes in asymptomatic patients that will not be identified on X-ray
- CT
  - Used in patients where MRI is contradicted or not tolerated by the patient

Management

CONSERVATIVE

- The aim of conservative treatment is to maintain the integrity of the joint, slow down the progression of the condition and improve function
- Maintain range of movement – passive and active exercises
- Suggest walking aids (crutches, frame, stick) to decrease weight-bearing through the hip and improve mobility
- Strengthen muscles around the hip
- Balance and proprioception exercises
- Hydrotherapy

MEDICATION

- Non-steroidal anti-inflammatory drugs (NSAIDs) where safe and tolerated
- Weak opiates with or without paracetamol if NSAIDs contraindicated, not tolerated or ineffective
- In the early stages, anticoagulants and cholesterol-lowering drugs may be prescribed to improve blood flow and prevent clotting

SURGERY

- Depending on the severity of pain and the stage of the condition at the time of diagnosis, various surgical options may be considered
- These include:
  - *Core decompression* – usually indicated in the early stages of hip AVN when the surface of the head of the femur is relatively undamaged. A core of necrotic bone is removed, which reduces pressure within the bone, promotes blood flow and stimulates the production of new bone tissue
  - *Bone graft* – bone tissue is harvested from another part of the body to replace damaged and necrotic bone and strengthen the area
  - *Osteotomy* – a small segment of necrotic bone is moved away from the weight-bearing surface, and an area of normal articular cartilage is brought into the weight-bearing area. This may delay the progression of the necrosis
  - *Total hip replacement* – in advanced cases, a complete hip replacement may be necessary

Knee

3.6.1　Anterior Cruciate Ligament

The anterior cruciate ligament (ACL) is a primary stabiliser of the knee, limiting the translation and rotation of the anterior tibia. It is the most injured ligament in the knee and is often associated with damage to other knee structures such as articular cartilage, meniscus, ligaments and bone. It commonly occurs during sports such as football, skiing, basketball, rugby and netball and is usually a non-contact injury, although it can be a result of direct trauma to the knee (i.e. a football tackle).

History

- The ACL can be injured in a number of ways:
  - An abrupt change in direction with the knee bent (pivoting, side stepping or cutting manoeuvre)
  - A sudden deceleration
  - A twisting movement with the knee in hyperextension and the foot fixed on the ground
  - Landing awkwardly from a jump and twisting or hyperextending the knee
- Due to the mechanism of injury, ACL tears are associated with other injuries, including:
  - Medial collateral ligament tear
  - Lateral collateral ligament tear
  - Meniscal tears
  - Osteochondral injuries
  - Tibial spine fracture
  - Epiphyseal fracture

Symptoms

- Immediate swelling and pain
- A 'pop' is sometimes heard or felt at the time of injury
- Knee feels unstable
- Episodes of 'giving way,' especially with twisting or pivoting movements
- Inability to continue with activity

Examination

- Acute swelling and effusion
- Widespread tenderness around the knee
- Loss of active and passive knee extension and flexion

Tests

- Lachman's test
- Anterior drawer test
- Pivot shift test

Differential Diagnosis

- Meniscal tears
- Osteochondral injuries
- Tibial spine fractures
- Other ligament injuries
- Epiphyseal fracture

Investigations

- X-ray
  - Will not reveal injury to ACL but is often requested to rule out an osteochondral fracture or Segond fracture (an avulsion fracture of the knee that is frequently associated with ACL rupture)
- MRI
  - Can accurately diagnose ACL injuries and will also identify concomitant injuries affecting the menisci, collateral ligaments, chondral structures and bone marrow
- CT
  - Can diagnose ACL rupture, but MRI is generally preferred. May be ordered when a fracture is suspected but plain radiographs are negative
  - Helps characterise an avulsion bone fragment when it is present

Management

CONSERVATIVE

- PRICE (Protect, Rest, Ice, Compression and Elevation) to control pain and swelling in the early stages
- Restore full knee extension and flexion – focus on passive extension initially
- Improve quadriceps strength

- Maintain patellar mobility
- Balance and proprioception exercises to improve knee stability
- Review gait, weightbearing and restore mobility

MEDICATION

- Non-steroidal anti-inflammatory drugs (NSAIDs) where safe and tolerated
- Weak opiates with or without paracetamol if NSAIDs are contraindicated, not tolerated or ineffective

SURGERY

- Surgery usually involves replacing the torn ACL with a substitute graft made of the tendon to restore its function after the injury
- The option of surgery is made on an individual basis but is usually considered in the following cases:
  - Active adults aged 18–35 years
  - Those that want to continue playing sports
  - Conservative measures have not helped
  - Body mass index <30 kg/m^2

3.6.2   Posterior Cruciate Ligament

Posterior cruciate ligaments (PCL) are injured far less frequently than anterior cruciate ligaments (ACL), and symptoms are often much less severe. As such, they often go undiagnosed. Due to the mechanism of injury, PCL tears are associated with other injuries to knee structures such as articular cartilage, meniscus, ligaments and bone.

History

- Direct blow to proximal tibia while the knee is flexed (dashboard injury)
- Forced hyperextension (missing a step)

Symptoms

- Pain and swelling of the knee – although less severe than those associated with ACL injury
- The knee feels unsteady or uncomfortable
- Difficulty walking

Examination

- Knee swelling
- May note bruising posteriorly

Tests

- Posterior sag sign
- Posterior drawer test

Differential Diagnosis

- ACL injury
- Medial collateral ligament injury
- Lateral collateral ligament injury
- Meniscal tears
- Posterolateral corner injury
- Talofibular ligament injury
- Bone contusion
- Avulsion fracture

Investigations

- X-ray
  - Will not reveal injury to PCL but is often requested to rule out an osteochondral or avulsion fracture
- MRI
  - Can accurately diagnose PCL injuries and identify concomitant injuries affecting the menisci, ligaments, chondral structures and bone marrow
  - Can identify indirect signs of PCL injury, such as bone bruises caused by forced posterior displacement of the tibia or hyperextension injuries

- CT
  - Can diagnose PCL rupture, but MRI is preferred. May be used when a fracture is suspected but plain radiographs are negative

Management

CONSERVATIVE

- PRICE (Protect, Rest, Ice, Compression and Elevation) to control pain and swelling in the early stages
- A short period of immobilisation in a brace or cast may be suggested following the initial injury
- Restore knee range of movement
- Improve muscle strength around the knee especially the quadriceps
- Balance and proprioception exercises to improve knee stability
- Review gait, weightbearing and restore mobility

SURGERY

- There is some debate as to whether PCL tears should be repaired surgically
- However, it may be considered when:
  - There is a grade III PCL tear (complete rupture)
  - Multiple ligaments have been injured
  - Knee instability has not responded to conservative treatment

3.6.3 Medial Collateral Ligament Injury

The medial collateral ligament (MCL) is the prime static stabiliser of the medial aspect of the knee as it resists valgus, rotational and anterior translation forces on the tibia. It is commonly injured while playing sports or following a fall.

Depending on the level of impact and integrity of the ligament, this results in one of three grades of injury:

- **Grade 1:** The ligament has been stretched with a minimal number of torn fibres
- **Grade 2:** The ligament has been stretched, and there is an increased degree of ligamentous disruption. Often referred to as a partial tear
- **Grade 3:** A complete tear of the ligament

History

- The patient may describe a contact or non-contact injury which may be due to:
  - Traumatic blow to the knee or upper leg while the foot is fixed to the ground (i.e. when playing rugby or football)
  - Large valgus force or tibial external rotation (or combination of both) exerted on the knee
  - Fall (particularly in the elderly population)
- A 'popping' sound may be heard or felt at the time of the injury – usually with a grade 2 or 3 injury
- Immediate onset of pain and swelling

Symptoms

- Localised pain around the medial border of the knee
- Swelling and bruising at the site of injury – mainly with grade 2 and 3 injuries
- Feeling of instability – mainly with a grade 3 injury
- Knee stiffness and difficulty bending and straightening the knee

Examination

- Pain on palpation of the medial joint line
- Swelling on the medial aspect of the knee
- Pain with weight bearing and putting load through the knee (i.e. walking, getting up and down from a chair and going upstairs)

Tests

- Abduction (valgus) stress test

Differential Diagnosis

- Medial meniscal tear
- Tibial plateau fracture
- Medial knee contusion
- Anterior cruciate ligament injury
- Pes anserinus bursitis

Investigations

- X-ray
  - A valgus stress X-ray of both knees (taken with the knee placed in 20° knee flexion with a foam pad underneath) will allow a comparison of the amount of medial compartment gapping in the injured and uninjured contralateral knee
  - The diagnostic accuracy is lower with grade 1 and 2 injuries than that with grade 3
  - X-rays are also useful when an X-ray is needed to rule out concomitant fractures to the tibial plateau, patella and femur
- MRI
  - Useful in diagnosing and determining the grade of the MCL tear
  - It can also provide a detailed view of the soft tissue surrounding the knee and identify whether there is an associated attachment avulsion or concomitant injury to the ACL, PCL and menisci
- Ultrasound
  - Used primarily in urgent care settings to make an immediate assessment or when MRI is not available

Management

CONSERVATIVE

- Isolated MCL tears are generally treated conservatively
- PRICE (Protect, Rest, Ice, Compression and Elevation) to control pain and swelling in the early stages
- Immobilisation and bracing if side-to-side instability present
- Maintain knee extension
- Progressive weight bearing on the affected limb
- Progressive range of movement exercises
- Strengthening exercises (quadriceps and hamstring)
- Balance and proprioception exercises to improve knee stability
- Review gait, weightbearing and restore mobility

MEDICATION

- Non-steroidal anti-inflammatory drugs (NSAIDs) where safe and tolerated
- Weak opiates with or without paracetamol if NSAIDs are contraindicated, not tolerated or ineffective

SURGERY

- Surgical repair or reconstruction of a grade 3 tear may warrant surgery if there is ongoing knee instability that has not responded to conservative treatment or if there are associated multi-ligament injuries or knee dislocations involving the MCL

3.6.4   Meniscal Injury

Meniscal tears can either be the result of acute trauma or due to degenerative changes. Acute injuries are often associated with sports involving side-step cutting, cross-step cutting and pivoting, such as football and basketball, while degenerative tears are associated with ageing or repetitive work-related activities such as kneeling, squatting or climbing stairs. In the older population, relatively minor trauma or stress through the knee can cause a tear or rupture. Medial tears are more common than lateral tears – except when there is a concomitant anterior cruciate ligament rupture, where lateral tears are more common.

History
TRAUMATIC ONSET

- A sudden twisting injury with the knee partially flexed or the foot firmly fixed on the ground
- Squat or kneel associated with a twist

DEGENERATIVE

- Little or no history of significant trauma
- Slow, insidious onset
- Older patients (>50 years old)
- More prevalent with increasing age
- Knee osteoarthritis (75%–90% have concomitant degenerative meniscus lesion)
- In the degenerative knee, the patient's symptoms are more likely to be caused by other degenerative changes rather than the meniscus itself

Symptoms
TRAUMATIC ONSET

- Immediate pain along the joint line
- A 'pop' is sometimes heard or felt at the time of injury
- Delayed or intermittent swelling

ACUTE AND DEGENERATIVE

- Mechanical symptoms – locking, clicking or catching
- Pain with rotational movements
- Pain will localise on the inside or outside of the knee joint depending on whether the medial or lateral meniscus has been torn
- Increased pain with knee flexion and extension
- Joint stiffness
- Pain when weight-bearing through the affected knee
- Eases with rest

Examination

- Knee effusion
- Tenderness to palpation along either medial or lateral joint line depending on the affected meniscus
- Pain with passive flexion
- Loss of passive extension

Tests

- Apley grind test
- McMurray's test
- Thessaly tests

Differential Diagnosis

- Anterior cruciate ligament injury
- Medial collateral ligament injury
- Lateral collateral ligament injury
- Osteochondritis dissecans
- Patellofemoral pain
- Osteoarthritis of the knee

Investigations

- MRI
  - MRI is used extensively to diagnose meniscal tears and guide management options in the early stage of injury
  - MRI is not normally indicated in middle-aged or older patients with degenerative meniscus lesions but may be ordered to identify other pathologies that may be contributing to symptoms
- Arthroscopy
  - Provides a direct view of the joint to review the level of damage, make a definite diagnosis and guide management options
- CT
  - Not generally used for diagnosing meniscal tears but may be used to rule out suspected fractures or diagnose associated ligamentous injuries

Management

CONSERVATIVE

- PRICE (Protect, Rest, Ice, Compression and Elevation) to control pain and swelling in the early stages
- Activity modification - avoid aggravating activities and prolonged inactivity
- Restore the range of movement in the knee
- Strengthen muscles that support and surround the knee
- Increase weight-bearing tolerance

- Normalise gait pattern
- Introduce balance exercises
- Progress exercise programme towards functional goals or return to sports

MEDICATION

- Non-steroidal anti-inflammatory drugs (NSAIDs) where safe and tolerated
- Weak opiates with or without paracetamol if NSAIDs are contraindicated, not tolerated or ineffective

INJECTION

- A corticosteroid injection may be considered when:
  - Surgery is not appropriate
  - Pain and inflammation are limiting the range of movement and function and preventing the patient from engaging with physiotherapy

SURGERY

- An arthroscopic partial meniscectomy or meniscus repair may be indicated when tears are causing mechanical symptoms such as locking of the knee or a significant reduction in the range of movement

3.6.5   Patellofemoral Pain Syndrome

Patellofemoral pain is a common disorder of the knee causing pain behind or around the patella that is worsened with increased load or stress through the knee. Although it is more prevalent in females and those who participate in sports involving frequent running, jumping or squatting, it can also occur in non-athletes.

History

- The condition is multifactorial and is associated with the following:
  - Overuse and overloading the patellofemoral joint
  - Muscle weakness and tightness
  - Biomechanical changes affecting gait and movement
- Normally affects active individuals involved in sports or activities where the knee is repeatably bent or loaded
- Onset is typically slow and progressive but can also be acute if there has been a sudden and significant increase in activity
- Typically non-traumatic

Symptoms

- Patient complains of diffuse, non-radiating retropatellar and/or peripatellar pain
- Pain is worsened with activities that load the knee, such as squatting, going up and down stairs, sitting with the knee flexed for prolonged periods, running, jumping and walking uphill

Examination

- Reproduction of anterior knee pain with squatting
- Pain on palpation of the distal pole and lateral and medial border of the patella
- Compression or grinding of the patella may increase pain

Tests

- Clarke's sign (patellofemoral grind test)
- Passive patellar tilt test
- Step up test

Differential Diagnosis

- Articular cartilage injury
- Bone tumours
- Chondromalacia patellae
- Hoffa's syndrome (infrapatellar fat pad irritation)
- Iliotibial band syndrome
- Septic arthritis
- Fractures
- Referral from hip or lumbopelvic region

Investigations

- Patellofemoral pain is primarily a clinical diagnosis that does not require specific imaging
- Imaging (X-ray, MRI) is mainly used as an adjunct to the clinical examination to review patellar alignment abnormalities and to rule out other causes of knee pain

Management

CONSERVATIVE

- Advice and information
- Activity modification - avoid aggravating activities and prolonged inactivity
- Relative rest in the early stages
- Strengthening of quadriceps and hip abductors, extensors and external rotators
- Lower limb and trunk stretches
- Patellar taping
- Foot orthoses
- Gait and movement retraining

MEDICATION

- Medication is not commonly used in managing patellofemoral pain in the long term. However, non-steroidal anti-inflammatory drugs may be used for short-term pain relief where safe and tolerated

SURGERY

- Surgery is very rarely indicated
- However, in severe cases where conservative treatment has failed to resolve symptoms, it may be considered
- Surgical options can include:
  - Arthroscopic debridement – involves removing damaged articular cartilage from the patella surface
  - Arthroscopic lateral release – the lateral retinaculum is loosened to correct an excessive patellar tilt and maltracking caused by tight lateral structures
  - Tibial tubercle transfer – the patellar tendon and a portion of the tibial tubercle are repositioned to realign the patella and improve tracking within the trochlear groove

3.6.6   Patella Tendinopathy

Patella tendinopathy is a common overuse disorder associated with sports and activities involving strenuous jumping, hopping or landing (e.g. basketball, volleyball, high jump, long jump, tennis, football).

History

- Patient may be involved in a sport or activity that entails repetitive loading of the patella tendon
- In most cases, patients report a non-traumatic, gradual onset

Symptoms

- Pain localised to the inferior pole of the patella
- Onset of pain when the knee is loaded or when performing an aggravating activity
- A decrease in pain when the load is reduced
- Normally no pain at rest

Examination

- Pain on palpation of the inferior pole or body of the patella tendon
- Increasing the load through the tendon produces a subsequent increase in pain intensity around the tendon (i.e. moving from a shallow squat to a deeper squat)
- Weak quadriceps
- Tight quadriceps and hamstring
- Possible tendon thickening

Differential Diagnosis

- Quadriceps tendinopathy
- Infrapatellar bursitis
- Hoffa's syndrome (infrapatellar fat pad irritation)
- Patella fracture
- Osteochondral lesions
- Osgood Schlatter's disease
- Meniscal tear
- Patellofemoral syndrome
- Chondromalacia patellar
- Patellar dislocation

Investigations

- Ultrasound
  - Ultrasound imaging is the mainstay of tendon imaging and can identify tendon thickening, loss of fibrillary pattern and neovascularity. It is also used to include or exclude other potential causes of anterior knee pain

- MRI
  - Used less frequently than ultrasound but can visualise thickening of the tendon, minor or complete tears and rule out other knee injuries

Management

CONSERVATIVE

- Relative rest in the early stages – complete rest needs to be avoided to prevent tendon and muscle atrophy
- A graded isometric and eccentric exercise programme to develop load tolerance of the tendon
- Progressive strengthening exercises to address lower limb deficits
- Stretching exercises
- Address biomechanical changes

MEDICATION

- A short course of non-steroidal anti-inflammatory drugs may be helpful, but long-term use can negatively impact tendon healing

INJECTIONS

- A corticosteroid injection may be considered when:
  - Pain and inflammation are limiting the range of movement and function and preventing the patient from engaging in rehabilitation
  - Corticosteroid injections are not routinely offered as there is a risk of the steroid weakening the tendon

SURGERY

- Rarely indicated, but surgery may be considered in late-stage patella tendinopathy when conservative measures have failed to resolve symptoms
- Surgical options include longitudinal splitting of the tendon, removal of abnormal tissue, resection and drilling of the inferior pole of the patella and arthroscopic tendon debridement with excision of the distal pole of the patella

3.6.7   Chondromalacia Patellae

Chondromalacia patellae (CMP) is a condition characterised by changes to the hyaline cartilage on the underside of the patella. In the early stages, the cartilage becomes soft, swollen and oedematous (hence its origins from the Greek words "chondro" meaning cartilage and "malakia" meaning softening). As the condition advances, there is subsequent tearing, fissuring and erosion of the patella cartilage. The condition is more prevalent in adolescents and young adults and affects females more than males.

The terms chondromalacia patella and patellofemoral pain syndrome (PFPS) are often used interchangeably when describing pain around the front of the knee. However, PFPS is seen as a separate entity from CMP. The main difference is that CMP is characterised by findings of patellofemoral cartilage damage on imaging or knee arthroscopy, whereas structural defects are not present in PFPS.

History

- Taking part in sports and activities that place large loads of stress on the knee (running, basketball, football, gymnastics, ballet or swimming breaststroke)
- Having an occupation that involves excessive kneeling or squatting (carpenters, plumbers)
- Previous trauma to the patella
- Previous dislocation or recurrent subluxations
- Malalignment of the patella due to:
  - Altered knee kinetics such as valgus knees, femoral anteversion (internal twisting of the femur), external tibial torsion (inward twisting of the tibia), increased Q angle, patella alta and excessive pronation
  - Structural abnormalities such as a laterally placed tibial tubercle, flattened lateral femoral condyle or osteochondral ridge
  - Imbalance of the quadriceps muscles

Symptoms

- Pain around the front of the knee
- Pain is increased with activities that load the knee, such as squatting, going up and down stairs, sitting with the knee flexed for prolonged periods, running, jumping or walking uphill
- Crepitus with knee flexion and extension
- Quadriceps wasting
- Knee swelling and stiffness may be present

Examination

- Pain on palpation of the lateral and medial border of the patella
- Quadriceps weakness (particularly vastus medialis)
- Palpable crepitus with knee movements
- Increased Q angle
- Pain with compression or rocking of the patella

Tests

- Clarke's test
- McConnell test for chondromalacia patella
- Step up test

Differential Diagnosis

- Hoffa's syndrome (infrapatellar fat pad syndrome)
- Synovial plica
- Osteochondritis dessicans
- Patellar tendinopathy
- Patellofemoral osteoarthritis
- Rheumatoid arthritis
- PFPS

Investigations

- X-ray
  - Although plain X-rays will not reveal chondral changes in the early stages of the condition, they may show patellofemoral joint space narrowing or osteophyte formation that may indicate the development of the condition. In the advanced stages, X-rays may show extensive cartilage loss, joint space loss and changes in the subchondral bone
- MRI
  - MRI is the investigation of choice as it is able to detect early changes in the patellar cartilage. It can also visualise soft tissue and osseous structures and may be ordered to rule out other knee pathologies
- CT
  - May not be able to pick up early chondral changes but, in the advanced stages, can be used to confirm focal cartilage loss

Management

CONSERVATIVE

- Relative rest
- Activity modification
- Strengthening and balancing the quadriceps muscles, especially the vastus medialis oblique
- Hamstring and quadriceps stretches
- Hip strengthening exercises
- Patella taping
- Patella stabilising brace
- Foot orthotics to decrease pronation

MEDICATION

- Non-steroidal anti-inflammatory drugs (NSAIDs) where safe and tolerated
- Weak opiates with or without paracetamol if NSAIDs are contraindicated, not tolerated or ineffective

SURGERY

- Surgery may be considered in the advanced stages when conservative treatment fails to alleviate significant pain and dysfunction
- Surgical options include:
  - Arthroscopic debridement of the patellar cartilage
  - Re-alignment procedures aimed at improving patellofemoral tracking by altering the position of the patellar (i.e. tibia tubercle transfer, lateral retinaculum release)
  - Articular resurfacing
  - Patellectomy (partial or total removal of the patella)

3.6.8 Knee Osteoarthritis

Knee osteoarthritis (OA) is a progressive joint disease characterised by the degeneration of the articular cartilage as well as the surrounding ligaments and joint capsule, synovial membrane inflammation and subchondral bone sclerosis. Symptoms vary between individuals but typically become more severe and debilitating over time.

History

- Gradual onset of knee pain
- Can be unilateral or bilateral
- Pain worsens with prolonged activity or after periods of inactivity (e.g. sitting)
- Difficulty with walking, bending down and going up and down stairs
- Pain and disability worsen over time
- Incidence increases with age

Symptoms

- Joint stiffness and swelling
- Morning stiffness – improves with movement and lasts less than 30 min
- Pain with movement
- Difficulty weight bearing on the affected side

Examination

- Knee swelling
- Muscle weakness and tightness, especially quadriceps
- Possible valgus or varus deformities
- Pain on palpation of the joint line
- Reduced range of movement
- Altered gait pattern
- Joint crepitus may be present

Differential Diagnosis

- Patellofemoral pain
- Iliotibial band syndrome
- Meniscal tear
- Anterior cruciate ligament tear
- Gout
- Septic arthritis
- Rheumatoid arthritis
- Anserine bursitis

Investigations

- X-ray
  - X-ray is the primary imaging technique for diagnosing knee OA
  - In the early stages of the condition, osteophytes, joint space narrowing, subchondral sclerosis or subchondral cysts are well visualised
  - It is important that X-rays are taken in standing to assess the extent of joint space narrowing
- MRI
  - MRI is able to visualise all the structures within the joint and can reveal evidence of cartilage degeneration, reactive bony oedema, inflammation of soft tissue around the knee and bony fragments within the joint
- CT
  - Can be used to identify OA changes, including subchondral cysts, bone sclerosis and osteophytes and their adjacent soft tissue
- Ultrasound
  - Ultrasound can detect and evaluate a wide range of structural abnormalities in the cartilage, bony cortex and synovial tissue and can identify tibiofemoral osteophytes and cartilage degeneration

Management

CONSERVATIVE

- Education and advice on managing the condition
- Activity modification – avoid aggravating activities and prolonged inactivity
- Weight management
- Exercise programme – aimed at strengthening and stretching exercises for the lower limb, increasing or maintaining range of movement and improving proprioception and function
- Hot and cold packs
- Hydrotherapy – if indicated and available
- Knee brace
- Walking aids

MEDICATION

- Non-steroidal anti-inflammatory drugs (NSAIDs) where safe and tolerated
- Weak opiates with or without paracetamol if NSAIDs are contraindicated, not tolerated or ineffective

INJECTIONS

- Intra-articular corticosteroid injections offer short-term pain relief and should be used in conjunction with other treatments to provide:
  - Pain relief
  - Reduce swelling
  - An opportunity to engage in rehabilitation

SURGERY

- Surgery may be indicated when:
  - Severe pain limits daily activity
  - There is ongoing pain, inflammation and swelling that does not respond to rest or medication
  - The knee has not improved with conservative treatment
- Surgical options:
  - *High tibial osteotomy* – a small wedge of bone is removed or added to the tibia to realign the joint and shift pressure and load away from the affected side and reduce wear and tear on that side. The procedure is aimed at delaying the need for partial or full knee replacement and is suited to young (less than 50 years old), active and non-obese patients committed to extensive postoperative rehabilitation
  - *Unicompartmental knee arthroplasty (partial knee replacement)* – a surgical procedure where only the arthritic compartment of the knee is removed. This is normally the medial or lateral compartment, but it can also be the patellofemoral compartment at the front of the knee. The procedure is less invasive with short recovery times but is only indicated for a small number of patients
  - *Total knee arthroplasty (total knee replacement)* – involves removing the arthritic ends of the tibia and femur and replacing each end with a prosthetic. The surgery is indicated for those with severe pain that has a significant impact on their daily lives and ability to function

3.6.9 Baker Cyst (Popliteal Cyst)

A Baker cyst is a growth that forms at the back of the knee due to the accumulation of synovial fluid within the popliteal bursa. They often occur independently in children. However, in adults the vast majority of cases are associated with pre-existing conditions such as osteoarthritis, rheumatoid arthritis, gout, meniscus or ligament tears.

History

- Development of a swelling or lump on the back of the knee
- Swelling behind the knee may appear more prominent when the leg is straightened
- Patient describes a diffuse ache in the back of the knee and a feeling of tightness around the knee
- Pain and stiffness around the knee may affect the ability to work or engage in activity

Symptoms

- Baker cysts are often asymptomatic – the presence and severity of symptoms are often related to the size of the cyst
- Pain around the back of the knee that can be aggravated by activities such as walking
- Loss of knee extension and flexion with larger cysts

Examination

- Palpable swelling or tenderness on the medial side of the popliteal fossa
- Pain is increased with full knee extension
- Swelling will feel firm when the knee is extended but soften or disappear when the knee is flexed (Foucher's sign)

Differential Diagnosis

- Deep vein thrombosis
- Synovial and ganglion cysts
- Phlebitis (superficial thrombophlebitis)
- Popliteal artery aneurysm
- Lipoma
- Lymphoma
- Sarcoma
- Abscess
- Haematoma
- Fascial tear with muscle herniation
- Soft tissue tumours

Investigations

- X-ray
  - Has limited diagnostic value as the cyst cannot be seen on X-ray. However, it may be ordered to identify associated joint pathology as part of a wider assessment

- Ultrasound
  - Used to confirm the diagnosis, evaluate the cyst and identify complications such as cyst rupture, haemorrhage, popliteal artery aneurysm or deep vein thrombosis
- MRI
  - Can diagnose the presence of the cyst and identify underlying joint pathology

Management

CONSERVATIVE

- Treatment is not always indicated if the Baker cyst is asymptomatic
- If symptomatic, the underlying cause of the cyst should be identified and managed, as it may be the primary source of pain, swelling and restricted movement
- Advise rest if symptoms are increased with activity or movement
- Advise regular ice packs to reduce swelling
- Maintain knee range of movement
- Improve muscle strength and flexibility around the knee

MEDICATION

- Non-steroidal anti-inflammatory drugs (NSAIDs) where safe and tolerated
- Weak opiates with or without paracetamol if NSAIDs are contraindicated, not tolerated or ineffective

INJECTION

- A steroid injection may be offered to reduce inflammation and pain

ASPIRATION

- Involves drawing excess fluid out of the cyst
- Procedure often carried out using ultrasound to guide the placement of the needle
- May include an intra-articular or intra-cystic corticosteroid injection for pain relief and to reduce swelling

SURGERY

- Surgery is rarely indicated
- Excision of the cyst may be considered for large cysts or where there are ongoing, severe symptoms that have not responded to non-surgical management
- Arthroscopy can also be considered for treating the underlying joint pathology (e.g. meniscal tears and ligament damage) that may be causing the cyst. This may result in the cyst resolving and not requiring excision

Foot and Ankle

3.7.1   Plantar Fasciitis (Plantar Fasciopathy)

Plantar fasciitis (PF) is a common cause of heel pain that affects both sedentary and active people. It is caused by repetitive overloading of the plantar fascia, a thick fibrous band of connective tissue that runs between the heel and the metatarsal heads. The plantar fascia has an important role in supporting the biomechanics of the foot, including arch support.

The condition is usually self-limiting and should resolve within 18 months without treatment. Only a minority present as 'recalcitrant' cases potentially requiring more invasive treatments.

History

Increased stress on the plantar fascia may be due to a number of factors:
- Being overweight (having a body mass index >25 doubles the risk)
- Age >40 years
- High or repeated impact activities (e.g. running)
- Abrupt change in training load, frequency or intensity of activity
- Prolonged standing – especially if on a hard surface
- Walking barefoot
- Calf tightness or limited dorsiflexion
- Overpronation
- Altered biomechanics:
  - Equinous – increased strain through plantar fascia if unable to get beyond 10° dorsiflexion
  - Pes planus (flat foot) may increase strain at the attachment into the calcaneus
  - Pes cavus (high arch) reduced shock absorption due to excessive supination

- Spondyloarthropathies (HLA-B27 +ve) – associated with enthesitis and PF
- Calcaneal spur
- Weak intrinsic muscles of the foot
- Poor footwear

Symptoms

- Pain may initially be diffuse heel or ankle pain before becoming more localised and is often described as 'knifelike'
- Pain with weight-bearing activities (e.g. difficulty walking up stairs)
- Pain with the first few steps of waking in the morning and after a period of inactivity (e.g. prolonged sitting)
- Pain improves with exercise but then worsens with extended activity
- Generally unilateral but may be bilateral in up to a third of cases – this should raise suspicion of a systemic driver for the problem (e.g. spondyloarthropathy)

Examination

- Focal tenderness at the origin of the plantar fascia on the medial tubercle of the calcaneus
- Pain with passive dorsiflexion
- Decreased dorsiflexion when the knee is extended
- Pain with dorsiflexion of the ankle joint and eversion of the subtler joint (Dorsiflexion-eversion test)
- Pain or an increase in pain with passive dorsiflexion of the metatarsophalangeal joint (Windlass test)

Differential Diagnosis

- Calcaneus stress fracture
- Tarsal tunnel syndrome
- Plantar nerve entrapment
- Baxter's neuritis
- Nerve root radiculopathy
- Achilles tendinopathy
- Posterior tibial tendinopathy
- Fat pad atrophy
- Retrocalcaneal bursitis
- Inflammatory arthropathy (ankylosing spondylitis, reactive arthritis, psoriatic arthritis)
- Tumours - primary bone tumours, lipoma, soft tissue sarcoma

Investigations

Not normally ordered for PF but may be considered if trying to rule out other causes of heel pain or if the patient is not responding to several months of conservative treatment.

- X-ray
  - To identify stress fracture of calcaneum
  - May also identify calcaneal spur (and possible features of seronegative arthritis)
- Ultrasound
  - Identifies thickening of the plantar fascia and possible features of enthesopathy, oedema and loss of the usual fibrillar structure

- MRI
  - To help identify soft tissue or bony mass
  - May find thickening of the plantar fascia with oedema around the insertion site
- Bone scan
  - Ordered if uncertainty around the presence of a possible stress fracture

Management

The majority of cases resolve within 6 to 18 months, and reassurance around the natural history is of value. A poorer prognosis is associated with bilateral presentations and those associated with seronegative spondyloarthropathy.

CONSERVATIVE

- Relative rest
- Activity modification – avoiding aggravating activities and prolonged rest and breaking up long periods of static loading
- Avoid walking barefoot, especially on hard surfaces
- Icing
- Gastrocnemius stretching
- Plantar fascia stretching
- Low die taping or strapping to offload the plantar fascia
- In-shoe orthosis, including heel pads and arch supports to maintain the medial longitudinal arch
- Foot splints at night – maintaining ankle dorsiflexion and toe extension may have a role for more persistent or hard-to-treat pain
- Weight loss, where relevant

MEDICATION

- A short course of non-steroidal anti-inflammatory drugs may help with pain and inflammation in the initial stages

INJECTION

- Corticosteroid
  - May provide short-term pain relief, but there is a small risk of fat pad atrophy, fascial rupture and infection

EXTRACORPOREAL SHOCK WAVE THERAPY

- May be considered in patients with significant heel pain and who are not responding to conservative treatment
- Creates local tissue disruption and neovascularisation with stimulation of growth factors

SURGERY

- Considered in chronic cases where pain persists, and function is significantly affected despite non-surgical therapy
- Surgery involves releasing the plantar fascia and can be either an open procedure or performed endoscopically

3.7.2   Hallux Valgus (Bunion)

Hallux valgus is the most common foot deformity and is characterised by a progressive lateral deviation of the first metatarsophalangeal joint (MTPJ), with a resultant movement of the great toe towards (and sometimes overlapping) the second toe.

This creates a bony prominence on the dorsomedial aspect of the first metatarsal head, with inflammation of the superficial bursa called a bunion.

History

- Can be seen in up to half of adults, where weaker intrinsic muscles may contribute to progressive deformity
- Also found in a small number of younger people and adolescents, usually with a family history of hallux valgus
- Tends to affect females more than males
- The rate of progression varies and may start off being unilateral before becoming bilateral
- Tight footwear, especially with a high heel, may enhance the progression of bunions
- There is an association with hypermobility syndromes (e.g. Ehlers Danlos syndrome, Down's or Marfan's syndrome) and severe pes planus (flat foot)
- There may be a history of preceding trauma to the foot or ankle (e.g. forced dorsiflexion or valgus injury of the foot)

Symptoms

- Pain around the first MTPJ
- Worse with weight-bearing or tight shoes
- Pain may affect other toes due to weight transfer away from hallux (lateral metatarsalgia)
- Foot deformity with difficulty getting normal footwear to fit and concerns over appearance
- Burning or numbness localised to the hallux may be described due to the involvement of the first digital nerve

Examination

- Valgus deformity at the first MTPJ
  - The angle is considered abnormal when it exceeds 14.5° and is considered severe if it exceeds 45°
- Pronation of the hallux (nail turning to face medially)
- The second toe may be bent at the interphalangeal joint (hammer toe deformity)
- Enlargement of the first metatarsal head with associated inflammation, thickening of the skin and/or ulceration
- Tenderness over the medial eminence
- Antalgic gait with external rotation of the foot or a tendency to bear weight on the lateral aspect of the foot
- There may be abnormal or excessive wear on the soles of shoes at the position of the first/second metatarsal heads
- Range of movement at the first MTPJ is generally preserved
- There may be an identifiable hind foot deformity (contributing to the forefoot deformity)

Differential Diagnosis

- Hallux rigidus (osteoarthritis first MTPJ)
- Septic arthritis
- Rheumatoid arthritis
- Gout

Investigation

Hallux valgus is primarily a clinical diagnosis. Further investigations (e.g. X-ray) may be ordered to help plan an intervention or if other pathologies are suspected.

Management

Principles focus on improving function by alleviating pain, preventing progression or surgical correction of the deformity.

CONSERVATIVE

- Advice and information:
- Footwear:
  - Looser fitting shoes to reduce friction or compression
  - Avoid high heels or tight shoes
  - Use soft shoes with a wide forefoot and a padded insole
- Orthotics:
  - Arch support for pes planus
  - Metatarsal pads
  - Medial posting – an insert in the midsole to reduce overpronation

MEDICATION

- Non-steroidal anti-inflammatory drugs (NSAIDs) where safe and tolerated
- Weak opiates with or without paracetamol if NSAIDs are contraindicated, not tolerated or ineffective

SURGERY

- There is a wide range of surgical procedures used to realign the anatomy, including:
  - *First metatarsal osteotomies* – where a wedge of bone is removed (and occasionally relocated) to correct the angle
  - *First MTPJ arthrodesis (fusion)* – generally in more severe cases with associated degenerative joint changes whereby the arthritic ends of the joints are removed and the bones joined together with plates or wires until they fuse
  - *Excision arthroplasty* - which involves cutting out the bunion and part of the joint at the base of the 1st metacarpal creating a flexible joint from the resulting scar tissue

3.7.3   Hallux Rigidus

A progressive, degenerative arthritis affecting the first metatarsophalangeal joint with a proliferation of osteophytes and altered joint biomechanics. This is one of the most common forms of arthritis in the foot causing pain, stiffness with a loss of dorsiflexion that can make it difficult to walk.

History

- Affects females more than males
- Usually unilateral but may progress to being bilateral – especially if there is a family history
- More common with increasing age
- May be found earlier in life in those with congenital deformities (e.g. altered shape of metatarsal head or phalanges, osteochondritis dissecans)
- Secondary to a range of possible factors, including:
  - Trauma – secondary changes following severe sprain or fracture
  - Repeated microtrauma (e.g. running)
  - History of inflammatory arthritis (e.g. gout)
  - Altered biomechanics (e.g. hallux valgus, tight Achilles tendon or gastrocnemius)

Symptoms

- Pain at the first metatarsophalangeal joint (MTPJ)
- Exacerbated by exercise, weight-bearing activities and unsupportive footwear (tight shoes or those with a significant heel increasing pressure across MTPJs)
- Lateral metatarsalgia – caused by altered weight-bearing or biomechanics
- Plantar foot pain – due to the involvement of sesamoid bones
- Stiffness – gradual limitation of dorsiflexion and plantarflexion
- Deformity – increased dorsal and medial prominence due to osteophytes
- Burning pain or paraesthesia if the digital nerve is affected

Examination

- Antalgic gait with pain at the push-off point
- Increased size of MTPJ due to osteophyte formation
- Superficial erythema from friction or pressure points
- Tenderness over the first MTPJ
- Loss of range of movement – usually decreased dorsiflexion
- Pain at the end range of movement (and throughout range in later stages)
- Joint crepitus

Differential Diagnosis

- Acute sprain
- Turf toe
- Hallux valgus
- Rheumatoid arthritis
- Gout
- Sesamoiditis
- Septic arthritis

Investigation

Hallux rigidus is primarily a clinical diagnosis. Further investigations (e.g. X-ray) may be ordered to help plan an intervention or if other pathologies are suspected.

Management

CONSERVATIVE

- Footwear:
    - Avoid tight or high-heeled shoes
    - Use soft shoes with a wide forefoot and a padded insole
    - Stiff soled shoes (alternatives include rocker sole or Morton's extension orthotic) to reduce motion through the first MTPJ

MEDICATION

- Topical or oral non-steroidal anti-inflammatory drugs (NSAIDs) where safe and tolerated
- Weak opiates with or without paracetamol if NSAIDs are contraindicated, not tolerated or ineffective

INJECTION

- A corticosteroid injection with a local anaesthetic may provide short-term relief of pain for up to three to six months
- May be both therapeutic and diagnostic

SURGERY

- Considered when conservative measures fail to address ongoing pain and functional limitation
- Usually undertaken under local (regional) anaesthetic
- May involve:
    - *Cheilectomy* – for mild to moderate cases and involves resection of osteophytes
    - *Arthrodesis (fusion)* – reduces pain but at the cost of joint mobility
    - *Osteotomy* – removal of a 'wedge' of bone to alter biomechanics through a joint
    - *Arthroplasty* – joint replacement

3.7.4 Morton's Neuroma

Morton's neuroma is an entrapment neuropathy on the underside of the foot characterised by fibrosis and degenerative changes of the interdigital nerve, most commonly in the third interdigital space.

History

- Affects females more than males
- Most commonly found in middle-aged women
- The exact cause is often uncertain, but it has been associated with the following:
  - History of forefoot trauma
  - Repeated irritation of the nerve with entrapment between metatarsal heads or ligaments
  - Changes in the biomechanics of the foot (e.g. forced dorsiflexion of toes in tight-fitting and/or high-heeled shoes)
  - Local factors (e.g. interdigital bursitis or ischaemia)

Symptoms

- May be asymptomatic
- Usually insidious in onset with acute, intermittent flares of pain gradually worsening over time
- Stabbing, burning pain localised at the plantar aspect of intermetatarsal space on weight-bearing
- May refer to other digits
- Often worse at night
- Exacerbated on wearing tight-fitting shoes
- Eased with rest or removing footwear
- May be associated with a tingling sensation or localised numbness
- Patients may describe that it feels like they are 'walking with a stone in their shoe' or similar

Examination

- Focally tender on the plantar aspect of the foot in relevant interdigital space
- Pain is reproducible upon applying pressure
- Swelling may be found in the interdigital space
- A click is felt on applying pressure across metatarsophalangeal joints whilst simultaneously applying pressure on the interdigital space from the plantar side (Mulder sign)

Differential Diagnosis

- Peripheral neuropathy
- Metatarsal stress fracture
- Lumbar radiculopathy
- Tarsal tunnel syndrome
- Rheumatoid nodule
- Osteoarthritis
- Plantar lipoma

- Metatarsal synovitis/capsulitis
- Intermetatarsal bursitis

Investigations

Morton's neuroma is primarily a clinical diagnosis that only requires further investigations if there is clinical uncertainty, if surgery is being planned or if other pathologies are suspected.

- Ultrasound
  - Is the imaging modality of choice for the majority and may show a mass usually proximal to metatarsal heads with neuromas >3 mm
- MRI
  - MRI is not commonly used but is sometimes ordered in atypical cases or in recurrent episodes to help confirm the diagnosis and exclude other pathologies

Management

CONSERVATIVE

- Education and information
- Advice on supportive footwear:
  - Avoid tight shoes and high heels
  - Use shoes with a wider toe box
  - Use a metatarsal pad

INJECTION

- Corticosteroid and local anaesthetic injection for pain relief but can be uncomfortable for several days afterwards
- A sclerosant injection of weak alcohol solution is used to break down fibrous tissue

RADIOFREQUENCY ABLATION

- Used in cases that do not resolve with less invasive measures, a radiofrequency probe is inserted into the neuroma using image guidance (fluoroscopy or ultrasound usually) under local anaesthetic and pulsed radiofrequency waves are passed down it, heating the tip of the probe causing localised thermal ablation, disrupting the neuroma

SURGERY

- Considered if conservative measures fail to resolve symptoms or there is a progression of symptoms
- Surgery involves excision of the neuroma, usually taking a dorsal rather than plantar approach

3.7.5 Medial Tibial Stress Syndrome (Shin Splints)

Medial Tibial Stress Syndrome (MTSS) describes an overuse or repetitive stress injury which is characterised by exercise induced pain over the anterior tibia which is commonly found in runners, military personnel and dancers. The cause of MTSS is unclear but it is thought to result from the tibia reacting to bone stress and/or repetitive muscle contractions pushing and pulling on the periosteum causing inflammation and pain.

History

- Woman are affected more than men
- Shin pain triggered in the early stages by weight-bearing exercise
- Pain is initially relieved by rest or may even settle during exercise, but in the later stages may progress and remain for hours after activity
- May feel worse in the morning
- Risk factors include:
  - Repetitive running or jumping activities, especially on hard or uneven surfaces
  - Hill running or running >20 miles a week
  - Previous history of MTSS or lower limb injury
  - Being overweight, underweight or malnourished may predispose to MTSS
  - Poorly fitting or poor-quality shoes
  - Biomechanical changes:
    - Hyperpronation of the foot
    - Leg length discrepancies
    - Foot arch abnormalities (pes planus)
    - Muscle imbalance between dorsiflexors and plantar flexors (causing decreased dorsiflexion)
    - Increased hip external rotation
  - Rapid increase in intensity, speed or duration of training

Symptoms

- Diffuse, dull pain located in the distal two-thirds of the posteromedial tibial border
- May be bilateral (seen in around half of the cases)
- There is normally no paraesthesia or numbness

Examination

- Diffuse tenderness over the medial tibial border (if in an area less than 5 cm, this may suggest a stress fracture)
- Pitting oedema may be evident, but bulging of the anterior compartment or any numbness would suggest compartment syndrome
- Non-tender to percussion (if pain is elicited with percussion, it may suggest a stress fracture)
- Pain may be reproduced with:
  - Stretching of soleus with passive ankle dorsiflexion
  - Resisted ankle plantar flexion
  - Standing toe raises

Differential Diagnosis

- Tibial stress fracture
- Exertional compartment syndrome
- Tendinopathy
- Lumbar radiculopathy
- Deep vein thrombosis
- Local nerve entrapment (e.g. common/superficial peroneal nerve)
- Malignancy
- Osteomyelitis
- Peripheral vascular disease

Investigation

- X-ray
  - Are generally used to exclude stress fracture, but a degree of hypertrophic bone in the area of pain may be seen in MTSS
- MRI
  - May identify signs of inflammation with bone marrow oedema, periosteal bone reaction, fascial or muscle inflammation
- Bone scan
  - May help differentiate between MTSS and fracture
  - MTSS may be normal or show a diffuse, linear uptake versus a focal uptake in the case of a fracture

Management

CONSERVATIVE

- PRICE (Protect, Rest, Ice, Compression, Elevation)
- Relative rest
- Activity modification
  - Reduced running volume and/or intensity
  - Switch to low-impact aerobic exercise (e.g., cross trainer)
  - Switch to a different training surface (avoiding harder surfaces)
- Supportive footwear – trainers should be replaced every 250–350 miles
- Taping or orthotics to manage overpronation
- Graded loading programme including stretching and strengthening of soleus, ankle dorsiflexors and plantar flexors and foot evertors and invertors

MEDICATION

- Non-steroidal anti-inflammatory drugs (NSAIDs) where safe and tolerated
- Weak opiates with or without paracetamol if NSAIDs are contraindicated, not tolerated or ineffective

SURGERY

- Use of surgery is extremely rare but may involve fasciotomy of the medial deep posterior compartment and periosteal stripping

3.7.6 Achilles Tendinopathy

Achilles tendinopathy (AT) primarily affects active sportspeople but can also occur in the less active population where there is an association with metabolic comorbidities. The diagnosis may be delayed as the early signs of the condition (mainly morning stiffness and mild discomfort) are often manageable and tend to be ignored. People may only seek help when the condition has progressed and pain starts to limit involvement in sports and activity.

There are two main types of AT:

- Insertional AT – where there is thickening and pain at the insertion of the tendon into the calcaneum and bone spurs may form at the back of the heel
- Non-insertional Achilles tendinitis – with swelling, thickening and pain along the middle fibres of the tendon, usually about 2–6 cm from the Achilles insertion

History

- Involvement in sports or activities that place repetitive or increased loading through the tendon
- Previous injury to the tendon or the surrounding area
- Being overweight or obese
- Risk factors:
  - Diabetes
  - Hypothyroidism
  - High blood pressure
  - Rheumatoid arthritis
  - Gout

Symptoms

- Localised pain above the insertion of the Achilles tendon to the calcaneum
- Morning pain and stiffness
- Stiffness after rest
- Pain worsens with weight-bearing activities and eases with rest
- Swelling along the tendon or the back of the heel

Examination

- Localised pain on palpation just above or around the Achilles tendon insertion
- Tendon enlargement or thickening
- Pain with weight-bearing or heel raise
- Pain with forced dorsiflexion or resisted plantar flexion
- Calf muscle atrophy
- Bone spur may be palpable

Differential Diagnosis

- Calcaneal fracture
- Retrocalcaneal bursitis
- Hagland deformity
- Posterior ankle impingement

- Plantar fasciitis
- Sever's disease
- Lumbar radiculopathy
- Deep vein thrombosis
- Os trigonum syndrome
- Ankle osteoarthritis
- Sural nerve irritation

Imaging

AT is primarily a clinical diagnosis that only requires further investigations if there is clinical uncertainty, to inform surgical planning or if other pathologies are suspected.

- X-ray
  - May reveal the presence of a posterior heel bone spur, which is indicative of an insertional AT
- MRI
  - MRI may be ordered to quantify the degree and site of the tendinopathy or to review other management options if conservative treatment has failed to resolve symptoms
- Ultrasound
  - Ultrasound can be used to confirm the diagnosis of AT, as it will show thickening and rounding of the affected part of the tendon
  - It may also inform management and can be used to monitor the outcome of treatment

Management

Management is aimed at reducing pain, improving lower limb strength, promoting tissue remodelling and increasing function.

CONSERVATIVE

- Relative rest
- Activity management
- Graduated loading programme
- Eccentric exercise programme
- Advice regarding weight loss, if appropriate

MEDICATION

- Non-steroidal anti-inflammatory drugs (NSAIDs) where safe and tolerated
- Weak opiates with or without paracetamol if NSAIDs are contraindicated, not tolerated or ineffective

INJECTION

- Corticosteroid injections are not recommended for AT as they may decrease tendon strength and increase the risk of rupture

SURGERY

- Surgery may be considered if the condition fails to respond to an extensive course of conservative treatment
- The type of surgery depends on the extent of damage to the tendon and its location
- Surgical options include:
  - Percutaneous tenotomy
  - Stripping of the tendon of peritendinous adhesions
  - Longitudinal tenotomies with debridement of the tendon

3.7.7 Peroneal Tendinopathy

Peroneal tendinopathy is characterised by pain, swelling, degeneration and thickening of the peroneal tendon around the posterolateral and inferior malleolar area of the ankle as a result of increased loading, repetitive movements and overuse. It is common in runners, dancers and activities involving rapidly changing direction and jumping e.g. basketball.

History

- Sudden increase in activity or training levels
- Trauma (e.g. repeated inversion ankle sprains)
- Running on a slope or uneven surface
- Wearing inappropriate or unsupportive footwear
- Lower limb muscle weakness and imbalance causing altered biomechanics
- Ankle instability

Symptoms

- Gradually worsening ankle pain
- Worse with activity (e.g. walking, running)
- Improves with rest
- Swelling or tenderness behind and below the lateral malleolus

Examination

- Tenderness on palpation of the peroneal tendon
- Hindfoot varus or pes cavus (high arches) can increase load and stress on the peroneal tendons
- Pain can be reproduced with:
  - Ankle eversion against resistance
  - Ankle dorsiflexion against resistance
  - Passive hindfoot inversion
  - Passive ankle plantar flexion

Differential Diagnosis

- Achilles tendinopathy
- Ankle sprain
- Peroneal subluxation
- Syndesmotic injuries
- Calcaneofibular ligament injury
- Talofibular ligament injury
- Ankle fractures – calcaneus or os perineum

Imaging

- X-ray
  - Are unable to diagnose peroneal tendinopathy but are often used as part of the assessment to rule out ankle fractures, avulsions, osteoarthritis, loose bodies and calcification of the tendon
- MRI
  - Is the imaging modality of choice to identify tendon pathology. Also used to evaluate the peroneal tendon and surrounding structures if surgery is being considered
- Ultrasound
  - Used to detect peroneal lesions and, where available, can assess dynamic stability

Management

CONSERVATIVE

- Relative rest
- Activity modification
- Ankle strengthening and stretching exercises
- Proprioceptive and balance training
- Soft tissue mobilisation
- Ankle strapping or brace, if appropriate
- Advice regarding footwear or orthotics

MEDICATION

- Non-steroidal anti-inflammatory drugs (NSAIDs) where safe and tolerated
- Weak opiates with or without paracetamol if NSAIDs are contraindicated, not tolerated or ineffective

INJECTIONS

- Corticosteroid injections may be offered to reduce pain or as a diagnostic tool, but the benefits need to be weighed against the risk of the steroid weakening the tendon and increasing the chance of a rupture

SURGERY

- If non-surgical treatment fails to resolve symptoms, surgery may be considered to debride and repair the tendon

3.7.8   Posterior Tibial Tendon Dysfunction

Posterior tibial tendon dysfunction is the most common cause of an acquired flatfoot deformity in adults. It occurs when the posterior tibial tendon, the primary stabiliser of the medial longitudinal arch of the foot, cannot provide support. As a result, there is a progressive collapse of the medial arch and an associated increase in pronation, heel valgus and forefoot abduction.

PTTD was initially classified by Johnson and Strom (1989) into three stages and modified by Myerson (1996), who added a fourth stage.

STAGE I

- The posterior tibial tendon length is preserved without deformity or collapse of the arch
- Patients present with medial foot and ankle pain and swelling, and mild weakness
- They may be able to perform a heel rise, but it is painful
- Degeneration is present

STAGE II

- A planovalgus deformity has developed, but it is passively correctable
- Patient exhibits 'too many toes' sign
- Posterior tibial tendon is functionally incompetent
- Progressive flattening of the arch
- Patient unable to a heel raise

STAGE III

- Degenerative changes in the subtalar joint
- The flat foot deformity becomes fixed

STAGE IV

- The most severe stage
- The deltoid ligament fails, resulting in a valgus tilt of the talus
- This leads to lateral tibiotalar degeneration

History

- More common in middle-aged females
- Prevalence increases with age
- There is a slow, insidious onset of flatfoot deformity
- Mainly unilateral
- Participating in sports that excessively load the tendon (e.g. football, tennis, hockey)
- Risk factors include:
  - Diabetes
  - Hypertension
  - Obesity
  - Previous surgery
  - History of foot or ankle trauma
  - Inflammatory joint disease
  - Corticosteroid injections in the area

Symptoms

- Pain on the medial aspect of the foot and ankle
- May or may not be accompanied by swelling
- Worse with prolonged activity (e.g. standing, walking)
- Aggravated by walking on uneven surfaces
- Pain on the lateral ankle in the advanced stage of the condition when, with increasing heel valgus deformity, the fibula comes into contact with the calcaneus

Examination

- Flat foot deformity – valgus heel, flattened arch and forefoot abduction
- Pain on palpation along the course of the posterior tibial tendon
- Swelling around the medial ankle
- Limited dorsiflexion – due to ankle stiffness and tight calf muscles
- Inability to single-leg heel raise
- May have a limp or impaired mobility
- Abnormal wear on shoes – associated with increasing foot deformity
- 'Too many toes' sign – when looking at the heel from behind, all four toes are visible. This occurs when the medial arch collapses down and causes the forefoot to abduct away from the midline. Normally only the little toe is seen

Tests

- Single-leg heel raise

Investigations

- X-ray
  - An X-ray is not necessary to diagnose PTTD
  - In the early stages of the condition, it will show normal findings or minimal changes of angular deformity. As the condition progresses, however, it will be able to quantify the changes in bony alignment and degree of deformity in the foot
- MRI
  - MRI can visualise the tendons, ligaments and other soft tissue around the ankle and diagnose PTTD. It can also detect bony changes, bony oedema and malalignment in the foot and ankle
- Ultrasound
  - Ultrasound can be used to assess signs of tendon damage and provide an accurate assessment of the posterior tibialis tendon

Management

CONSERVATIVE

- In the initial stages (Stages I and II)
  - PRICE (Protect, Rest, Ice, Compression and Elevation)
  - Relative rest – a cast or walking boot may help to rest the tendon
  - Activity modification
  - Stretching and strengthening exercises

- Balance and proprioception exercises
- Brace or orthotics – to stabilise and support the ankle

INJECTION

- A corticosteroid injection may be offered to reduce inflammation and pain

MEDICATION

- Non-steroidal anti-inflammatory drugs (NSAIDs) where safe and tolerated
- Weak opiates with or without paracetamol if NSAIDs are contraindicated, not tolerated or ineffective

SURGERY

- In Stages III and IV, surgery may be considered if the patient experiences persistent pain with or without significant deformity
- A number of surgical options are available to correct alignment and support the arch, including tendon transfers, osteotomy, arthrodesis and tendon repair or debridement

3.7.9   Ankle Sprain

Ankle sprains are very common, especially in sports. Although they can be thought of as an acute or traumatic injury, they may often present in the subacute phase or with longer-term sequelae. Early and appropriate management is important to reduce the risk of longer-term problems and recurrence, which is increased for 6 to 12 months after the initial injury. It is worth noting that sprains refer to an injury of a ligament, whereas a 'strain' describes the involvement of muscle or musculotendinous junction.

Ankle sprains can be classified according to the structures involved:

- Lateral ligament sprains – are associated with inversion injuries. They are far more common than eversion injuries due to the differences in relative strengths of the lateral versus medial ligaments as well as lateral joint instability
- Medial ligament sprains – are associated with eversion injuries. Because of the stronger structure, injuries to the medial ligament involve a greater force and may be associated with fractures (medial malleolus, talar dome or joint surface). They often take longer to rehabilitate
- Inferior tibiofibular ligaments – are generally associated with a more severe injury, often including an ankle fracture

History

- There is a wide range of risk factors for ankle sprains that include:
  - Previous history of ankle sprain – affecting proprioception, strength and integrity of stabilisers
  - Participation in sports (e.g. basketball, ice skating, volleyball and football) or activities involving the following:
    - Rapid change of direction (lateral ligament)
    - Activity on uneven surfaces
    - Jumping activities
  - Congenital abnormalities of the foot:
    - Pes planus
    - Joint laxity
    - Limited dorsiflexion of the foot

Symptoms

- Acute onset of pain
- Located over the medial or lateral aspect of the ankle, depending on the mechanism and which ligament(s) are involved
- Usually able to partially bear weight immediately after injury – complete inability to bear weight would raise suspicion of more significant injury
- Swelling and bruising – may take 24 h or more to develop – note that any deformity of the joint or lower limb may suggest a fracture
- Stiffness of the ankle joint
- Ankle instability – the degree of instability relates to the severity of the injury

Examination

- Swelling and/or bruising – corresponding to the region affected
- Reduced range of movement with reproduction or worsening of pain
- Loss of active range of movement helps to identify the degree of functional deficit
- Loss of passive range of movement may identify injury
  - Loss of inversion suggests lateral ligament injury
  - Loss of eversion suggests medial ligament injury
  - Loss of plantar flexion and inversion suggests talofibular ligament injury
- Impaired proprioception – inability to single-leg stand with eyes closed
- Tenderness over the base of the fifth metatarsal may signify an associated avulsion fracture
- Grading of sprain describes the degree of injury and can guide treatment
  - Grade I: microscopic injury with no abnormal ligament instability and mild symptoms or signs
  - Grade II: macroscopic injury to the ligament, but it remains intact with some instability on testing and retains a firm endpoint
  - Grade III: complete rupture of a ligament – gross laxity with no discernible end point (may be less painful than grade II)

Special Tests

- Anterior draw test
- Talar tilt test
- Squeeze test

Differential Diagnosis

- Osteochondral lesion of talus
- Ankle impingement
- Tarsal tunnel syndrome
- Sinus tarsi syndrome
- Fracture
- Dislocation
- Tendon rupture (tibialis posterior, peroneal tendon)
- Complex regional pain syndrome
- Syndesmosis sprain

Investigation

- X-ray
  - Informed by Ottawa ankle rules (ankle injury)
  - Refer for an X-ray if there is:
    - Pain in the malleolar area (lateral or medial) and
    - Bone tenderness at the posterior tip of the lateral (and/or) medial malleolus or
    - Patient was unable to bear weight at the time of the injury, and when seen

- MRI
  - May be useful to identify osteochondral lesions
- CT/bone scan
  - May be used if MRI contraindicated

Management

Principles focus on early rehabilitation, and avoiding prolonged immobilisation, as inadequate or incomplete rehabilitation increases the likelihood of a poorer outcome.

CONSERVATIVE

- Protect, Rest, Ice, Compression and Elevation (PRICE)
- Initial non-weight-bearing (in first 24 h) followed by gentle weight-bearing and mobilisation.
- Range of movement exercises
- Muscle strengthening and conditioning
- Proprioceptive work – start early and progress as able
- Functional exercises – once pain-free and sufficient strength and range of movement have been regained
- Taping and bracing if appropriate

MEDICATION

- Non-steroidal anti-inflammatory drugs (NSAIDs) where safe and tolerated
- Weak opiates with or without paracetamol if NSAIDs are contraindicated, not tolerated or ineffective

SURGERY

- Is usually reserved for grade III injuries, although conservative rehabilitation may achieve similar results
- Surgery involves ligament reconstruction, where the remaining ligament is shortened and reattached to the bone

Regional Musculoskeletal Conditions: Shorts

Anterior Interosseus Syndrome

Anterior interosseus syndrome describes the entrapment of the anterior interosseous nerve (the motor branch of the median nerve) in the forearm. This can be spontaneous or traumatic e.g. following a forearm fracture or penetrating injuries such as stab wounds.

The condition is characterised by motor loss with weakness in the thumb and index finger pincer movement. As a result, the patient is unable to make an 'OK' sign with their hand. It may also be hard to make a fist due to loss of flexion in the second and third fingers giving the characteristic 'sign of Benediction.' There are no sensory symptoms but it may sometimes be associated with pain in the proximal, volar aspect of the forearm. Recovery may be spontaneous or require surgical exploration and decompression.

Cervical Arterial Dysfunction

Cervical artery dysfunction (CAD) is an umbrella term describing interruption of the blood supply to the brain via the anterior (internal carotid) or posterior (vertebrobasilar) arteries causing symptoms of a transient ischaemic attack (TIA).

This can be caused by intermittent arterial occlusion associated with underlying problems, including atherosclerosis, compressive lesions, dissection or a subclavian steal (a stenotic lesion in the subclavian artery causing a reversed flow of blood in the vertebral artery associated with increased arm activity).

Signs and symptoms of CAD include:
- **5 Ds:**
  - **D**ysarthria – slurred/slow speech
  - **D**ysphagia – swallowing difficulties
  - **D**izziness
  - **D**rop attacks – sudden collapses
  - **D**ouble vision
- **3 Ns:**
  - **N**ystagmus – repetitive, uncontrolled eye movement
  - **N**ausea
  - **N**umbness – facial
- **2 As:**
  - **A**taxia – difficulties with coordination and balance
  - **A**nhydrosis – loss of sweating on the face

Of note, Horner's syndrome is seen in more than 80% of cases. This syndrome is characterised by ptosis (drooping eyelid), miosis (constricted pupil) and anhydrosis (loss of sweating on the face).

CAD may be acute in onset (e.g. following trauma) or chronic. Intermittent or insidious presentations can come with signs of a TIA, acute onset head pain, ipsilateral face or neck pain and lower cranial nerve dysfunction (IX-XII).

Assessment includes screening for cardiovascular risk factors (e.g. smoking, family history, hypertension, diabetes, hypercholesterolaemia) and may include positional testing. Patients with significant pain and/or peripheral neurological deficit or episodes of transient brain ischaemia need to be referred to neuro-vascular surgeons. This should be treated as an emergency if there are any objective features of a cerebrovascular accident with evidence of a persistent neurological deficit.

Charcot Joint

This term describes damage to a joint due to the progressive loss of sensation most commonly associated with diabetic neuropathy or, more rarely, due to syphilis or syringomyelia. This can cause ulceration and infection and potentially lead to amputation.

Charcot joint usually affects the midfoot (tarsometatarsal joints) and, less commonly, the forefoot or rear foot. It may present in the early stages with mild pain and inflammation before progressing to joint subluxation and dislocation with subsequent ankylosis and new bony growth. This leads to a characteristically painless, deformed joint.

Unlike diabetic neuropathy, Charcot joints preserve heat and light touch sensation. X-rays may show dislocation, subluxation of the joint with calcification and potentially extensive joint destruction. Treatment is generally conservative and includes splints or casts as well as managing the underlying condition (e.g. diabetes).

Cubital Tunnel Syndrome

Cubital tunnel syndrome is commonly seen as an overuse injury in repeated overhead throwing sports (e.g. javelin) as well as a range of other causes including trauma, space occupying lesions and anatomical variance. Patients present with medial elbow pain, hand weakness with clawing of the 4th and 5th fingers and paraesthesia in the medial forearm. Wrist flexion remains unaffected.

Inflammation of the ulnar nerve is caused by compression at the cubital tunnel, where it can be trapped between the two heads of flexor carpi ulnaris.

Symptoms include numbness and paraesthesia in the ring and little fingers and occasionally the ulnar aspect of the palm or forearm. There can be pain in the region of the cubital tunnel. In the advanced stage it can cause wasting of the muscles in the hand with loss of grip strength and clumsiness.

An examination may show evidence of clawing of the ring and little fingers (known as the Duchenne sign) due to paralysis of hand muscles (lumbricals and interossei). Further tests include a positive Tinel's sign over the ulnar nerve at the elbow and Froment's sign, which shows evidence of weakness in adductor policis.

Treatment may include activity modification or surgery, but this tends to address progression rather than recovering function.

Developmental Dysplasia of the Hip

Developmental dysplasia of the hip (DDH) is a term used to describe abnormal hip development that affects the ability of the femoral head to be contained within the acetabular cavity. The presentation of DDH ranges from minor hip instability to acetabular dysplasia, hip subluxations and frank dislocation. Originally referred to as 'congenital dislocation of the hip,' the term was changed to reflect that many of the findings are not present or identified at birth. Early diagnosis and treatment are essential to prevent early osteoarthritis (OA) and functional limitations (a limp) and improve treatment outcomes.

Treatment options depend on age at presentation and may include use of a pelvic harness, traction or use of casts before the age a child starts walking. Treatment options after this stage are subject to debate but may include physical therapy and, potentially, surgery.

Diffuse Idiopathic Skeletal Hyperostosis (DISH)

DISH usually affects the thoracic spine and is a relatively common condition in older people (a variant of spondylosis). It is caused by calcification or ossification of soft tissues, entheses and ligaments (primarily the anterior longitudinal ligament of the spine). Diagnosis is based on finding these changes in four or more spinal levels with preserved disc space and no signs of inflammation. It is associated with metabolic derangements, diabetes, hyperlipidaemia, hypertension and obesity.

DISH may be asymptomatic or cause reduced range of movement (side bending of the thoracic spine), stiffness and pain. Patients may also describe additional features, including hyperostosis of other entheses (elbows, hips, shoulder and ankles), spur formation (elbow, heel, knee), hypertrophic osteoarthritis (shoulder and elbow), swallowing difficulties and voice changes (osteophytes causing impingement in the throat), lumbar stenosis and cervical myelopathy.

Treatment options include managing metabolic comorbidities, analgesia, physical therapy for mobility and, very rarely, surgical decompression or stabilisation.

Dupuytren's Disease (Contracture)

Dupuytren's disease is a benign, slowly progressive condition characterised by the thickening of the palmar fascia (not the tendons). Starting within the superficial fascia and dermis, it initially causes skin pitting or puckering followed by the development of thick cords running between the palm and fingers and palpable nodules formed by fibrosis of the palmar aponeurosis. Actual contracture of the plantar fascia is seen in the later stages of the disease. This can eventually cause proximal interphalangeal joint (PIPJ) and metacarpophalangeal joint (MCPJ) contracture, typically in the ring and little fingers.

The presence of a fixed flexion deformity separates it from trigger finger, where any flexion deformity can be overcome by straightening the finger.

There is a genetic susceptibility, more prevalent in males and white Europeans, and it is associated with heavy alcohol use, smoking and diabetes mellitus. It can coexist with nodular fibromatosis in the knuckle pads (Garrod's disease), feet (Ledderhose disease) and penis (Peyronie's disease).

Treatments are not curative but aim to manage the contractures. Referral from primary care would be indicated when there is an MCPJ contracture of 30° or more at the MCPJ and/or 10° at PIPJ.

Treatments include:
- Injections of clostridial collagenase, causing lysis and rupture of cords
- Needle fasciotomy
- Surgery – fasciectomy

Femoroacetabular Impingement

Femoroacetabular impingement (FAI) occurs as a result of anatomical abnormalities of the femoral head and the acetabulum. As a result of these structural deformities, there is early contact between the femoral head and the acetabulum, which limits movement – mainly hip flexion, adduction and rotation. As well as limiting movement, the repetitive contact between the femoral head and acetabulum may damage the labrum and articular cartilage and lead to the early development of hip osteoarthritis (OA). The condition may be caused by a combination of genetic and environmental factors and be present from birth (congenital) or may develop in later life (acquired).

Three types of impingement may occur:
- Cam impingement – due to aspherical deformation of the femoral head
- Pincer impingement – due to abnormal prominence of the outer rim of the acetabulum
- Mixed – a combination of cam and pincer impingement

Patients typically present with anterior or anterolateral hip or groin pain and limited range of movement, especially hip internal rotation.

Diagnosis is usually confirmed with imaging (X-ray, MRI and/or CT scan) to identify acetabular or femoral head structural abnormalities and the presence of hip OA and can rule out other causes of hip pain.

In the early stages, management involves relative rest, functional training, movement pattern training, postural correction, patient education and hip strengthening exercises. Patients should be encouraged to avoid aggravating movements such as squatting, sitting cross-legged, twisting or using combined movements (hip flexion, adduction and internal rotation) during everyday activities.

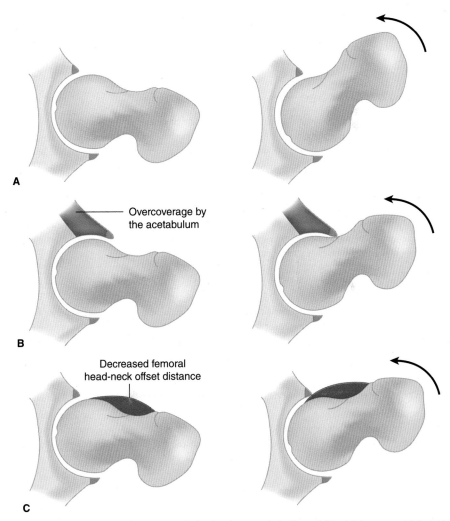

Fig 3.8.3 Cam and pincer femoroacetabular impingement A Normal hip joint – unrestricted hip motion B Pincer-type femoroacetabular impingement – abnormal prominence of the outer rim of the acetabulum C Cam-type femoroacetabular impingement – aspherical deformation of the femoral head.

Surgical treatment of FAI is aimed at improving the mechanics of the hip joint and preventing the early onset of hip OA. Arthroscopic hip surgery is used to trim and correct the shape of the acetabulum and femoral head and address any intra-articular damage.

Ganglion Cyst of the Wrist

A very common, benign lesion of the wrist with no clear predisposing factors. They are usually found at the dorsal or volar aspect of the wrist. A ganglion is a cyst filled with a thick fluid forming a non-tender mass communicating with the wrist joint. It is normally asymptomatic but can cause local pain and some neuromuscular compromise if big enough. Ultrasound or MRI may be used if the diagnosis is in doubt.

Management may consist of keeping it under observation, or it may need to be aspirated with a large bore needle with or without corticosteroid injection. Although this can be effective, it can be associated with recurrence. Surgical excision is the most successful treatment, but they can still recur. The historic suggestion of hitting them with a bible is more likely to cause damage to other structures in the wrist and is probably best avoided.

Kienböck's Disease

Kienböck's disease describes avascular necrosis of the lunate bone, one of the key carpal bones in the wrist involved in wrist mobility. Seen more often in younger males, it is associated with repeated loading or trauma (e.g. in sports people with repeated wrist impacts) as well as in people with congenital anatomical differences such as negative ulna variance (a shortened ulna compared to radius).

Symptoms include activity-related dorsal wrist pain and weakness. Swelling may be found above the lunate alongside some localised tenderness and reduced wrist extension.

In the late stages of the condition, X-rays may show a smaller than expected lunate with increased radio-opacity (increased bone density). An MRI or radio-isotope bone scan can be used to aid diagnosis. Conservative treatment includes immobilisation, while surgical options include radial osteotomy in the early stages or wrist arthrodesis in the later stages.

Mallet Finger

Mallet finger describes the characteristic flexion deformity of a fingertip (into a mallet or hammer shape) usually caused by a distal extensor tendon rupture or extensor avulsion fracture.

It usually follows a forced flexion injury at the distal interphalangeal joint (e.g. when attempting to catch a hard ball), although, in older patients, it can involve injuries with less force.

Examination shows a disruption of the extensor mechanism with no active extension of the fingertip, but passive movement is retained. Diagnosis is based on history and clinical findings. An X-ray may be helpful to exclude fractures.

Treatment is usually conservative, with a mallet splint for six weeks. The splint holds the distal interphalangeal joint extended but enables movement at the proximal interphalangeal joint. Surgery may be indicated if there is an associated fracture or it fails to respond to conservative approaches.

Osgood-Schlatter Disease

Osgood-Schlatter disease (OSD) is a common cause of knee pain amongst active, growing adolescents. It is caused by repeated tractioning of the patellar tendon at its insertion on the tibial tuberosity (apophysis), causing inflammation and irritation. This leads to focal tenderness and swelling over the tibial tuberosity. The condition is more prevalent in males and those participating in sports such as running, jumping, football and gymnastics, although it can also affect less active adolescents.

Treatment usually consists of icing or non-steroidal anti-inflammatory drugs (NSAIDs) for pain relief, stretching and strengthening of quadriceps and hamstrings, relative rest and activity modification. The condition usually resolves once bone growth is completed (apophysis fuses), though, in a small percentage of patients, symptoms may persist. Patients with OSD often display a more prominent bump around the tibial tuberosity.

Osteoarthritis of the Ankle

Despite the ankle being subjected to significant loads, primary osteoarthritis (OA) of the ankle is rare. OA tends to be associated with previous trauma, malalignment, erosive arthropathies (e.g. gout or rheumatoid arthritis) and rare conditions such as haemophilia, which causes bleeding into the joint.

Usually unilateral, symptoms include swelling, crepitus and stiffness with insidious onset of ankle pain that is worse on weight-bearing and eased by rest.

There is tenderness at the anterior joint line, and there may be a decreased range of movement (dorsiflexion/plantarflexion). It is worth noting deformity and swelling of the ankle joint in the absence of pain might suggest a Charcot joint.

Imaging (X-ray) may show loss of joint space, osteophytes, deformity, sub-chondral sclerosis and evidence of past trauma.

Conservative treatments include NSAIDs, weight management, shoe modifications (cushioned heel, rocker-bottom sole), exercise therapy (including swimming, elliptical bike) and intra-articular corticosteroid injections. Surgical options include arthroscopic debridement, arthrodesis (joint fusion) or arthroplasty (joint replacement).

Osteoarthritis of the Base of Thumb (First Carpo-Metacarpal Joint)

Osteoarthritis of the base of thumb is a very common condition seen in primary care and may present in the context of generalised osteoarthritis (OA) or as a result of occupational overuse. The patient complains of pain at the base of the thumb and, as it progresses, loss of range of movement, a decrease in grip strength and difficulty in performing dexterous tasks.

An examination may reveal characteristic squaring deformity at the base of the thumb due to osteophytic lipping at the base of the metacarpal and can be associated with profound wasting of the thenar muscles. Passive movements of the joint will be painful. Axial compression combined with the rotation of the thumb (grind test) elicits the patient's pain.

It is important to differentiate this condition from De Quervain's disease. Management can be conservative and may include referral to an occupational therapist for functional support, topical NSAIDs, splints, corticosteroid injection and surgery.

Osteoarthritis of the Fingers

Osteoarthritis of the fingers may be described as 'nodal' osteoarthritis (OA) and tends to involve the distal more than the proximal interphalangeal joints, with swelling of the joint(s) and pain. This may settle, leaving a bony swelling around the joint. These are called Heberden's nodes at the distal interphalangeal joint and Bouchard's nodes at the proximal interphalangeal joints.

There may be a degree of deformity alongside pain and stiffness, often with a marked impact on function. The use of topical non steroidal anti-inflammatory drugs (NSAIDs) alongside input from hand therapists and the use of aids may significantly improve quality of life. Surgical treatment, including fusion of affected joints, is rare.

Osteochondral Lesion of Talus

Osteochondral lesion of talus describes a compression fracture of a section of the talar dome. This is usually found in the superomedial region of the talar dome due to compression by the tibia. It often occurs alongside an ankle sprain with a mode of injury that includes compressive forces (e.g. landing awkwardly from a jump).

It may present with persistent pain, especially on weight-bearing, with tenderness felt over the talar dome when rotated out of the ankle joint in plantar flexion (though this may be too painful to do in practice). There may be clicking, locking and loss of range of movement with associated loose bodies.

If the lesion is undisplaced, treatment may be conservative with immobilisation, physical therapy and protective braces. If displaced, treatment may involve arthroscopic excision of the lesion.

Osteochondritis Dissecans

Osteochondritis dissecans (OCD) is a relatively common cause of activity-related knee pain among children and adolescents (juvenile OCD) but can also occur in adults (adult OCD). It arises when a small segment of subchondral bone begins to separate from the surrounding healthy bone due to a lack of blood supply. This may result in the separation of the associated articular cartilage, leading to mechanical symptoms (locking of the knee), pain, swelling and, in some cases, the formation of loose bodies. If untreated, it can lead to degenerative changes.

OCD can occur in a number of joints, including the ankle, elbow, shoulder and hip but mainly affects the posterolateral aspect of the medial femoral condyle of the knee. In most children and adolescents, the condition will resolve on its own with rest from vigorous activities. If the condition fails to resolve with conservative measures, surgery to improve vascularisation, tether loose bodies or graft new bone and cartilage in the damaged area may be an option.

Patellar Dislocation (Traumatic)

Acute patellar dislocations are primarily due to a twisting, non-contact injury to the knee or as a result of a direct blow to the medial aspect of the knee. The patella is forced out of the trochlear groove, resulting in damage to the medial patellofemoral ligament and the development of hemarthrosis (bleeding into the knee joint). The dislocation normally resolves spontaneously, though a small percentage of patients may require reduction.

Initial treatment involves immobilising the knee for a few weeks and starting to bear weight as soon as pain allows. Rehabilitation is aimed at restoring movement, strengthening and stretching of the quadriceps, hamstrings and adductors and improving knee stability. Surgery may be necessary with recurrent dislocations.

Plica Syndrome

Plica syndrome is a common source of knee pain among young athletes involved in repetitive flexion-extension activities such as rowing, cycling, jumping, swimming and running. The synovial plica are membranous inward folds of the synovial lining of the joint capsule that can become irritated and inflamed as a result of direct injury or overuse.

In the knee, the medial plica is most prone to injury, and patients complain of pain and tenderness around the medial patellar area above the joint line as the plica catches or impinges between the surface of the patellar and femur. Patients may also present with crepitus and swelling. Presentation is similar to a medial meniscal tear, which would need to be ruled out as part of the differential diagnosis.

Treatment consists of icing and non steroidal anti-inflammatory drugs (NSAIDs) for pain relief, stretching and strengthening hamstrings and quadriceps, modifying activity and relative rest. A corticosteroid injection may be considered if the pain is severe and prevents engagement in exercise therapy. If conservative treatment fails to resolve symptoms, arthroscopic surgery may be necessary to remove thickened or fibrosed plica that may be causing ongoing impingement.

Pronator Teres Syndrome

Pronator teres syndrome describes median nerve entrapment at the elbow. It tends to be an overuse injury (e.g. musicians or factory workers) with compression of the median nerve as it passes through two heads of the pronator muscle at the elbow.

Symptoms include pain in the proximal and ventral aspect of the forearm with paraesthesia of the thumb, index, middle finger and radial half of the ring finger. There is also sensory loss over the thenar eminence and a lack of night symptoms, which helps distinguish it from carpal tunnel syndrome. Resisted pronation of the forearm elicits localised tenderness, pain and weakness. Tinel's test is negative at the wrist but positive over the proximal forearm.

Conservative management may include corticosteroid injection or surgical decompression.

Radial Nerve Lesions

Radial nerve lesions result from a range of factors that include fractures to the humerus, stab wounds to the antecubital fossa, forearm or wrist, compression in the axillae (e.g. with the use of crutches – 'crutch palsy'), tight plaster casts, prolonged surgical tourniquet time, falling asleep with an arm hanging over back of a chair ('Saturday night palsy') or with the arm underneath someone ('honeymoon palsy').

Symptoms include sensory loss over the posterior arm, forearm and dorso-radial aspect of the hand. Associated weakness in wrist extensors (brachioradialis and supinator components of the posterior compartment of the forearm) can cause a characteristic wrist drop. There may also be weakness in the elbow, thumb and metacarpophalangeal joint extension.

Radial tunnel syndrome (posterior interosseous nerve entrapment) shows milder symptoms where it can be trapped and compressed by a range of anatomical structures and may be hard to differentiate from extensor tendinopathy.

Treatment may include conservative approaches such as soft tissue and exercise therapies or may require surgical decompression.

Scaphoid Fracture

Scaphoid fracture is the most common carpal bone injury, but it is easy to miss as there is often no bruising or deformity to be seen. Key symptoms include localised tenderness and swelling in the anatomical snuff box with pain on the dorsiflexion of the wrist and when gripping. There may also be grip weakness.

Standard hand and wrist X-rays may not show evidence of fracture, so 'scaphoid views' are required when a fracture is suspected.

Treatment includes immobilisation in a cast for un-displaced fractures or reduction and internal fixation for displaced fractures. Failure to identify and treat scaphoid fractures can lead to non-union, avascular necrosis and advanced osteoarthritis (OA) of the wrist.

Scheuermann's Disease

Scheurmann's disease, also known as juvenile kyphosis, is found in adolescents and describes the defective growth of the vertebral cartilage endplate. This causes wedging of the vertebrae of varying degrees and mainly affects the thoracic or thoracolumbar spine. Its cause is uncertain, with theories including genetics, abnormal ossification of the endplates and mechanical stress during the growth of the spine.

Scheuermann's disease tends to be diagnosed in the teenage years and affects men more than women. It may cause reduced flexibility and back pain with varying degrees of kyphosis. It can be asymptomatic in some cases. Formal diagnosis requires the presence of 5° wedging in three or more adjacent vertebrae on an X-ray.

The prognosis is generally good, with pain resolving at skeletal maturity in most cases. However, it increases the risk of developing back pain as an adult. Treatment in children with significant symptoms includes physical therapy (stretching, postural advice, activity modification, exercise and education), bracing and analgesia. Surgery may be considered in children with kyphosis >75° or significant pain or neurological compromise.

In adults, treatment is conservative with exercise therapy and pain management.

Sinding-Larsen and Johansson Disease

Sinding-Larsen and Johansson disease is a condition that typically affects early adolescents (between 10 to 14 years old) involved in regular activity or sport. It is caused by repetitive traction on the proximal patella tendon as it inserts into the patella causing irritation and inflammation. This leads to focal tenderness and swelling around the inferior pole of the patellar. Treatment consists of icing and non steroidal anti-inflammatory drugs (NSAIDs) for pain relief, stretching and strengthening exercises, relative rest and activity modification (avoiding activities such as kneeling, jumping, ascending stairs and running). A patellar band around the knee may be trialled to see if it reduces symptoms. The condition is self-limiting and usually resolves once bone growth is complete. X-rays of the knee may show a spur at the inferior pole of the patella.

Sinus Tarsi Syndrome

Sinus tarsi syndrome refers to pain arising in the anterolateral aspect of the ankle and sinus tarsi (the channel that runs between the talus and calcaneus bones) with multiple possible underlying pathologies.

It most commonly follows a significant sprain (classically an ankle inversion injury) or overuse injury. It involves a degree of ligamentous laxity, synovitis and fibrosis in the sinus tarsi causing pain in the lateral ankle that is worse in standing or walking (especially over uneven ground). Pain is often accompanied by a degree of instability with an increased range of motion of the subtalar joint. Localised tenderness and reproduction of pain with passive plantar flexion and supination are characteristic of the condition.

X-rays may be used to exclude fracture, while MRI scans may detect soft tissue changes to the ligaments and degeneration in the subtalar joint. Corticosteroid injections have a diagnostic as well as therapeutic role. Conservative treatments include strengthening and sensorimotor training, non steroidal anti-inflammatory drugs (NSAIDs), taping and bracing. Arthroscopic surgery may be considered to address issues with the subtalar joint or for debridement of the sinus tarsi.

Snapping Hip Syndrome (Coxa Saltans or Dancer's Hip)

Snapping hip syndrome (SHS) occurs when a tendon or muscle slips over bone or other structure, creating a characteristic snapping or popping sensation. It can be felt or heard when the hip is flexed and extended during activity (i.e. when walking, getting up from a chair, going up stairs) and commonly affects those involved in activities that require repetitive hip movements, such as dancers, footballers, weightlifters and runners.

Patients will often be able to describe the sensation and point to the area where it occurs. The sensation is often palpable and can be reproduced with certain movements.

SHS is classified as either an external, internal or intra-articular snapping hip, depending on the structures that are responsible for the snapping sensation.

- External:
  - The iliotibial band snaps over the greater trochanter
  - The proximal hamstring tendon subluxes over the ischial tuberosity
  - The fascia lata moves over the greater trochanter
  - The psoas tendon rolls over the iliac muscle
- Internal:
  - The iliopsoas tendon snaps over anatomical structures such as the iliopectineal eminence, the anterior hip capsule, the femoral head or the iliofemoral ligament
- Intra-articular:
  - Patients may also describe a clicking or catching sensation in the hip joint. This may be due to intra-articular causes such as labral tears, ligementum teres tears or loose bodies within the joint

Diagnosis is mainly made through clinical examination and patient history, but imaging may be ordered to rule out other hip pathology and identify soft tissue changes (i.e. thickened iliotibial band or gluteus maximus muscle) or anatomical variations that may be causing the condition. Dynamic ultrasonography may be used to examine the movement of the iliotibial band over the great trochanter.

SHS that is intermittent and asymptomatic will not require treatment. When the condition is painful and affects performance and function, it can be managed conservatively with activity modification, stretching, strengthening, self-myofascial release (foam roller) and soft tissue mobilisation.

Non steroidal anti-inflammatory drugs (NSAIDs) and corticosteroid injections may be indicated where inflammation is an issue. Surgery to lengthen or release the iliopsoas or iliotibial band is rarely indicated and is only considered in severe cases where conservative treatment has failed.

Spina Bifida

Spina bifida is a neural tube defect resulting from the incomplete closure of the vertebral canal during foetal development. Causes are uncertain but are associated with low levels of maternal folic acid.

There are two main types

Spina Bifida cystica (open) – where the meningeal sac and contents protrude through a midline opening of the skin

Variants include:
- Meningocele
  - Cystic cerebrospinal fluid (CSF)-filled cavity lined with meninges but no neural tissue
  - Usually repaired early with a good prognosis
- Meningomyelocele
  - Sac contains elements of nerves and the cord itself
  - Causes a range of disabilities and potential longer-term impairment

Spina Bifida occult (closed) – where the skin is closed over the defect. There is often a visible dimple, skin pigmentation (naevus) or patch of hair above it. There is usually a defect in the posterior vertebral arch of L5 and S1, but this rarely causes symptoms. Further investigations are indicated if there are gait changes, deformities in the feet or urinary problems

Spondylolisthesis

Spondylolisthesis describes the abnormal displacement of one vertebra relative to the vertebra below it. This most commonly occurs in the lumbar spine but is also seen in the cervical spine. It rarely occurs in the thoracic spine.

It is caused by a range of factors, including fracture of pars interarticularis (more commonly seen in athletes such as fast bowlers in cricket), degenerative changes in the spine, congenital changes, trauma and pathological weakening of pars (due to tumours or osteoporosis).

Features include backache, reduced range of movement, a distinct step on palpation of the spine and signs of nerve root irritation. An X-ray of the spine may show a forward shift of the vertebra, facet joint degeneration and a pars fracture (seen on oblique views). Spondylolistheses are graded according to the percentage slip of one vertebra over the other:

- Grade I=<25%
- Grade II=25-50%
- Grade III=50-75%
- Grade IV=75-100%

Treatment can be conservative (with relative rest and graded rehabilitation) or involve surgery such as spinal fusion if it is more disabling and/or there is evidence of neurological compromise.

Tailors Bunion (Bunionette)

Tailors bunion is common but often asymptomatic bony prominence around the fifth metatarsal head that may be accompanied by bowing of the fifth metatarsal and/or widening of the fourth or fifth inter-metatarsal angle. These may be idiopathic, related to sports activity (e.g. running and skiing), rheumatoid arthritis or congenital abnormalities.

When symptomatic, it can cause pain and difficulty with tight or restrictive footwear. There may be a visible prominence around the fifth metatarsal head with overlying thickening of the skin (a 'corn') with ulceration and infection in some cases.

Treatment is initially conservative with changes to footwear, orthoses and chiropody. The option of surgery may be considered for recalcitrant cases and may include osteotomy and metatarsal head resection.

Tarsal Tunnel Syndrome

Tarsal tunnel syndrome is the most common entrapment neuropathy of the foot. It involves compression of the tibial nerve as it passes through the tarsal tunnel, which sits behind the medial malleolus and beneath the flexor retinaculum. This may be idiopathic, related to trauma (fracture or dislocation of the talus, calcaneus or medial malleolus), due to local structural changes (e.g. osteophytes caused by rheumatoid arthritis, tenosynovitis or arthritis) or due to space-occupying lesions (e.g. ganglions, tumours, fibrosis)

Symptoms include medial heel or ankle pain (burning or shooting in nature) that may radiate distally. It is generally worse on prolonged standing or walking and eased with rest. It may be associated with numbness along the plantar aspect of the foot, localised oedema, varicosities and with weakness and/or loss of function and atrophy of the plantar foot muscles.

Clinical signs include a positive Tinel's sign (percussion over the course of the tibial nerve causing proximal or distal paraesthesia) and a positive compression test (ankle plantar flexion and eversion of ankle reproducing symptoms). Nerve conduction studies and electromyography (EMG) may show prolonged tibial motor latency and slowing of conduction velocities across the flexor retinaculum. Imaging, including ultrasound and MRI, may show structural deformities or space-occupying lesions.

Treatment may be conservative and includes analgesia, taping, orthotics and local steroid injections. Surgical options include decompression, excision of space-occupying lesions or correction of deformities.

Triangular Fibrocartilage Complex (TFCC) Injuries

A common cause of chronic wrist pain, the TFCC acts as a stabiliser for the wrist and can be damaged during a distal radial-ulnar fracture or after significant, compressive loads to the wrist in ulnar deviation (e.g. baseball and gymnastics).

Patients may describe ulnar-sided wrist pain that is worse with activity associated with weakness in the grip and 'clicking' on movement. Tenderness and swelling may be localised to the dorsal ulnar region. TFCC compression or the 'Press' test (the patient lifts themselves out of a chair with their wrists in an extended position, reproduction of pain indicates a positive test) may be helpful in diagnosing the condition.

Imaging includes MRI and ultrasound to detect tears. Treatment may be conservative with relative rest, bracing, activity modification and physical rehabilitation. Surgical options are considered when conservative measures fail and include arthroscopic debridement, repair and shortening of the ulnar where relevant.

Ulnar Nerve Palsy at the Wrist (Cyclist's Palsy)

Ulnar nerve palsy at the wrist involves ulnar nerve compression as it passes through Guyon's canal at the wrist to enter the hand. This is usually triggered by a combination of vibration and direct pressure over the canal with prolonged wrist flexion and ulnar deviation. In cyclists, this is exacerbated by cycling downhill, having the saddle set too high or tilted too far down, which increases pressure on the wrists.

Symptoms can vary and may include paraesthesia, numbness in the ring and little fingers and weakness in the thumb and hand. Nerve conduction studies and electromyography (EMG) can help locate the lesion and inform prognosis.

Treatments involve correction of any contributory factors (e.g. change ride position, seat height and handlebars) as well as the use of non steroidal anti-inflammatory drugs (NSAIDs), splints and corticosteroid injection or decompression surgery for cases not responding to conservative measures.

Systemic Conditions

Rheumatoid Arthritis

Rheumatoid arthritis (RA) is a chronic inflammatory arthritis causing progressive joint pain and deformity with significant disability if left untreated. It is characterised by the production of autoantibodies including rheumatoid factor affecting the synovium of joints (classically the small joints of the hands and feet) causing hypertrophy and subsequent destruction. There may also be extra-articular involvement of other systems, including the kidneys, lungs and skin.

History

- Classically starts early in life (30s)
- It is more common in women than men
- Higher incidence in certain populations (e.g. Native Americans)
- Genetic component with an association with the HLA-DR4 marker
- Factors associated with increased risk include:
  - Smoking
  - Obesity
  - Epstein Barr Virus infection

Symptoms

- Joint pain usually in a symmetrical pattern affecting the small joints of the hands, wrists and feet and, more rarely, larger joints
- May present as an insidious onset of symmetrical polyarthritis or a more acute mono-arthropathy or palindromic (flares of joint pain that return to normal between episodes)
- Morning stiffness (>30 min) and loss of function
- Sleep disturbance – may wake with pain in the early hours of the morning
- Neck pain with involvement of the cervical spine (atlanto-axial+/-subluxation) but not normally of the thoracolumbar spine
- Fatigue
- Weight loss
- Carpal tunnel syndrome (and other entrapment neuropathies) secondary to synovial hypertrophy and joint subluxation
- Amyloidosis secondary to chronic inflammation – this involves a build-up of protein in the kidneys, causing renal failure. Look for leg oedema, renal function changes and protein in the urine
- Chest pain (pain worse on deep breath) – from lung disease or pericarditis
- Scleritis or uveitis – dryness, redness and pain in the eye

Examination

- Synovitis
  - Tender joints, boggy swelling

- Rheumatoid changes to the fingers include:
  - Boutonniere deformity of thumb (flexion at proximal interphalangeal joint [PIPJ] and extension at distal interphalangeal joint [DIPJ])
  - Swan neck deformity of fingers (flexion at DIPJ extension at PIPJ)
  - Ulnar deviation of metacarpophalangeal joints (MCPJs)
  - Rheumatoid nodules – firm, non-tender nodules usually found over the dorsal side of the hand
  - Subluxation of MCPJs
- Skin
  - Rheumatoid nodules
  - Peripheral vasculitis
  - Leg ulcers
- Eye
  - Features of uveitis, scleritis – i.e. erythema, corneal ulceration, eye dryness
- Cardiac
  - Pericardial effusion/pericarditis – causing chest pains, pericardial rub
- Peripheral neuropathies
  - Pain, paraesthesia, sensory and/or motor deficits

Test

- Lateral compression (squeezing) of the MCPJ or metatarsophalangeal joint (MTPJ) causes tenderness (Squeeze test)

Investigations

Rheumatoid arthritis is a clinical diagnosis with no single test or investigation making a definitive distinction. Up to a third of people with RA will have normal blood tests

- Blood tests
  - Rheumatoid factor – may be positive, but up to 30% of patients with RA will have a negative result
  - Anti-CCP – may be positive (although up to 30% of patients with RA will have a negative result, it is more specific to RA when found and may be positive where rheumatoid factor is negative)
  - Full blood count – normochromic, normocytic anaemia as chronic inflammation can reduce the production of red cells
  - ESR/CRP – often raised (but not always)
- X-ray
  - May show periarticular erosions and joint space narrowing
  - Also used for disease monitoring
  - Radiographs of hands and feet may be done as part of the initial work up
- Ultrasound
  - May identify synovitis (e.g. at wrist and fingers)

Management

Early diagnosis and treatment are essential, and a referral to rheumatology at the first presentation of symptoms may help achieve better outcomes. Delays contribute to significant morbidity and mortality. Treatment involves a 'treat to target' approach based on assessing disease activity (used validated scores, e.g. DAS 28) and treating with disease modifying drugs to reduce and maintain low disease activity.

DISEASE ACTIVITY SCORE (e.g. DAS 28)

- Is a score based on the number of swollen joints (out of 28 joints), number of tender joints (out of 28 joints), functional status and inflammatory markers
- Determines disease activity and assesses prognosis
- A DAS 28 of greater than 5.1 suggests active disease, less than 3.2 suggests low disease activity, and less than 2.6 is indicative of remission

CONSERVATIVE

- Holistic, multidisciplinary team care including primary care, secondary care, third sector and others
- Education, signposting and onward support
- Exercise to help improve strength, flexibility and specific hand exercises where relevant
- Lifestyle changes
  - Diet
  - Weight management
  - Smoking cessation – important due to high lifetime risk of cardiovascular disease
- Occupational therapy
  - Support with functional activities and hand function
- Long term monitoring
  - Monitoring disease activity and flare-up management
  - Identifying and managing comorbidities (e.g. anxiety, depression, fibromyalgia and supporting access to psychological interventions
  - Be aware of increased risks of infection, cardiovascular disease and skin cancer
  - Screening for long term effects of medication (e.g. retinal screening if on hydroxychloroquine for bulls-eye retinopathy)

MEDICATION

- Steroids (oral) - may be used to rapidly reduce inflammation or to manage acute flares
- Disease modifying drugs (DMARDs) work to suppress the immune/inflammatory response, aiming for remission or low disease activity
  - Conventional DMARDs
    - Such as methotrexate, hydroxychloroquine, sulfasalazine
  - Biologic DMARDs
    - Anti-TNF drugs (e.g. etanercept, infliximab)
    - Others (e.g. rituximab, tocilizumab)
  - Targeted synthetic DMARDs
    - Such as baricitinib, tofacitinib
- NSAIDs (including COX-2 specific) for managing flares

INJECTION

- Corticosteroids
  - Intramuscular or intra-articular
  - May be used for symptom management and bridging therapy (i.e. until more definitive treatment has started or is starting to take effect, which may be 2–3 months)

SURGERY

- Considered if:
    - Persistent pain
    - Synovitis with joint damage
    - Worsening function
    - Progressive deformity
    - Tendon rupture
    - Nerve compression
    - Stress fracture
- May include joint replacement, arthrodesis, osteotomy and tendon surgery

Systemic Lupus Erythematosus (SLE)

Systemic lupus erythematosus (SLE) is a chronic connective tissue disease causing inflammation and tissue damage in multiple organs and systems. Characterised by the production of autoantibodies (e.g. anti-nuclear antibodies) that can cause widespread inflammation and damage. Precise causes are uncertain, but a combination of genetic and environmental factors are likely to be involved.

SLE is one of a cluster of connective tissue diseases (CTDs) that include Sjögren's syndrome, dermatomyositis, polymyositis and systemic sclerosis (scleroderma), which can exist in isolation, in combination (overlap), or that present in a way that is not clearly definable (undifferentiated).

History

- More common in young women and those of non-white ethnicity (Afro-Caribbean, Asians)
- A family history of a CTD is a risk factor
- Multiple environmental triggers have been suggested, including:
  - Medication (e.g. terbinafine, carbamazepine, phenytoin, hormone therapy)
  - Infection (e.g. Epstein Barr Virus and HIV)
  - UV light

Symptoms

- Fatigue
- Rash
  - Malar rash (butterfly-shaped rash on face)
  - Photosensitive rash
  - Discoid rash
  - Non-scarring alopecia (hair loss)
- Joint pain
  - Normally affecting two or more small joints, with hand and wrist joints most commonly affected
  - Rarely affects large joints
- Morning stiffness >30 min
- Neurological features:
  - Seizures, psychosis, mononeuritis, myelitis, neuropathy, confusion
- Respiratory features:
  - Serositis – causing pleural effusions (shortness of breath, pleural rub)

- Cardiac features:
  - Pericardial effusion (chest pains)
- Gastrointestinal features:
  - Oral ulcers, abdominal pain, nausea, weight loss
- Vascular features:
  - Vasculitis, Raynaud's phenomenon, livido reticularis, thrombosis (venous or arterial)
- It can also present in teenage years with growing pains, migraine and glandular fever in the context of a family history that may include thyroid disease, fatigue, ME
- In women there may be recurrent miscarriages

Examination

- Rash
  - May be a butterfly-shaped rash across the cheeks (malar) and bridge of the nose with features of photosensitivity (which can come with itch) or a discoid rash with red, raised patches with thickened or scaly surface
- Synovitis
  - Tenderness, swelling, effusion
- Cardiovascular signs
  - Pleural rub
  - Hypertension
- Lymphadenopathy
  - Cervical or axillary – but may be a sign of infectious disease
- Oral or nasal ulceration

Investigations

- Blood tests
  - Full blood count – may show anaemia (may be haemolytic in SLE), low white cells and platelets
  - ESR – may be raised
  - CRP – often normal
  - U&E – abnormal (nephritis is seen in many SLE patients)
  - Rheumatoid factor – may be positive
  - Antinuclear antibody (ANA) – usually positive (raised titre >1:160 consistent with autoimmune disease)
  - Anti-dsDNA – may be positive (high specificity to SLE)
  - Extractible nuclear antigens (ENA) – anti-Ro, Sm and RNP may be found
  - Creatinine kinase (CK) – raised in polymyositis
  - Complement proteins C3/C4 – may be used to monitor activity
- Urine dipstick test
  - Screening for blood/protein indicative of nephritis and renal failure
- Chest X-ray
  - If there are any cardiopulmonary symptoms, it is used to screen for signs of pleural effusion
- ECG
  - May show signs of pericarditis (ST segment elevation, PR depression)

Management

Early recognition and referral of suspected cases to rheumatology is important. Treatment is aimed at remission or low disease activity to prevent organ damage and improve long term survival.

CONSERVATIVE

- Reduce sun exposure
  - Sunscreen, clothing and avoidance to reduce photosensitive rash
- Manage increased cardiovascular risk
  - Smoking cessation
  - Maintain cardiovascular fitness, screen for hypertension
- Psychological support
  - Specialist cognitive behavioural therapy (CBT), mindfulness-based interventions and peer groups
- Maintain physical activity and encourage regular exercise

MEDICATION

- Non-steroidal anti-inflammatories (NSAIDs)
  - First line for joint pains and stiffness where appropriate and tolerated
- Hydroxychloroquine
  - Used for the majority of people with SLE – modulates the immune system, reducing flares and protecting against organ damage
  - Can cause 'bullseye retinopathy' so regular eye exams are recommended (fundoscopy)
- Corticosteroids
  - Used for flares and occasionally as maintenance
- Other disease modifying anti-rheumatic drugs (DMARDs)
  - Steroid sparing agents (e.g. methotrexate, azathioprine, mycophenolate)
  - Biologics (e.g. belimumab, rituximab)
- Topical agents (often in conjunction with oral agents)
  - Topical corticosteroids for rash
- Antipsychotics and antidepressants
  - Targeted to neuropsychiatric manifestations when present

Sjögren's Syndrome

Sjögren's disease is an autoimmune condition characterised by infiltration of glands that produce tears, saliva, and other fluids. This causes dry eyes and mouth (sicca symptoms) and also affects other organ systems such as the skin, lungs, joints, stomach, nerves, etc.

It can be primary or secondary, where the sicca symptoms co-exist with systemic lupus erythematosus or another systemic autoimmune condition such as rheumatoid arthritis, primary biliary cirrhosis or systemic sclerosis.

History

- Precise causes are uncertain
- Younger women are affected far more than men

Symptoms

- Sicca symptoms
  - Dry, itchy, or gritty eyes (keratoconjunctivitis)
  - Dry and/or burning mouth, which may affect eating (xerostomia)
- Synovitis
- Fatigue
- Rash
  - Vasculitic rash described as 'palpable purpura' (purplish–red spots)
- Myositis
- Lung disease
  - Due to reduced chest secretions causing chronic bronchitis and interstitial lung disease
- Renal disease
  - Nephritis
- Peripheral neuropathies
  - Usually sensory or autonomic

Examination

- Dry eyes, dry mouth and other mucous membranes (e.g. atrophic vaginitis)
- Corneal ulceration
- Parotid or other salivary gland enlargement – found in the majority of primary Sjögren's but less common in secondary Sjögren's disease
- Vasculitic skin rash – may find red-purple lesions or small bruises, though many patients only ever have a single episode of rash
- Dental caries, missing teeth
- Signs of bronchitis or active chest infection (e.g. chest crepitations, reduced air entry)
- Peripheral neuropathy
- Palpable lymph nodes (lymphadenopathy)
- Enlarged spleen (splenomegaly)

Investigation

- Blood tests
  - Full blood count – low white blood cells
  - ESR – may be raised significantly in Sjögren's
  - CRP – often normal in Sjögren's
  - U&E – acidosis with hypokalaemia may be found
  - Rheumatoid factor – often positive
  - Anti-nuclear antibodies – often positive
  - Extractable nuclear antigens – anti-SSa and anti-Ro may be found
- Schirmer test
  - Uses special paper strips to identify a lack of tear production in the eye
- Biopsy
  - Of lacrimal and salivary glands showing T and B cell (lymphocytes) and dendritic cell infiltration
  - Of the rash
- Urinalysis
  - May show haematuria/proteinuria

Management

Is usually under the care of rheumatologist and based on treating symptoms and complications (e.g. infections, corneal ulceration and chest infections)

CONSERVATIVE

- Treat sicca symptoms
  - Artificial tears and saliva
  - Eye lubricants
  - Pilocarpine – cholinergic drug that stimulates tear secretion
  - Avoid drugs that make symptoms worse (e.g. anti-cholinergics, antihistamines and diuretics)
- Fatigue management
- Pacing and graded approaches to activity
- Smoking cessation advice where relevant

MEDICATION

- Simple analgesia (e.g. weak opiates with or without paracetamol for joint pains)
- DMARDs (e.g. hydroxychloroquine may be used to reduce organ damage and manage joint pain)
- Corticosteroids – taken orally may be used for flares of joint pain and vasculitic skin rashes
- Immunoglobulin therapy (intravenous) - may be used for vasculitis and peripheral neuropathy (which may also help peripheral neuropathy) for rashes
- Potassium replacement for renal tubular acidosis causing hypokalaemia

Spondyloarthropathy

Spondyloarthropathies are a group of inflammatory arthropathies, including ankylosing spondylitis, psoriatic arthritis, reactive arthritis and enteropathic arthritis.

They share the following characteristics:

- Sero-negativity: spondyloarthropathies tend to be negative to rheumatoid factor, autoantibodies and anti-CCP, which is their main distinguishing characteristic to rheumatoid arthritis
- Association with human leukocyte antigen B27 (HLA-B27)
- Asymmetrical large joint arthritis - often lower limb oligoarthritis (usually <5 joints)
- Axial involvement – including sacroiliac joint (SIJ) involvement
- Enthesitis – plantar fasciitis, Achilles tendinitis (with bursitis)
- Dactylitis – inflammation of a digit (either a finger or toe)
- Extra-articular features such as:
  - Anterior uveitis (iritis) – seen in up to 40% of AS patients
  - Oral ulcers
  - Aortic valve incompetence
  - Inflammatory bowel disease

Axial Spondyloarthritis

Axial spondyloarthritis (AS) is a type of inflammatory arthritis affecting the joints and entheses (the junction where tendons, ligaments, or joint capsule attach to the bone) of the spine. It can be classified as either:

- **Non-radiographic** – the earlier stages of AS where there are symptoms, but there are no bony changes on X-ray visible. Inflammation may be visible on MRI, or symptoms are present
- **Radiographic** – where, in the later stages of the condition, there are visible changes on X-rays of the spine and sacroiliac joints (also described as ankylosing spondylitis)

History

- AS is often misdiagnosed as mechanical back pain and should be considered in anyone whose back pain started before 45 years of age and has continued for more than three months
- Typical onset is in the late teens to the early 20s
- Affects men more than it affects women
- Risk factors include:
  - Family history of AS (first degree relative)
  - Past or current history of psoriasis, uveitis, iritis or enthesitis
  - HLA-B27 gene present

Symptoms

- Back pain
- Buttock pain that may alternate from one side to the other
- Morning stiffness >30 min
- Pain eased with movement and not relieved with rest
- Improvement of pain with NSAIDs (within 48 hours of taking)
- Pain may wake patient in the early hours
- Symptoms develop gradually with progressive loss of spinal movement
- Fatigue
- Enthesitis (e.g. patella tendon insertion, plantar fasciitis, insertional achilles tendinitis)
- Uveitis/iritis – red, painful eye, sensitive to light with blurred or altered vision (of note acute uveitis requires assessment under ophthalmology)
- Inflammatory bowel disease – Crohn's disease or ulcerative colitis
- Although predominantly a spinal condition, asymmetrical large joint arthritis may sometimes be seen – more often in the lower limb

Examination

- Examination may be relatively normal in early stages but, as the condition progresses, the following may be seen:
  - Sacro-iliac joint tenderness
  - Iritis/uveitis – red eye, reduced visual acuity, photophobia
  - Costochondritis
  - Reduced lumbar range of movement
  - Kyphosis and loss of lumbar lordosis
  - Reduced chest expansion (<5 cm)
  - Peripheral joint arthritis (e.g. hips)

Psoriatic Arthritis

Psoriatic arthritis (PsA) is type of inflammatory arthritis seen in 10-40% of patients with psoriasis (an inflammatory skin condition characterised by scaly plaques on the skin). It overlaps with other types of spondyloarthropathy.

Before the development of skin features, a pattern of presentation can be seen that includes:
- Asymmetrical and oligoarticular arthritis
- Swollen and painful distal interphalangeal joints (characteristic of PsA but not that common)
- Dactylitis
- Low back pain and sacroiliitis (in 20% of patients)
- Conjunctivitis and anterior uveitis (but less often than in AS)

Reactive Arthritis

Reactive arthritis (ReA) is an aseptic arthritis that develops after an infection elsewhere in the body, usually the gastrointestinal or genitourinary tract.
- Post–gastrointestinal infection (e.g. Campylobacter, Salmonella, Yersinia)
- Post–sexually transmitted disease (e.g. chlamydia)
- Viral–(e.g. Arbovirus)

Symptoms normally develop one to three weeks after infection and, in epidemics of Salmonella and Yersinia, reactive arthritis is found in up to 7% of individuals (this rises to 20% in HLA-B27 positive people)
The pattern of symptoms usually consists of:
- Asymmetrical oligoarthritis (up to four joints in six months)
- Enthesitis
- Dactylitis
- Extra articular features may include:
  - Conjunctivitis (normally bilateral and painful)
  - Anterior uveitis (unilateral and often with conjunctivitis so it can be hard to differentiate)
  - Urethritis (dysuria and urethral discharge)
  - Skin changes that include circinate balanitis and keratoderma blennorrhagicum (painless papular eruption on the palms of the hands or soles of the feet)
- 60–90% of affected patients are positive for HLA-B27 antigen. The main differential diagnosis is septic arthritis, so a joint aspirate and culture are recommended where possible
- Most cases last two to three months with the presence of HLA-B27, increasing the chances of axial involvement and chronicity

Enteropathic Arthritis

Enteropathic arthritis (EnA) is an inflammatory arthritis associated with inflammatory bowel disease (IBD); usually ulcerative colitis or Crohn's disease
It tends to follow two distinct patterns:
- Type 1
  - 5% of patients with IBD
  - Peripheral arthritis – oligoarticular, mainly in the knees
  - Is normally self-limiting and does not lead to joint deformity
  - Joint symptoms can start before bowel symptoms
  - Enthesitis (e.g. Achilles), plantar fasciitis and dactylitis can occur
- Type 2
  - 3% of patients with IBD
  - Polyarticular arthritis can include:
    - Metacarpophalangeal joints, knees, ankles, elbows, shoulders, wrists, proximal inter-phalangeal joints and metatarsophalangeal joints
    - It can also move from joint to joint
  - Sacroiliitis and spondylitis is seen in around 20% of patients with IBD

Investigations

- X-ray
  - May be normal and not usually recommended to investigate AS
  - Changes on X-ray may include:
    - Erosions
    - Sclerosis and squaring of the vertebrae
    - Syndesmophytes (bony growths in spinal ligaments)
    - Facet joint fusion (where the spine appears as a continuous column. Also called a 'Bamboo spine')

- MRI
  - May be indicated for people with suspected AS
  - Changes may include:
    - Radiographic sacroiliitis
    - Squaring of vertebrae and 'shiny' corners of vertebrae
- Blood tests
  - HLA-B27
  - Positive in around 90% of case (but present in 10% of the normal population)
  - ESR/CRP
    - May be raised (prognosis worse if ESR >30)

Management

AS is usually managed under the care of rheumatologists with medication and rehabilitation aimed at reducing pain and improving or maintaining spinal movements, posture, function and mobility.

CONSERVATIVE

- Structured exercise programme
  - Reduce the impact of the disease
  - Reduce pain and fatigue
  - Improve or maintain mobility
  - Improve function and quality of life
  - Enable self-management
  - Education and signposting of peer support and self-help
  - Lifestyle changes (e.g. dietary advice, smoking cessation)

MEDICATION

- NSAIDs where safe and tolerated
  - NSAIDs are usually avoided in enteropathic arthritis due to their potential for exacerbating inflammatory bowel symptoms
- Paracetamol with or without a low dose of codeine as an adjunct
- Oral, intra-articular, or intramuscular corticosteroids may be considered to reduce inflammation and pain (e.g. in sacroilitis)
- Sulphasalazine/methotrexate if peripheral joint involvement
- Biologics
  - TNFα blockers (e.g. etanercept, adalimumab)
  - Interleukin (IL 27/23) inhibitors (e.g. secukinumab, ixekizumab)

Polymyalgia Rheumatica and Giant Cell Arteritis

Both polymyalgia rheumatica (PMR) and giant cell arteritis (GCA) are forms of inflammatory disease. PMR causes proximal muscle pain, and GCA is a form of vasculitis causing inflammation of the vessels supplying the head and neck.

They have overlapping features and tend to affect the same population, so it is worth considering both pathologies together as patients with PMR can develop symptoms of GCA and vice versa.

History

- Usually affects an older population with peak onset between 70–80 years old
- Rarely seen in people under the age of 50
- Women are affected more than men by a ratio of 2:1
- Higher rates in northern European population
- The underlying causes are uncertain but are likely to be multifactorial, with a combination of genetic and environmental triggers involved including:
  - Infection
    - Mycoplasma, Chlamydia, Parvovirus, Herpes and others
  - Genetics
    - Familial patterns and racial differences in prevalence seen with links to HLA-DR4
  - Immune
    - Increased levels of circulating cytokines have been seen

Symptoms

PMR	GCA
Rapid (sub-acute) onset over days to weeks.	New onset headache (normally around side of head), but this is absent in 25% of cases.
Age >50, normally >65.	Age >50.
• Pain and stiffness affecting proximal muscles of shoulder and pelvic girdle	• Scalp tenderness (brushing hair, putting on glasses)
• Worse at night and first thing in the morning	• Jaw claudication (pain in jaw on chewing)
• Difficulty raising arms above head (reaching high shelves, getting out of a chair, walking up stairs)	
Fatigue	Fatigue

Continued on following page

PMR	GCA
Low grade fever.	Visual disturbances – may be unilateral or bilateral (amaurosis fugax, diplopia, blurred vision, visual field loss and sudden onset blindness most serious potential consequence).[1]
Weight loss.	Palpable 'nodular' change in late stage in temporal artery region and visibly dilated temporal artery with a bounding pulse.
Depressed mood	Different blood pressure reading between both arms – GCA affecting aorta and its branches with aneurysms and stenosis as late-stage feature.
Polyarthritis and synovitis can be present	

[1]Singh, A. G., Kermani, T. A., Crowson, C. S., Weyand, C. M., Matteson, E. L., Warrington, K. J. (2015). Visual manifestations in giant cell arteritis: trend over 5 decades in a population-based cohort. *The Journal of Rheumatology, 42*(2), 309-315.

- Weakness is not normally seen and should raise suspicion of myositis
- Tenderness of muscles can be seen but may be suggestive of fibromyalgia

Investigations

- Blood tests
  - Full blood count
    - Normochromic, normocytic anaemia can be seen
    - Raised platelets may be seen in GCA
  - ESR
    - Raised in over 95% patients
    - Generally >40 in PMR and >50 in GCA and has better sensitivity and specificity than CRP
  - CRP
    - Raised in over 95% patients
  - LFT
    - ALP may be raised
- Temporal artery biopsy for GCA
  - Can be negative due to 'skip' lesions (patchy distribution of change in artery wall)
  - Useful if done just before treatment is started or within 24 hours. Chance of seeing a positive result drops a week after starting steroids but can remain positive for up to a year
- Ultrasound
  - Can now often be used as a pre-biopsy screen in GCA looking for oedema around the vessel

Management of PMR

- PMR is usually managed in primary care, but referral to outpatient rheumatologist for review is advised if:
  - Age <60
  - Diagnostic uncertainty
  - Suspicion of other rheumatological diagnosis
  - Normal or very high acute phase proteins (ESR/CRP)

MEDICATION

- Steroids (e.g. prednisolone)
  - A trial of prednisolone should produce a marked reduction in symptoms and is a useful diagnostic
- Bisphosphonates, calcium and vitamin D may be used to manage fracture risk if on longer term steroids
- Aspirin has been used to reduce risk of strokes but has an increased risk of gastric bleeds
- Monitoring
  - Patient should be issued a steroid user card
  - Response to treatment with ESR/CRP
    - CRP is helpful in discerning between age related changes when tapering as less likely to be raised with age
  - For signs they are developing GCA
  - For diabetes, obesity, or hypertension secondary to steroids, treatment is advised
  - Chest X-rays every two years (for life) to screen for thoracic aortic aneurysms

Management of GCA

- Patients with symptoms of GCA and visual disturbance need a same day specialist assessment and treatment to avoid permanent loss of vision. This usually involves high dose steroids under the care of ophthalmology but depends on local pathways
- Early intervention with high dose oral steroids and referral to rheumatology in cases without visual disturbance is standard

4.6

Fibromyalgia

Fibromyalgia syndrome (FMS) is a condition characterised by persistent, widespread pain and sensory amplification. As a primary pain processing disorder, it is characterised by symptoms including hyperalgesia (an increased or disproportionate response to a painful stimulus), allodynia (a pain response to a non-painful stimulus) and expansion of the receptive field.

It can occur in isolation as a chronic primary pain disorder or as a secondary phenomenon associated with other conditions (e.g. rheumatoid arthritis, osteoarthritis and chronic back pain).

History

- Although the exact cause of fibromyalgia is unknown, it has been linked to inflammatory, immune, endocrine, genetic and psychosocial factors including:
  - Depression and/or a history of adverse childhood events
  - Central and peripheral nervous system sensitisation - with abnormal function and connectivity between areas of the brain (seen on fMRI studies) and inflammation increasing synaptic transmission in peripheral nerves
  - Genetics - you are more likely to have FMS if someone else in your family has it
- Factors that may be associated with a poor prognosis include abnormal health beliefs, social withdrawal/isolation, work related problems such as bullying, dissatisfaction at work and ongoing compensation claims, low levels of patient activation (i.e. low participation in treatment) and an overprotective family or spouse

Symptoms

- Reported symptoms may fluctuate and evolve over time. Symptoms vary between individuals but may include:
  - Back pain
  - Temporomandibular joint pain
  - Headache
  - Musculoskeletal chest pain
  - Myalgia
  - Arthralgia
  - Fatigue
  - Depression
  - Anxiety
  - Dizziness
  - Cognitive dysfunction – poor memory and/or concentration
  - Urinary dysfunction
  - Stiffness
  - Sleep dysfunction
  - Irritable bowel syndrome
  - Dyspepsia (indigestion)

Investigations

There are currently no definitive diagnostic tests for fibromyalgia. Instead, diagnostic tests are used to rule out other conditions that may be causing the patient's symptoms.

- Blood tests
  - No blood tests diagnose fibromyalgia, but they may be used to help exclude other pathologies (e.g. full blood count to exclude anaemia, ESR to identify possible inflammatory disease), thyroid function tests to exclude hypothyroidism, bone profile to identify hypercalcaemia and bone metabolic disorders (e.g. Paget's disease), Hba1c/fasting glucose to exclude diabetes
  - Further testing (e.g. ANA, rheumatoid factor, anti-CCP, vitamin D) may be justified if there are symptoms or signs that suggest they are relevant

The American College of Rheumatology Criteria 2016 provide an objective scale to assess symptoms to enable a diagnosis of fibromyalgia (see below).

Pain Location			Symptoms	
Region	Left	Right	Symptom	Score
Neck			Fatigue*	0 1 2 3
Jaw			Waking unrefreshed*	0 1 2 3
Shoulder			Cognitive symptoms*	0 1 2 3
Upper arm			Headache	Yes = 1 No = 0
Lower arm			Abdominal pain	Yes = 1 No = 0
Chest			Depression	Yes = 1 No = 0
Upper back			*Score guide 0=No problem 1=Mild problem (may be intermittent) 2=Moderate problem often present 3=Severe, pervasive, life disturbing	
Lower back			**Total symptom severity score (SSS) (0-12)**	/12
Hip			**Combined scoring and interpretation**	
Abdomen			WPI	
Upper leg			SSS	
Lower leg			Total	
Total widespread pain index (WPI) score	/19		**Scores suggesting diagnosis of fibromyalgia** **WPI ≥7 + SSS ≥5** **OR** **WPI ≥3 + SSS ≥9**	

Management

FMS cannot be cured, but supportive management focusses on improving quality of life and functional outcomes.

CONSERVATIVE

- Information and education for patients, relatives and clinicians to manage misconceptions and better understand the diagnosis and prognosis
- Exercise programmes and physical activity
  - Supervised exercise programmes
  - Combined exercise and relaxation programmes including T'ai chi, yoga, and water-based therapies
- Psychological therapies including acceptance and commitment therapy (ACT) or cognitive behavioural therapy (CBT)
- Sleep – supported self-management including sleep hygiene
- Combinations of the above are often used in multidisciplinary, multimodal rehabilitation programmes (Pain Management Programme) that are central to most chronic pain services

MEDICATION

- Options are limited, and care should be taken to avoid creating dependence and causing harm
- SSRIs (e.g. citalopram/fluoxetine/duloxetine) or TCAs (e.g. amitriptyline)
- Gabapentin or pregabalin are sometimes used

Hypermobile Ehlers–Danlos Syndrome (hEDS)

Hypermobile EDS is a heritable connective tissue disorder caused by abnormalities in collagen production and structure. As a result, the tensile strength of the connective tissue is impaired, causing characteristic signs of joint hypermobility. Whilst many cases of joint hypermobility are benign, it can be associated with significant disability and distress.

The diagnostic criteria for hEDS (and all other types of EDS) were revised by the International EDS Consortium in 2017, and there is broad recognition of the spectrum existing from benign joint hypermobility to hEDS. Although most types of EDS are considered rare conditions, hEDS is much more common and accounts for the majority of EDS diagnosed.

History

- Family history of hEDS
- More common in women
- Associated with other conditions including:
    - Postural orthostatic tachycardia
    - Irritable bowel syndrome
    - Autonomic dysfunction
    - Anxiety
    - Depression
    - Chronic fatigue
    - Sleep disorders

Symptoms

- Generalised joint hypermobility
    - Beighton score:
        - 6 for children and adolescents
        - 5 for men and women up to the age of 50
        - 4 for those >50 years of age
    - Positive family history (one or more first degree relative with confirmed hEDS)
    - Extra-articular features may include:
        - Mild skin hyperextensibility – defined as stretching over 1.5 cm at distal forearms and the dorsum of the hands; 3 cm at neck, elbow and knees; and 1 cm on the palm of the hand
        - Smooth, velvety skin that bruises easily
        - Atrophic (wide or flat) scars in at least two sites
        - Unexplained stretch marks (striae)
        - Soft, skin-coloured papules found on the heels (Piezogenic papules)
        - Recurrent abdominal hernias
        - Prolapse of the pelvic floor, rectum or uterus

- Dental crowding and high/narrow palate
- Arachnodactyly
- Arm span to height ≥1.05
- Mitral valve prolapse
- Aortic root dilatation
- Musculoskeletal features may include:
  - Pain for more than three months affecting two or more limbs
  - Chronic widespread pain for more than three months
  - Atraumatic recurrent dislocations or instability of joints

Investigations

- hEDS is primarily a clinical diagnosis based on history, examination and further investigations if there is clinical uncertainty or other pathologies are suspected
- Diagnosis is based on excluding other types of EDS (features of unusual skin fragility would raise suspicion), autoimmune disease, connective tissue disorders, rare hereditary or neuromuscular disorders with hypermobility as an additional feature
- Genetic testing is only undertaken for the rarer types of EDS

Management

Treatment needs to be tailored to the individual, focussing on managing acute manifestations, preventing deterioration, and will likely involve multidisciplinary team input, including pain management.

CONSERVATIVE

- Suspected hEDS may suit a referral to Rheumatology, where the diagnosis is normally clinical based on signs and symptoms
- Education and behavioural modification with a focus on maintaining normal activities and active lifestyle
- Treatment of any acute injuries or soft tissue lesions
- Supports or splints have a role, especially in acute phase of injury
- Balance, coordination, and proprioception exercises reduce risk of falls and injuries
- Low resistance exercise to improve core and peripheral muscle quality and improve joint stability and maximise bone strength
- Mobility aids, including wheelchairs, may help offload lower limb
- Surveillance, including bone density scans, may be indicated

MEDICATION

- Simple analgesia (NSAIDs, paracetamol, weak opioids) may have a role as short term adjuncts but, as with other chronic pain conditions, the evidence suggests that medication provides limited benefits in the longer term

Gout

Gout is the most common type of inflammatory arthritis. It is caused by an excessive build-up of uric acid in the blood leading to its precipitation out of the solution and forming urate crystals in the joints and soft tissues. These then trigger an immune inflammatory response.

Uric acid is a breakdown product of purines and levels in the blood increase due to an under-secretion via the kidneys or increased intake of purines in the diet. Other sources of raised purines/urate include breakdown of red cells due to blood cancers or chemotherapy and genetically inherited over-production of urate. Gout can be a primary abnormality (a heritable condition caused by an overproduction/under-secretion of uric acid) or secondary to disorders like leukaemia (causing red cell breakdown releasing uric acid into the blood), medication, excessive dietary intake of purines or problems excreting urate via the kidneys.

History

- Men are affected more than women
- Age usually between 35–50 years
- Risk factors include:
  - High purine diet – especially meat and shellfish
  - Alcohol – especially beer (contains high amounts of purines)
  - Sugary drinks containing fructose
  - Renal insufficiency – most urate is excreted through the kidneys
  - Family history – genetic inheritance
  - Medication – diuretics, chemotherapy agents, salicylates
  - Obesity
  - Pregnancy
  - Hypothyroidism
  - Malignancies – especially leukaemia/lymphoma, which causes high cell turnover

Symptoms

- Acute onset of joint pain that may be 'excruciating'
- Most commonly affecting great toe or knee (also ankle, wrist, elbows, fingers)
- Pain usually starts overnight or in the early morning
- Pain builds to crescendo after six to twenty four hours and can last up to two weeks
- Joint appears red, swollen and exquisitely tender
- Possible difficulty in weight bearing and mobilization on affected foot or limb
- There may be a history of acute episodes with full recovery (remission) of weeks or months before symptoms return
- Repeated episodes of gout can damage the joint causing a secondary osteoarthritis

Examination

- The affected joint is usually swollen, erythematous and warm to touch
- Joint effusion may be found (e.g. in the knee)
- Joint tenderness on palpation - may be severe in acute cases
- Mild fever
- Altered gait and difficulty walking
- Hardened deposits of uric acid called tophi may be found in the tissues on the elbows, Achilles tendon or ears with chronic gout. These can rupture and cause infections

Investigations

- Diagnosis is generally clinical, but joint aspiration or blood tests can be helpful to confirm the diagnosis
- **Blood tests**
  - Urate – may be raised but usually low or normal in an acute attack. It is best measured one to two weeks after an acute attack has settled
  - ESR/CRP – may be raised
  - Liver function tests – may be abnormal if prolonged, heavy user of alcohol
  - U&Es – may identify renal disease leading to an accumulation of urate
  - Full blood count – may identify diseases causing breakdown of blood cells; white cell count may be slightly raised in gout
- Joint aspirate and microscopy
  - Urate crystals described as 'negatively birefringent' when examined by microscopy under polarised light
  - Of note is that pseudogout (calcium pyrophosphate crystal deposition) has positive birefringent crystals seen on microscopy
- X-ray
  - Findings may include soft tissue opacities, bone erosions and osteophytes at the edge of erosions
- Ultrasound
  - Not usually used but may show evidence of erosions, tophi and the 'double contour' sign, which is a sonographic sign specific for gout

Management

Aims to treat acute episodes and prevent further episodes by reducing levels of uric acid in the blood and prevent poly-articular gout and joint damage. Specialist (rheumatology) advice may be required in cases of diagnostic uncertainty, resistance to treatment, significant kidney disease or organ transplants.

CONSERVATIVE

- PRICE (Protection, Relative rest, Icing, Compression, Elevation) in acute flares
- Dietary advice and education
  - Reduce purine-rich foods (meat/seafood)
  - Limit sugary drinks
  - Reduce alcohol (beer especially)

MEDICATION

- Treating an acute attack
    - Non-steroidal anti-inflammatory drugs, where safe and tolerated
    - Colchicine
    - Oral steroids
    - Urate lowering therapy
        - Allopurinol
        - Febuxostat

INJECTION

- Intramuscular or intra-articular corticosteroid injection may be considered to reduce inflammation and pain where oral therapy is ineffective or contra-indicated

SURGERY

- Joint replacements may be considered when there is severe joint destruction with functional loss and uncontrolled pain

Pseudogout

Pseudogout is an inflammatory arthritis caused by the deposition of calcium pyrophosphate dihydrate crystals (CPPD) in the joints. It most commonly affects large joints like the knees, causing an acutely painful synovitis that is often mistaken for gout. It can present in a number of patterns:

- Asymptomatic
  - Crystals are deposited into the cartilage (called chondrocalcinosis) and can be seen on X-ray in the absence of any symptoms. This may be a precursor to active symptomatic disease
- Acute inflammatory pattern of joint pain (commonly knee or wrist)
  - Occurs when crystals form in the joint space, causing a response similar to that of gout
- Chronic form
  - Marked joint destruction and polyarthritis that mimics other forms of arthritis (e.g. rheumatoid arthritis)

History

- Risk factors identified include:
  - Family history of pseudogout
  - Increasing age
  - Long term steroid use
  - Dialysis
- Associations with a range of other medical conditions including:
  - Diabetes
  - Gout
  - Osteoarthritis
  - Hyperparathyroidism
  - Haemochromatosis
  - Hypomagnesaemia
  - Acromegaly
- The relevance of genetic links and lifestyle choices is uncertain

Symptoms

- Painful, tender joint(s)
- Acute on chronic pattern of pain
- Acute calcific tendinitis, most commonly affecting the shoulder region in younger adults, has been described as another variant of pseudogout

Examination

- Hot, erythematous joint(s)
- Focal tenderness

- Joint effusion
- Low grade fever and malaise in older patients
- Severe destruction of joints that can mimic a Charcot joint
- Tendinitis

Investigations

- Joint aspiration
  - Identifying *positively* birefringent rhomboid shaped crystals when the aspirate is examined under polarised light can be very helpful to differentiate from the *negatively* birefringent crystals seen in gout
  - Will also help exclude septic arthritis
  - Can be therapeutic as well as diagnostic, especially when teamed with corticosteroid injection (which tends to be first line treatment of acute attack)
- Blood tests
  - Are not used to diagnose CPPD but help to exclude other diagnoses and may include FBC, ESR, CRP, calcium, parathyroid hormone, magnesium, iron studies
- X-rays
  - May show calcification of cartilage or tendons, which is relevant only in the presence of symptoms
  - There may be rapid joint degeneration with characteristic hook shaped osteophytes and bony collapse
- Ultrasound
  - May help identify smaller calcium deposits in cartilage that X-rays may miss
  - May be useful to consider if there is high clinical suspicion but normal X-rays
- CT scans
  - Rarely used, may also pick up smaller calcium deposits

Management

- The focus is on managing acute flares as there is little evidence that any approach reduces the crystal load and prevents attacks
- Symptomatic measures include rest, ice and elevation of the affected limb

MEDICATION

- Non-steroidal anti-inflammatories (NSAIDs) where safe and tolerated
- Oral corticosteroids to reduce pain and inflammation (e.g. prednisolone)
- Colchicine

INJECTION

- Intra-articular corticosteroid injection may be considered to reduce inflammation and pain if symptoms are not resolving with conservative measures or in acute attacks

SURGERY

- Joint replacements may be considered when there is severe joint destruction with functional loss and uncontrolled pain

4.10

Osteoporosis

Osteoporosis (OP) is a progressive condition characterised by the loss of bone mass along with defects in the bony architecture, making it more brittle and increasing the risk of fracture. It is usually associated with age-related loss of bone density and the loss of oestrogen after menopause, but it can also be secondary to a range of medical conditions including malignancy, metabolic bone disease or the effects of medication (e.g. steroids, SSRIs, anticonvulsants, proton-pump inhibitors).

History

- Prevalence increases with age as bone mass starts decreasing after the 20s
- Affects women considerably more than men
- Factors involved in causing secondary osteoporosis can be remembered by the mnemonic **SHATTERED**
  - **S**teroid use
    - More than 5 mg daily for longer than three months (450 mg of steroid in total)
  - **H**yperthyroidism
    - Causes an acceleration of bone turnover and loss of mineral density
  - **A**lcohol use
    - Slows down bone turnover as it has an effect on osteoblasts (cells that synthesise bone)
  - **T**hin (BMI<18.5)
    - Mixed hormonal changes (loss of oestrogen) and reduced load bearing
  - **T**estosterone
    - There is an increased risk of OP in men when reduced (e.g. with anti-androgen therapy in prostate cancer)
  - **E**arly menopause
    - Due to loss of oestrogen
  - **R**enal or liver failure
    - Disordered vitamin D, calcium, phosphate metabolism
  - **E**rosive or inflammatory bone disease
    - Including myeloma, rheumatoid arthritis
  - **D**ietary calcium
    - Reduced due to malabsorption or poor intake

Symptoms

- Osteoporosis is asymptomatic with symptoms relating to the fragility fractures it causes
- Vertebral fractures are the most common fragility fracture but are often asymptomatic or undiagnosed with a significant risk of further fracture if left untreated
  Symptoms of vertebral fractures include:
  - Back pain and tenderness
  - Restricted range of spinal movement

- Loss of height
- Change in the contour of the spine (e.g. kyphosis)
- Hip fractures are the second most common fragility fracture
- Other fractures often relate to low energy falls (e.g. distal radial fracture)
- New onset of bone pain in an individual at risk should be considered as a possible fracture, even in a low energy injury (e.g. stepping off a pavement)

Examination

May identify the consequences of osteoporosis (i.e. fractures or risk factors for falls)
- May identify associated features that increase the risk of, or explain a fall, such as:
  - Frailty
  - Poor vision
  - Gait changes
  - Lower limb weakness
  - Balance difficulties
- Signs of vertebral fracture
  - Loss of height
  - Increasing kyphosis and progressive rounding of shoulders (dowagers hump)
  - Focal spinal pain and tenderness on palpation of spinous process
  - A step deformity may be apparent
  - Features of acute fracture:
    - Pain
    - Focal tenderness
    - Bruising and/or swelling
    - Deformity

Investigations

- Blood tests (investigating for secondary causes of osteoporosis)
  - Full blood count – anaemia (myeloma)
  - ESR – inflammatory pathologies, malignancy
  - Bone profile – hypercalcaemia in malignancy, metabolic bone disease
  - U&E – renal failure
  - Liver function tests – liver disease
  - Prostate specific antigen (PSA) – prostate cancer
  - Thyroid function tests – hyperthyroidism
  - Serum protein electrophoresis – monoclonal (paraprotein) band in myeloma
  - Serum free light chain assay – abnormal ratio (myeloma)
- Q-Risk/FRAX score
  - Designed to help evaluate the risk of fracture in patients
- DEXA scan (dual energy X-ray absorptiometry)
  - T score at or below -2.5 SD is diagnostic of osteoporosis

Management

This focusses on prevention to reduce bone loss and reduce the risk of falls and treatment to reduce the risk of fragility fractures.

CONSERVATIVE

- Information, education and support around the diagnosis, risks and prevention
- Smoking cessation, where relevant
- Alcohol reduction, where relevant
- Weight bearing, resistance and balance exercises
- Balance exercises and falls prevention strategies
- Advising a diet rich in calcium and vitamin D

MEDICATION

- Calcium and vitamin D supplements
  - May be used if calcium and/or vitamin D deficient
- Bisphosphonates (e.g. alendronate, risedronate)
  - Work by decreasing osteoclast activity
  - However, prolonged bisphosphonate therapy is associated with abnormal calcium deposition that may cause atypical (sub-trochanteric) hip fractures
- Strontium ranelate
  - Decreases osteoclast activity and increases osteoblast activity
  - May be used when bisphosphonates not tolerated
- Teriparatide
  - Increases osteoblastic activity significantly and reduces the relative fracture risk of vertebral and non-vertebral fractures
- Hormone replacement therapy
  - May be used to reduce risk of osteoporosis, especially in women with early menopause
  - Reduces fracture risk and treats menopausal symptoms
- Denosumab
  - Reduces bone resorption
  - Given as an injection (subcutaneously) every six months

Osteomalacia

Osteomalacia is characterised by bone becoming weaker and more likely to fracture. If present in childhood (where it is called rickets), it can lead to marked deformities. It is usually the result of a lack of one or more factors required for creating healthy bone, such as phosphates or, more commonly, vitamin D.

History

- Vitamin D deficiency is most commonly seen in:
  - Dietary deficiency
  - Darker skin – melanin absorbs more UV light, meaning less is available for vitamin D synthesis
  - Lack of exposure to sunlight (e.g. housebound, institutionalised or using full body covering)
  - Malabsorption (e.g. coeliac disease)
  - Pregnancy or prolonged breastfeeding – increased requirements to fuel foetal growth and production of breast milk
  - Liver disease – failure of liver to help metabolise vitamin D to its usable form as well as links to malabsorption of vitamin D
  - Renal osteodystrophy – chronic kidney disease leading to a problem with vitamin D metabolism
- Drug induced
  - Anticonvulsants – these induce liver enzymes and break down the precursor to vitamin D

Symptoms

- May be asymptomatic in the early stages
- Bone pain usually in lower limbs, spine or pelvis
- Leg weakness
- Fragility fractures

Examination

- Proximal muscle wasting – waddling gait
- Symptoms relating to contributory conditions:
  - Malabsorption syndromes (e.g. low weight, diarrhoea, abdominal pains)
  - Features of liver cirrhosis
- Note that there may be little to see on examination

Investigations

- Blood tests
  - Vitamin D – likely to be low
  - Bone profile – low calcium and phosphate
  - Liver function tests – increased alkaline phosphatase
- X-rays
  - May show transverse lucencies with sclerotic borders going part way through bone (Looser's zones)
  - Fractures of vertebrae, ribs, pubic rami and femoral neck
  - Bowing of long bones
- Bone biopsy
  - Evidence of decreased bone turnover and increased, unmineralized bone matrix (osteoid)

Management

- Replacement of any deficiency (e.g. vitamin D and the correction of any underlying cause)

Paget's Disease

Paget's disease, also called osteitis deformans, is driven by increased turnover and remodelling of bone. This affects the integrity of the bone as newer bone tends to be thicker but more brittle and irregular than normal bone. This is often asymptomatic but can lead to pain from micro-fractures and nerve compression as well as bone deformities and hearing loss.

History

- It is more common with age (above the age of 50)
- It can be mistaken for osteoarthritis
- A family history of Paget's disease increases the risk of developing the condition
- Infections (e.g. measles) have been identified as a risk factor

Symptoms

- Asymptomatic in the majority of cases
- May be an incidental finding on a blood screening (finding a raised alkaline phosphatase [ALP] on blood tests) or on seeing characteristic X-ray findings
- Bone pain – may affect hips, pelvis, lumbar spine, skull, femur and tibia
- Change in shape of limbs and posture due to bone deformities
- Pain worse on weight bearing (long bone involvement) and at night
- Fractures
- Radicular pain – nerve compression from bone overgrowth
- Hearing loss – due to bone density changes in the hearing apparatus of the skull (cochlear)
- Cardiac failure (rare) – increased vascularity of bone causing ventricular hypertrophy

Examination

- Bony deformity
  - Bowed 'sabre' tibia and femur
  - Bone enlargement
  - Pathological fractures
  - Kyphosis
  - Skull thickening (frontal bossing and thickening of dome of skull)
  - Appearance of a short neck – shortening of skull base
- Localised increase in temperature due to increased metabolic activity and vascularity

Investigations

- Blood tests
  - Bone profile – may show raised ALP with normal calcium and phosphate

- X-rays
  - Findings may include localised bone enlargement, cortical thickening and deformity
- Bone scan
  - Shows extent and location of lesions

Management

Treatment focusses on reducing osteoclastic activity, decreasing bone turnover and enabling normal bone growth. It always requires referral to secondary care.

CONSERVATIVE

- Exercise regimen promoting range of motion, improved strength and mobility
- Orthoses and/or walking aids – if long bone deformities
- Diet rich in calcium and vitamin D

MEDICATION

- Bisphosphonates – reduces the bone turnover
- Calcitonin – if bisphosphonates are not tolerated or contraindicated
- Calcium and vitamin D supplementation
- Simple analgesia where appropriate

SURGERY

- Managing complications (e.g. pathological fracture or nerve decompression)

Hypercalcaemia

Hypercalcaemia describes raised levels of calcium in the blood that can cause a range of symptoms including abdominal pain, kidney stones and confusion. Very high levels of calcium in the blood can be life threatening.

Abnormal levels may relate to problems with its hormonal control via the action of parathyroid hormone (PTH) and vitamin D, but it is also the most common metabolic abnormality found in cancer patients and is a generally a poor prognostic sign as it often indicates extensive disease.

History

- Commonest causes:
  - Primary hyperparathyroidism
    - The majority of cases in the community
    - Usually a non-cancerous tumour (adenoma) in the parathyroid gland oversecreting PTH
    - Affects women more than men, often in a younger age group
  - Malignancy
    - Accounts for most of the rest of the cases
    - May be either localised disease with increased osteoclast activity or tumours releasing parathyroid hormone related peptide (PTHrp)
    - A history of a cancer that metastasises to bone is a significant risk (e.g. breast, prostate, lung, thyroid, kidney, myeloma)
- Uncommon causes:
  - Overdosing of vitamin D
  - Familial benign hypercalcaemia
  - Sarcoidosis – causes increased production of vitamin D
  - Hyperthyroidism – thyroid hormones increase osteoclast activity
  - Milk-alkali syndrome – excessive dietary milk or antacids (e.g. calcium carbonate)

Symptoms

Symptoms of hypercalcaemia are often described using the mnemonic **"Bones, stones, groans and psychic moans"**
- Skeletal **(Bones)**
  - Bone pain, skeletal deformities
  - Osteoporosis and fragility fractures
- Renal **(Stones)**
  - Kidney stones – renal colic (intense spasms of loin to groin pain)
  - Increased frequency of urination (polyuria), increased thirst (polydipsia) and dehydration

- Gastrointestinal **(Groans)**
  - Nausea, vomiting, anorexia, weight loss
  - Constipation, abdominal pain
  - Peptic ulcer, pancreatitis (both rare)
- Neuromuscular and neuropsychiatric **(Psychic moans)**
  - Drowsiness, delirium, coma, fatigue, lethargy, insomnia
  - Impaired concentration and memory, confusion
  - Depression, anxiety, irritability, psychosis
  - Muscle weakness
- Cardiovascular
  - Hypertension
  - Shortened QT interval, prolonged PR interval on electrocardiogram (ECG)
  - Cardiac arrhythmias such as ventricular fibrillation (rare)

Investigations

- Blood tests
  - Bone profile – raised calcium. ALP may be increased in primary hyperparathyroidism, Paget's disease, myeloma or bone metastases
  - PTH – typically raised in primary (and tertiary) hyperparathyroidism and suppressed or undetectable in malignancy-related hypercalcaemia or non PTH-dependent causes
  - Vitamin D – may be raised
  - Full blood count, U&E, ESR/CRP, myeloma screen and thyroid function tests – may be used to screen for causes and assess impact

Management

Depends on the severity. Treatment in a hospital setting is required if moderate or severe
- Identify and treat underlying cause
- Reduce or stop medication likely to exacerbate hypercalcaemia (e.g. lithium, thiazide diuretics, vitamin D)
- Maintain adequate hydration and salt intake
- Facilitate excretion via kidneys – this may require intravenous fluids and a loop diuretic (e.g. furosemide)

MEDICATION

- Bisphosphonates – in cases of increased osteoclastic activity
- Plicamycin – inhibits osteoclastic synthesis and decreases bone resorption
- Calcitonin – inhibits osteoclastic bone resorption and enhances excretion

SURGERY

- Surgery may include parathyroidectomy if a parathyroid adenoma is found

Diabetes Mellitus

Diabetes mellitus is a common, chronic, multisystem disease characterised by a lack of insulin or of insulin becoming less effective. Insulin is a hormone produced by the pancreas that enables the cells of the body to absorb glucose from the bloodstream and use it as fuel. There are a range of significant metabolic and structural consequences of diabetes mellitus, and it is a common comorbidity found with, and contributing to, many musculoskeletal pathologies.

History

There are two types of diabetes mellitus – Primary and Secondary
Primary:
- Type I diabetes
  - An autoimmune condition usually seen in younger people due to the production of antibodies that target the insulin secreting cells (β-cells) in the pancreas causing a complete absence of insulin
  - Caused by a mixture of genetic and environmental factors
- Type II diabetes
  - Is a chronic, metabolic condition caused by a mixture of genetic and environmental factors including obesity, lack of exercise and excessive consumption of sugars causing two key problems:
    - Reduced production of insulin
    - Insulin resistance – where tissues are unable to respond to insulin
- Maturity onset diabetes of the young (MODY) – a rare form of the disease
Secondary:
- Causes include steroid use, some medication (e.g. HIV medication and antipsychotics), pancreatic dysfunction from surgery, pancreatitis, trauma, cancer, Cushing's disease, pregnancy, acromegaly and hyperthyroidism

Symptoms

Patients may be asymptomatic or present with acute or more chronic features of hyperglycaemia that may include:
- Polyuria (increased urination due to the osmotic effects of excess glucose being excreted by the kidneys and drawing fluid from the tissues as it does so)
- Polydipsia (thirst – from dehydration)
- Unexplained weight loss
- Blurred vision
- Thrush (repeated oral/genital thrush)
- Lethargy
- Diabetic ketoacidosis – drowsiness/lethargy, abdominal pain, nausea/vomiting with dehydration and raised blood sugar on finger prick testing and ketones on dipstick testing of their urine – may be life threatening

Investigations

Diabetes is diagnosed on the basis of history, clinical signs and some bedside and laboratory tests
- Raised blood glucose levels including on a glucose tolerance test
- Raised Hba1c in some (but not all) types of diabetes
- Urine tests may show evidence of ketones (more commonly in type I diabetes)
- Auto-antibodies – positive antibody test (anti-GAD, insulin autoantibodies [IAA] and islet cell antibodies [ICA]) – indicative of type I diabetes

Management

CONSERVATIVE

- Education and advice
- Routine reviews – proactive care and screening (e.g. for diabetic retinopathy, neuropathy and renal disease)
- Management of cardiovascular risk (e.g. hypertension, hyperlipidaemia)
- Diet focussed on low intake of carbohydrates
- Exercise

MEDICATION

- Metformin – increases insulin sensitivity and helps with weight loss (can cause diarrhoea but does not cause hypoglycaemia)
- Sulphonylureas (e.g. gliclazide) – stimulates insulin secretion by pancreatic cells (can cause hypoglycaemia and weight gain)
- Glitazone – increases insulin sensitivity (can cause hypoglycaemia, fluid retention, fractures and abnormal lung function tests. Avoided in heart failure and osteoporosis)
- DPP4 inhibitors/gliptins (e.g. sitagliptin) – work by blocking the action of DPP-4, an enzyme that destroys the hormone incretin, which helps the body produce more insulin only when it is needed and reduces the amount of glucose being produced by the liver when it is not needed
- Selective sodium glucose co transporter-2 (SGLT-2) inhibitor (e.g. empagliflozin) – blocks reabsorption of glucose in the kidneys, thereby increasing its excretion
- Insulin – short-, medium- or long-term acting preparations normally injected to replace endogenous insulin

Hypothyroidism

Hypothyroidism is a condition characterised by decreased production and secretion of thyroid hormones by the thyroid gland. The thyroid gland produces two hormones, triiodothyronine (T3) and thyroxine (T4), which influence body thermoregulation, growth and development, metabolism and heart rate via their influence on the basal metabolic rate and sympathetic nervous system.

Hypothyroidism carries an increased risk of cardiovascular disease, osteoporosis, cognitive dysfunction and lipid disorders. It is often seen alongside other autoimmune disorders (e.g. diabetes) as well as in genetic disorders such as Down's and Turner's syndromes. Hypothyroidism is an important part of the differential diagnosis for chronic pain or chronic fatigue presentations.

History

- Primary (the vast majority of cases)
  - Autoimmune thyroiditis (e.g. Hashimoto's thyroiditis)
  - Iatrogenic (e.g. following radio-ablation of the thyroid in hyperthyroidism or after surgery)
  - Iodine deficiency – iodine is essential for making thyroid hormones
  - Drug induced
    - Inhibitors of T3/T4 production (e.g. lithium, iodine, amiodarone)
    - Drug induced thyroiditis (e.g. interferon, disease-modifying antirheumatic drugs, antiretrovirals for HIV)
- Secondary hypothyroidism (very rare)
  - Hypopituitarism leading to reduced production of thyroid stimulating hormone (TSH)
  - Hypothalamic dysfunction – post surgery, genetic defects and associated with inflammatory disease (e.g. sarcoidosis)
  - More common in women than men

Symptoms

- Often slow, insidious onset
- Tiredness
- Depressed mood
- Cold intolerance
- Dry and/or thin skin and hair
- Cold hands
- Reduced memory/cognitive function
- Menstrual changes (heavy periods and infertility)
- Weight gain
- Myalgia
- Cramps and weakness
- Severe conditions from undertreated hypothyroidism may include pericardial or pleural effusion and hypotension. When extreme can cause a coma (myxoedemic coma)

Examination

- Goitre – an enlargement of the thyroid (can be benign), seen mostly in Hashimoto's thyroiditis
- Slow relaxing reflexes
- Ataxic gait
- Dry skin/hair
- Round, puffy face, obesity
- Constipation
- Ileus – a temporary lack of the normal muscle contractions of the intestines
- Low heart rate, angina, cardiac failure

Investigations

- Blood Tests
  - TSH – increased
  - T4 – reduced
  - Autoantibodies – thyroid peroxidase antibodies (positive in many cases)
  - FBC – may see a normochromic anaemia
  - Lipids – raised cholesterol and triglycerides may be seen
- Ultrasound
  - May be used to assess any goitre

Management

- Centres around the use of thyroid hormone replacement with levothyroxine
  - Treatment is usually advised if TSH >10 mU/L
  - Factors taken into account for initiating treatment for lower levels of TSH include pregnancy, presence of thyroid autoantibodies, presence of goitre, age <65 with associated abnormal lipids or cardiovascular risk factors

Hyperthyroidism

Hyperthyroidism describes the overproduction and secretion of thyroid hormones by an overactive thyroid gland. It is much rarer than hypothyroidism but causes effects.

These can present more dramatically than hypothyroidism, with agitation and palpitations being a common feature.

History

- Grave's disease accounts for the majority of cases
  - Caused by the production of autoantibodies (thyroid stimulating hormone [TSH] receptor antibodies) that drive the thyroid gland to enlarge and overproduce thyroid hormones
  - Affects women more than men, usually in their 40–60s
  - There is a genetic predisposition
- Thyroiditis
  - Inflammation of thyroid and overproduction of thyroid hormones caused by:
    - Viral infection of the gland (de Quervain's thyroiditis)
    - Post-partum – usually six to twelve weeks after birth
    - Drug induced (e.g. amiodarone, iodine, lithium)
- Toxic multi-nodular goitre – caused by over secreting nodules in the thyroid, seen more in elderly patients
- Toxic adenoma – a benign tumour of the thyroid producing thyroid hormones
- Thyroid cancer
- Iodine excess from diet or contrast media
- Overdose of thyroxine

Symptoms

- Diarrhoea (and increased frequency of motions)
- Sweating
- Weight loss
- Heat intolerance
- Palpitations
- Tremors
- Menstrual changes (irregular/infrequent periods)
- More rarely psychosis, panic, itching

Examination

- Fast, irregular pulse (atrial fibrilliant or ventricular tachycardia)
- Tremors
- Sweats

- Thin hair
- 'Staring' appearance to eyes due to eyelid retraction with proptosis (bulging eyes) – specific to Grave's disease
- Enlarged thyroid (goitre) might be seen

Investigations

- Blood tests
  - TSH – reduced (<0.1mU/L)
  - T4 and T3 – increased
  - Full blood count – mild normochromic anaemia
  - ESR – may be raised in thyroiditis
  - Thyroid autoantibodies – thyrotrophin receptor antibodies
- Radio-iodine uptake test
  - Shows an increased uptake in Grave's disease and toxic multi-nodular disease but very low in thyroiditis
- Ultrasound
  - Identifies nodules, differences in colour-flow Doppler can distinguish between Grave's disease and thyroiditis and features of malignancy (e.g. calcification, irregular borders)

Management

Dependent on cause but can include:

MEDICATION

- Anti-thyroid drugs (e.g. carbimazole)
- Symptom control
  - Beta-blockers – for increased heart rate
  - Corticosteroids or NSAIDs may be used for thyroiditis

SURGERY

- Total thyroidectomy may be used if:
  - Enlargement of the thyroid is causing compression of local structures
  - Suspected thyroid malignancy
  - No response to radio-iodine or antithyroid drugs

RADIO-IODINE TREATMENT

- First line for Grave's disease
- Considered for toxic multi nodular goitre or toxic adenoma
- Can cause post-treatment hypothyroidism requiring thyroid hormone replacement

Hyperparathyroidism

Hyperparathyroidism is an endocrine disorder characterised by an excessive release of parathyroid hormone (PTH) from the parathyroid glands. PTH is vital in the homeostatic of calcium. Increased levels of PTH cause bone resorption and subsequent hypercalcaemia.

Hyperparathyroidism can be classified as:

- Primary
  - Parathyroid adenoma – a benign, secretory tumour of the parathyroid glands that causes the majority of cases of hyperparathyroidism
  - Multiglandular hyperplasia – enlargement of the parathyroid glands
  - Parathyroid carcinoma
  - Due to medication – thiazide diuretics, lithium, anticonvulsants, steroids, isoniazid, rifampicin
- Secondary
  - Chronic renal failure
    - Failure of the kidney to excrete phosphate and reabsorb calcium
    - Failure of endocrine function of the kidney
  - Malabsorption and vitamin D deficiency
- Tertiary
  - Created by prolonged or untreated secondary hyperparathyroidism causing the glands to change and not return to normal even after the cause of secondary hyperparathyroidism has resolved
- Malignant hyperparathyroidism
  - Caused by the release of parathyroid hormone-related peptide (PTHrp) by some tumours (e.g. breast, lung and renal cancers)

History

- Family history – associated inherited diseases include multiple endocrine neoplasia (MEN)
- Primary hyperparathyroidism is more common in women than in men and increases with age
- Past lithium treatment increases the risk
- Possible links to past radiotherapy of the head and neck

Symptoms

- Asymptomatic – may be an incidental finding on blood tests
- Mood disturbance – confusion, anxiety, fatigue, depression
- Fragility fractures – osteoporosis or osteopenia from bone resorption
- Kidney stones
- Abdominal pain
- Constipation
- Vomiting
- Polyuria/polydipsia
- Fatigue and sleep disturbance – the mechanism is uncertain

Investigations

- Blood tests
  - Bone profile/PTH – raised calcium with high (unsuppressed) parathyroid hormone levels
  - Phosphate – low or low-normal in primary hyperparathyroidism
  - U&E – there may be impaired renal function
  - Vitamin D – may be low
  - Alkaline phosphatase (ALP) - may be raised in the absence of other raised liver function tests due to increased bone turnover
- DEXA scan
  - May reveal osteopenia or osteoporosis
- MRI/USS
  - To identify parathyroid adenoma
- X-ray
  - Increased sclerosis of end plates in vertebrae with increased lucency may be found in thoracic radiographs. Subperiosteal and subchondral resorption of bone may be seen in the phalanges, acromioclavicular, sternoclavicular and sacroiliac joints as well as 'pepper pot' changes in the skull

Management

MEDICATION

- Bisphosphonates – may increase the bone mineral density
- Calcimimetics (e.g. cincalcet) – mimics calcium, binds to calcium receptors and reduces PTH levels
- Vitamin D replacement

SURGERY

- Parathyroidectomy for symptomatic patients (primary) or for those with end-organ changes (osteoporosis, fractures, reduced renal function)

Motor Neurone Disease

Motor neurone disease (MND) refers to a group of degenerative conditions affecting the brain and spinal cord. It characteristically causes muscle weakness due to the degeneration of motor neurones but no sensory loss (a useful way to distinguish MND from other neurological conditions).

The presentation varies and can include upper and lower motor neurone signs and symptoms, often in the same limb.

The main types include:

- Amyotrophic lateral sclerosis (ALS)
    - The most common type of MND
    - Lower motor neurone muscle wasting and upper motor neurone hyperreflexia
    - Causes characteristic atrophy in the arm, leg, neck or diaphragm but may also spread to the body and face
- Progressive muscular atrophy (PMA)
    - Has a better prognosis than that of ALS as it only has lower motor neurone signs
    - Affects the cervical region, leading to the atrophy of the muscles of the hand. Involvement spreads to the arms and shoulder girdles and may spread to the legs
    - It affects distal motor groups before it affects proximal groups
- Progressive bulbar palsy
    - Only affects cranial nerves IX-XI. Affects swallowing, speaking, chewing and causes weakening of the jaw, facial muscles and tongue as well as progressive speech loss

History

- Cause is uncertain with a range of suggested possible environmental and genetic factors, with few patients having a family history of MND
- It generally has a poor prognosis, with short life expectancy after the diagnosis
- Onset tends to be insidious, with symptoms evolving over months
- Men tend to be more affected than women are, with a peak age of onset in their 60s

Symptoms

- Lower limb
    - Gait disturbances (e.g. stumbling, falling)
    - Proximal muscle weakness
    - Stiffness
    - Foot drop
- Upper limb
    - Weakness
    - Stiffness
    - Wrist drop
- Fasciculation of skeletal muscle
- Painful muscle spasms

- Bulbar signs (lower cranial nerves)
  - Difficulty in swallowing, weak tongue and jaw muscles with speech changes (slurred, hoarse or nasal sounding), drooling and choking (may lead to aspiration pneumonia)

Examination

- Upper motor neurone signs
  - Spasticity
  - Brisk reflexes
  - Upward plantar reflex
- Lower motor neurone signs
  - Wasting
  - Fasciculation
  - Muscle weakness
  - Muscle atrophy
- Memory loss
  - Fronto-temporal dementia is found in a significant proportion of patients with MND
- Bulbar signs
  - Flaccid fasciculation of tongue
  - Absent jaw jerk

Investigations

- Electromyography (EMG) and nerve conduction studies (NCS)
  - Shows characteristic changes including:
    - Spontaneous fibrillation – spontaneous discharges of motor units
    - Evidence of disorganised or reduced functional motor units
- MRI
  - May show hyperintensity in corticospinal or corticobulbar tracts (moreso in ALS)
  - Cerebral atrophy may be found in patients with cognitive impairment

Management

There is currently no cure for MND, so treatment is focussed on maximising survival and managing the symptoms with multidisciplinary team management. Referral to neurologist should be made for diagnosis and treatment advice if MND is suspected.

CONSERVATIVE

- Occupational therapy – support independence and assistance with functional activities
- Speech and language therapy - advice for swallowing difficulties. Percutaneous endoscopic gastrostomy (PEG) may be required for support with feeding as disease progresses
- Physical rehabilitation and support may include:
  - Standing and positioning support (frames, treadmill training)
  - Active exercises and exercise programmes to help improve the range of motion, prevent contractures and reduce stiffness and discomfort
- Respiratory therapists – help with breathing and secretion clearance
- Psychological support – counselling and psychological therapies
- Splinting and orthotics to improve stability and function

- In the later stages, standing and positioning support may be needed, and as movement decreases patients may require constant positioning management and pressure area monitoring
- Mechanical ventilation support, usually via tracheostomy for respiratory failure, is a common feature of progression and may be life threatening

MEDICATION

- Disease modifying therapy – antiglutamates (e.g., riluzole) are used to extend life and delay the need for mechanical ventilation
- Quinine, baclofen, dantrolene, tizanidine or gabapentin for spasticity
- Anticholinergics (e.g. amitriptyline, glycopyrrolate) for drooling
- NSAIDs for pain relief where safe and tolerated
- Opiates may be used for pain relief, with an additional role for managing respiratory symptoms

4.19

Multiple Sclerosis

Multiple sclerosis (MS) is the most common neurological disorder in young adults and is the greatest cause of non-traumatic disability in this group. It is characterised by inflammation within the central nervous system (CNS), causing patchy demyelination 'plaques' in nerves. These cause characteristic visual and sensory disturbances with bladder and bowel disruption, limb weakness and gait disturbance. The peripheral nerves are unaffected.

History

- The cause of MS is uncertain but is likely due to a combination of genetic and environmental factors
- It typically presents in the late 20s
- Affects women more than men
- Is the most common cause of transverse myelitis (myelopathy)
- The majority of cases have a pattern of relapsing-remitting MS with acute attacks ('relapses') with recovery between symptomatic episodes. However, some follow a steadier progression of symptoms, known as progressive MS, either from the beginning (primary progressive MS), or following a relapsing-remitting pattern (secondary progressive MS)

Symptoms

- Symptoms are based on the area of the CNS affected and may include:
  - Visual changes
    - Optic neuritis – pain on eye movement and loss of central vision
    - Double vision
    - Visual field loss
  - Bladder and bowel problems
    - Urgency
    - Incontinence and increased frequency
  - Sensory changes
    - Abnormal sensations (e.g. transient paraesthesia that may spread up the leg and resolve within a few days)
    - Trigeminal neuralgia – severe, 'shock-like' facial pain
  - Cerebellar signs
    - Ataxic gait (unsteady or staggering)
    - Intention tremor
    - Speech changes (e.g. slurred speech)
  - Sexual dysfunction
    - Erectile dysfunction
    - Loss of orgasm

Examination

- Wide based gait
- Cerebellar signs – ataxia, nystagmus and dysarthria (slurred or slow speech that may be hard to understand)
- Spasticity (increased muscle tone, stiffness, spasms and involuntary contractions)
- Motor signs
  - Limb weakness
  - Spasticity
  - Hyperreflexia
  - Clonus
- Fundoscopy may show a pale optic disc
- Sensory changes
  - Loss of vibration sense
- Trigeminal neuralgia may be associated with facial weakness and sensory loss

Investigations

- MRI
  - Identifies plaques of demyelination in the CNS
  - Excludes other causes of upper motor neurone symptoms such as other causes of myelopathy or cord compression
- Cerebrospinal fluid (CSF)
  - Signs of inflammation
  - Presence of autoantibodies
- Nerve conduction studies
  - Visual evoked potentials – shows delayed nerve conduction along the optic nerve due to demyelination
  - Auditory and sensory evoked potentials are also affected

Management

Treatment aims to reduce the severity of symptoms and how often they occur with support to improve function and quality of life and to reduce disability. Referral should be made to a neurologist for the diagnosis of MS if suspected.

CONSERVATIVE

- Multidisciplinary team management
- Lifestyle advice including smoking cessation where relevant, dietary modification and stress reduction
- Identify and avoid triggers of trigeminal neuralgia (e.g. food, drinks, cold, stress)
- Standing and positioning support (frames, treadmill training)
- Splinting and orthotics to improve stability and function
- Exercise and balance programmes to maintain and improve mobility and postural control
- In the later stages, standing and positioning support may be needed; moreover, as movement decreases, patients may require constant positioning management and pressure area monitoring
- Intermittent self-catheterisation for some with loss of bladder control

- Psychological therapies including acceptance and commitment therapy (ACT) or cognitive behavioural therapy (CBT)

MEDICATION

- Steroids (e.g. methylprednisolone) – mainstay of treatment of relapses to help shorten and reduce the severity
- Disease modifying drugs (e.g. beta-interferon) – immunomodulators aiming to reduce severity and frequency of relapses
- Carbamazepine for the management of trigeminal neuralgia
- Baclofen, dantrolene, benzodiazepines for spasticity
- Gabapentinoids and botulinum toxin for focal areas of increased tone
- Anticholinergics (e.g. oxybutynin or amitriptyline) for urinary urgency
- Antidepressants may play a role for managing depression
- Amantadine can be used for fatigue

Peripheral Neuropathy

Peripheral neuropathy (PN) describes a group of conditions caused by damage to the peripheral nerves, usually resulting in pain, sensory changes and weakness in the arms and legs, typically in a glove and stocking distribution.

There are more than 100 types of PN that can affect single nerves (mononeuropathy) or multiple nerves (polyneuropathy). They can either be inherited or acquired due to systemic disease (diabetes), toxins (including alcohol), trauma (e.g. car accidents), falls, sports injuries or caused by infections or autoimmune disorders. Most cases of PN are caused by diabetes and heavy or prolonged alcohol use.

History

- Diabetes
- Toxins
  - Alcohol – direct effects and associated with nutritional (B12) deficiency
  - Medication – chemotherapy agents, statins, fluoroquinolones, amiodarone, colchicine, lithium, phenytoin
  - Heavy metal poisoning (e.g. lead, mercury, thallium)
- Kidney failure – PN is common in patients requiring dialysis
- Acromegaly – overproduction of growth hormone can lead to enlargement of joints and localised nerve compression
- Hypothyroidism – may be due to fluid retention around nerves
- B12/folate deficiency (e.g. vegan diet, malabsorption)
- Autoimmune disease (e.g. rheumatoid arthritis, connective tissue disease)
- Inflammatory neuropathies such as:
  - Guillain-Barre syndrome
  - Chronic inflammatory demyelinating polyneuropathy (CIDP)
  - Multifocal motor neuropathy that exclusively affects the motor nerves
- Malignancies
  - Direct compression or widespread nerve disruption from multiple benign tumours, such as neurofibromatosis (multiple fibromas), as well as benign tumours of the nerves themselves (neuroma)
  - Paraneoplastic syndrome – antibody mediated peripheral neuropathy sometimes seen in advanced lung or breast cancer
  - Myeloma and monoclonal gammopathy of undetermined significance (MGUS) causing paraprotein mediated neuropathy, amyloidosis and hyperviscosity
- Family history of heritable neuropathy (e.g. Charcot-Marie Tooth disease)
- Time course can indicate possible cause:
  - Acute onset neuropathies (less than four weeks) include:
    - Ischemic neuropathy
    - Nerve compression (direct compression, haemorrhage, swelling)
    - Trauma, penetrating wounds, iatrogenic (e.g. injection), thermal injury

- Subacute onset over days to weeks (four to twelve weeks) may be caused by:
  - Rheumatoid arthritis
  - Toxic and metabolic neuropathies (e.g. diabetes, alcohol related)
- Chronic course over months to years (>12 weeks) may be caused by:
  - Hereditary neuropathy
  - CIDP
- Relapsing remitting course is seen with Guillain-Barre syndrome

Symptoms

Symptoms vary widely according to the underlying pathology and nerves affected but may include:
- Motor nerve
  - Muscle weakness
  - Cramps
  - Fasciculations
  - Muscle wasting
- Sensory nerve
  - Neuropathic pain may be described as 'burning,' 'stinging,' 'shooting' and can be independent of stimulus or worsened by touch (e.g. contact with bed sheets or shoes)
  - Progressive loss of sensation dependent on which nerves are affected
    - Large fibre loss – reduced touch and vibration sense
    - Small fibre loss – reduced pain and temperature sensation
- Autonomic nerves
  - Includes problems digesting food (diarrhoea, constipation, bloating), increased urinary frequency, low blood pressure, dizziness, problems with sweating and sexual dysfunction (erectile dysfunction, lack of ejaculation/anorgasmia)

Examination

- Sensory loss most commonly in the hands and feet in a 'glove and stocking' distribution
  - Loss of pin-prick or thermal sensation
- Muscle weakness
- Muscle atrophy
- Absent deep tendon reflexes
- Hyperalgesia and allodynia are possible but rare
- There may be altered sensation in the trunk in some diabetics (intercostal nerve involvement)
- In small-fibre neuropathy (some diabetics, amyloid), motor function, tendon reflexes, proprioception, joint position sense and coordination may be normal
- Reflexes are usually reduced or absent
- Wider examination for other signs of systemic disease including:
  - Connective tissue disease – rash, lymphadenopathy, synovitis
  - Vasculitic rash
  - Skeletal deformities or lesions causing entrapment
  - Signs of liver failure (e.g. enlarged liver)

Investigations

- Blood tests
  - May help identify the underlying cause and include:
    - Full blood count – macrocytic anaemia seen in B12 and folate deficiency and alcoholism
    - ESR – may be raised in inflammatory or autoimmune conditions

- Vitamin B12 and folate – low in nutritional deficiencies and pernicious anaemia
- Fasting blood sugar (or HbA1C) – to identify diabetes
- U&E – renal failure
- Liver function tests – liver disease (e.g. alcoholic liver disease)
- Thyroid function tests – low T4 and raised TSH in hypothyroidism
- Additional blood tests may include
    - Serum protein electrophoresis – myeloma
    - Autoantibodies – (e.g. Sjögren's, SLE, etc)
    - Serology (e.g. Lyme disease, HIV)
    - Heavy metal toxin screen
- Nerve conduction studies and electromyogram
    - May show evidence of demyelination or axonal loss with altered conduction velocities, amplitude and reduced muscle activity that can help locate the site of any lesion, assist in identifying the nature of the pathology and assess its severity
- Nerve biopsy
    - Usually reserved for rarer types of asymmetrical polyneuropathy (e.g. with vasculitis, amyloidosis or sarcoidosis)
- MRI
    - May identify space occupying lesions, anomalous structures and other abnormal anatomy (e.g. bone spurs, constrictions, hypertrophy) that may be a source of nerve entrapment
- Chest X-ray
    - If features suggestive of malignancy
- Urine dipstick
    - For glucose/protein – suggestive of diabetes, renal disease

Management

Is based around treating any underlying cause of the neuropathy as well as providing information and advice on the signs of progression and understanding the cause. Regular monitoring is important to prevent potentially serious consequences such as infection or ulceration.

CONSERVATIVE

- Managing any reversible lifestyle factors including alcohol consumption
- Supplementing any vitamin deficiencies
- Foot care – important in at risk groups (e.g. diabetics)
- Non-pharmacological approaches for pain management include acupuncture, TENS and percutaneous electrical nerve stimulation (PENS)
- Holistic management with multidisciplinary specialist pain services with MDT input when indicated

MEDICATION

- Management of neuropathic pain may include:
    - Tricyclic antidepressants (e.g. amitriptyline, nortriptyline)
    - Topical capsaicin cream
    - Selective noradrenaline re-uptake inhibitors (e.g. duloxetine, venlafaxine)
    - Anti-epileptics (e.g. gabapentin or pregabalin)
    - Tramadol

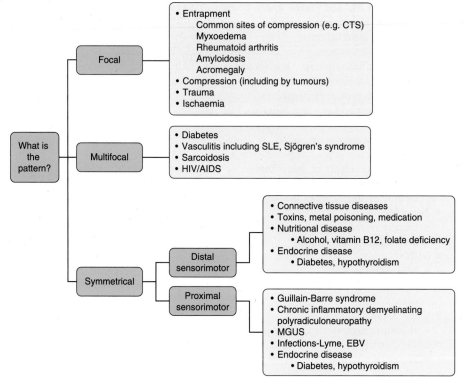

Fig 4.20.1   Patterns of peripheral neuropathy

4.21

Multiple Myeloma

Multiple myeloma is a cancer of plasma cells (lymphocytes) in the bone marrow that in turn produce large amounts of non-functioning immunoglobulins (antibodies) called 'paraproteins.' As the abnormal cells proliferate, they can create a mass known as a plasmacytoma as well as localised lysis of bone causing characteristic painful lesions and fragility fractures. The loss of healthy bone marrow causes a reduction in red cells, white cells and platelets, often leading to anaemia and impaired defence against infection. Paraproteins, or parts of them, spill into the blood from the bone marrow, increasing the plasma viscosity and damaging the kidneys and peripheral nerves. Different types of myeloma are classified by the antibody produced (or part of antibody i.e. light chains).

History

- Risk factors include:
  - Increasing age – most commonly seen around the age of 70
  - Affects men more than women
  - Afro-Caribbean origin
  - Obesity
  - Diet low in fish and green vegetables
  - Family history of myeloma
- Symptoms

Key signs and symptoms can be remembered by the mnemonic **CRAB.**

- Hyper**C**alcaemia
  - Causing confusion, polydipsia (excessive thirst), polyuria (excessive urination), constipation, anorexia (reduced appetite). If excessive, then it can cause seizures, coma, cardiac arrythmia and death
- **R**enal impairment
  - Normally asymptomatic, but it can cause low urine output (oliguria) or high levels of urea in the blood (uraemia)
- **A**naemia
  - Low haemoglobin may be found with low white cells (leucopoenia) and low platelets (thrombocytopaenia)
- **B**ony lesion
  - Lytic lesions (areas of bone destruction, especially the back or ribs)
  - Spontaneous fractures or spinal deformity
- Other features include:
  - Signs of immunocompromise (i.e. recurrent infections)
  - Bleeding (e.g. nosebleeds or bruising) – due to low platelets
  - Peripheral neuropathy – distal sensorimotor and focal (e.g. carpal tunnel syndrome)

Examination

- Weakness and sensory changes in the lower limbs – secondary to vertebral compression fractures
- Weight loss
- Fever
- Bone tenderness
- Hepatomegaly
- Rarely lymphadenopathy and/or splenomegaly
- Distal, symmetrical or focal sensorimotor nerve abnormalities

Investigations

- Blood tests
  - Serum protein electrophoresis (SPE) – may show a 'paraprotein band'
  - Serum free light chain assay – may show raised free light chain and/or an abnormal ratio (can be with a normal SPE in light chain disease)
  - Urinary electrophoresis – urinary free light chains ('Bence Jones proteins')
  - Full blood count – may show anaemia, low platelets and white cells
  - ESR often increased (with a normal CRP)
  - Bone profile – hypercalcaemia
  - U&Es – may show signs of renal failure secondary to myeloma
- X-ray
  - May show evidence of localised bony erosions (lytic lesions), osteopenia, fractures or vertebral collapse
- Bone marrow aspirates and biopsy
  - Monoclonal plasma cell infiltrates – the amount informs management and prognosis
- MRI
  - May identify focal lesions and bone marrow infiltration

Management

MEDICATION

- Chemotherapy with cytotoxic agents (e.g. doxorubicin, vincristine, melphalan)
- Non-chemotherapy agents (e.g. thalidomide, lenalidomide)
- Bisphosphonates – for bone pain and osteolytic bone disease
- Corticosteroids (e.g. dexamethasone, prednisolone) – often in conjunction with chemotherapeutic agents for pain

OTHER TREATMENTS

- Plasmapheresis (removal and replacement of a patient's blood plasma to manage hyperviscosity and for rehydration)
- Stem cell transplant
- Radiotherapy for painful bony lesions
- Blood transfusions

Primary Bone Cancer

Primary bone cancers are those that originate in bone rather than metastasising to them. They are caused by abnormal growth and division of any of the cells that are found in bone. They most usually cause bone pain and swelling and are one of the more common causes of cancer in children and adolescents.

There are three main types of primary bone cancer that make up the majority of cases.

- Osteosarcoma – most common form in young people (due to abnormal osteoblast cells)
- Ewing's sarcoma – second most common form (affects bones or tissues around bones)
- Chondrosarcoma – most common in adults (arise from cartilage cells)
- Rarer forms include chordoma, adamantinoma, angiosarcoma of the bone, giant cell tumour of the bone and spindle cell sarcoma of the bone

History

- Mostly found in teens to those in their 20s
- Men are affected more than women
- Osteosarcoma and Ewing sarcoma affect a younger age group (10–25-year-olds)
- Osteosarcomas are more commonly found in the lower end of the femur, upper end of humerus and in pelvic bones
- Chondrosarcoma and chordomas tend to affect those over the age of 40
- Risk factors include:
  - Previous history of bone tumour
  - Radiotherapy
  - Genetic predisposition
  - Underlying bone abnormalities – people with conditions such as Paget's disease of the bone are more likely to develop primary bone cancer
  - Gene translocation – a non-inheritable gene change seen in Ewing's sarcoma

Symptoms

It is worth noting that symptoms can be very generalised and mimic sports injuries or musculoskeletal pathologies. Possible symptoms include:

- Bone pain that is initially intermittent but becomes more constant
- Pain that may not respond to analgesia or usual therapies
- Pain that can be worse at night
- Focal bony tenderness on palpation
- Lump or mass – may be palpable but not if the tumour is within the confines of the bone
- Altered gait – with lower limb tumours
- Reduced mobility
- Systemic features
  - Malaise
  - Weight loss

- Muscle atrophy
- Loss of muscle tone
- Pathological fracture is a late-stage sign

Investigations

- Blood tests
  - ESR – increased
  - Bone profile – may show raised lactate dehydrogenase (LDH) and alkaline phosphatase (ALP)
- X-ray
  - Useful first line investigation (the full length of the bone needs to be imaged)
  - May show features of bone destruction, new bone formation, periosteal and/or soft tissue swelling
- CT
  - May show a bony mass with central calcification and destruction of cortical bone
- MRI
  - May show a mass with extension into soft tissue (low signal T1 weighted, high signal T2 weighted) with vascularity identified using gadolinium enhancement
  - Useful for staging and guiding treatment
- PET/bone scan
  - Shows a 'hot' signal at the tumour site and may be helpful to identify metastatic disease
- Bone biopsy
  - Is the diagnostic investigation of choice

Management

Usually occurs under the care of specialist services with treatment usually involving chemotherapy in combination with surgery and sometimes radiotherapy to cure, treat the symptoms or prolong and maintain the quality of life.

SURGERY

- Surgery may involve amputation or limb sparing procedures including resection of localised tumour and replacement with prosthetics or bone grafts

Metastatic Bone Cancer

Secondary or metastatic cancers are caused by the spread of cancerous cells from other 'primary' cancers to the bone marrow where they grow and proliferate, creating 'secondary' tumours that disrupt the bony structure. This distinguishes between cancers of the bone (primary bone cancers) and cancers that have spread to the bone (secondary bone cancers).

History

- The symptoms of metastatic bone cancer may be the first signs of an underlying primary cancer
- History of a cancer that metastasises to bone is a clear red flag for someone presenting with bone pain. The cancers that metastasise to bone are:
  - Breast
  - Prostate
  - Lung
  - Thyroid
  - Kidney
  - Bowel (rare)
- Breast and prostate cancer represent the origins of over two thirds of all bone metastases

Symptoms

- Weight loss
- Loss of appetite
- Night sweats
- Fatigue
- Bone pain – severe and unremitting, usually localised to the site of metastasis
- Can affect any bone, but common sites include vertebrae, ribs, pelvis, femur and skull
- Pathological fracture – if there is significant destruction of the bone. In the spine this may be accompanied by metastatic spinal cord compression or nerve root compression (with features of radiculopathy)
- Hypercalcemia – the most common metabolic abnormality in cancer, causing confusion, polydipsia (excessive thirst), polyuria (excessive urination), constipation, anorexia (reduced appetite). If severe, can cause seizures, coma, cardiac arrythmia and death

Type of Cancer	Possible Signs and Symptoms
Breast	Breast – breast lump, skin changes (rash, dimple, nipple inversion or discharge) Lung – breathlessness (pleural effusion) Liver – enlarged liver, jaundice
Bowel	Change in bowel habit, bleeding, rectal mass

Continued on following page

Type of Cancer	Possible Signs and Symptoms
Bronchus (Lung)	Lung-cough, chest pain, blood in sputum (haemoptysis), hoarse voice (if recurrent laryngeal nerve affected), Horner's syndrome – a left apical lung tumour (Pancoast tumour) causing ptosis (drooping of the upper eyelid), miosis (constriction of pupil) and anhydrosis (decreased sweating)
Prostate	Lower urinary tract symptoms – hesitancy, poor stream, urgency, nocturia, terminal dribbling
Thyroid	Rapidly enlarging thyroid mass, hoarse voice, pain on swallowing
Kidney	Blood in the urine (haematuria), flank pain and palpable mass

Investigations

- Blood tests
  - Non-specific
    - Full Blood count – anaemia, low white cells, low or high platelets
    - ESR/CRP – may be increased
    - Calcium and alkaline phosphatase (ALP) – may be raised
    - U&E/liver function tests – abnormal if involvement of kidneys or liver
  - Specific
    - Prostate specific antigen – may be raised in prostate cancer
    - Serum protein electrophoresis – monoclonal (paraprotein) band in myeloma
    - Serum free light chain analysis – abnormal ratio in myeloma
    - Urinary electrophoresis – light chains (Bence Jones proteins) in myeloma
- X-ray
  - May show evidence of erosions or pathological fractures but are very limited in identifying bone metastases and should not be used to rule out cancer
- MRI
  - Soft tissue masses, nerve root involvement or spinal cord compression and features such as oedema
- CT
  - Where MRI is unsuitable (e.g. metalwork or pacemaker in situ)

Management

The primary objective is to achieve remission or cure of the underlying cancer according to its origin and staging. The following are treatments specific to the management of pain from bony metastases.

CONSERVATIVE

- Offloading and rest
- Activity modification
- Walking aids where appropriate

MEDICATION

- Non-steroidal anti-inflammatories (NSAIDs) where safe and tolerated
- Opioids (e.g. morphine)

- Neuropathic painkillers if nerve pain a feature
- IV bisphosphonates – may be useful as an adjunct and given mainly to increase stability and reduce the risk of fractures than to reduce pain

RADIOTHERAPY

- May be used to reduce bony pain, even in frail patients

SURGERY

- Treatment of fractures
- Prophylactic to prevent pathological fracture

4.24

Lymphoma

Lymphoma is a cancer of white cells (lymphocytes), predominantly within the lymphatic system (bone marrow, lymph nodes, spleen and thymus gland). This causes symptoms including bone pain and fatigue, so it is a rare but important part of a differential diagnosis for non-specific musckuloskeletal presentations.

Prognosis depends on stage at presentation, but is generally good compared to those of other malignancies

There are two main types:

- Non-Hodgkin's lymphoma
  - With many subtypes according to which white cells (B cells, T cells) are affected
- Hodgkin's lymphoma
  - Characterised by the presence of a specific cell type called Reed Sternberg cells
    - Subcategorised into different types including nodular sclerosing, mixed cellularity, lymphocyte rich, lymphocyte depleted and nodular lymphocyte predominant Hodgkin's lymphoma (NLPHL)

History

- Non-Hodgkin's lymphoma
  - Has been linked with viral and bacterial infections as well as environmental causes
  - It affects men more than women
  - Usually >50 years old
  - It can be graded as low, intermediate or high
- Hodgkin's lymphoma
  - Affects younger patients with peak age range 15–35 years
  - It affects men more than women

Symptoms

Related to the location and spread and can be limited to the lymph nodes (nodal) or may be more widespread (extra-nodal features).

- Inflammatory symptoms (sometimes called 'B-Symptoms') are associated with a poor prognosis. They include:
  - Night sweats (may be drenching, requiring them to change clothes)
  - Weight loss
  - Fever (>38°C)
- Other symptoms
  - Fatigue
  - Breathlessness – lung involvement, mediastinal mass and/or anaemia
  - Bone/back pain – spread to bones or epidural space
  - Headache, confusion, dizziness or ataxia – CNS/meningeal involvement

- Jaundice, itch – liver involvement
- Abdominal pain

Examination

- Painless lymphadenopathy – enlarged lymph nodes in the neck, abdomen, armpits or groin
- Splenomegaly – enlarged spleen
- Hepatomegaly – enlarged liver

Differential Diagnosis

- Infection
  - Epstein-Barr virus
  - HIV
  - Cytomegalovirus
  - Toxoplasmosis
  - Brucellosis
  - Tuberculosis
  - Hepatitis
- Sarcoidosis
- Leukaemia
- Systemic lupus erythematosus
- Rheumatoid arthritis

Investigations

- Blood tests
  - Full blood count – low platelets, raised white cell count or low white and red cell count (pancytopenia). Seen in bone marrow involvement
  - Blood film – immature white cells (blasts) may be seen
  - ESR – may be raised (poor prognosis)
  - U&E – abnormal if end organ damage
  - LFT – abnormal with raised LDH
- Lymph node/bone marrow biopsy
  - Looking for cancerous cells
- X-ray
  - May show widened mediastinum, suggesting mediastinal mass (enlarged mediastinal nodes)
- PET scan
  - Increased uptake at involved sites
  - Helps stage the cancer

Management

- Involves care under the haematologists and/or oncologists in secondary care
- Treatment may include:
  - Active surveillance – in slow developing/non-aggressive types
  - Chemotherapy
  - Radiotherapy
  - Bone marrow or stem cell transplant

4.25

Leukaemia

Leukaemia is a cancer of the blood-forming cells in the bone marrow that may also be found within the bloodstream (distinct to lymphoma, which mostly affects the lymph nodes). It is the most common cancer in children, but it is more prevalent in the elderly. Symptoms are related to the loss of functional bone marrow with anaemia, fatigue and increased risk of bleeding and infection.

It is categorised according to whether it is acute or chronic, whether it affects the precursors of myeloid cells (granulocytes, monocytes, erythrocytes or platelets) or lymphoid cells (lymphocytes – B and T cells) and the degree of their differentiation from immature to mature abnormal cells.

History

- The cause is unknown but is likely a combination of genetic (there is an association with Down's syndrome) and environmental factors (including radiation exposure)
- Presentation is dependent on the subtype:
  - Acute lymphocytic leukaemia (ALL)
    - Most common in children
    - Involves a rapid proliferation of cancerous cells (immature white cells) with bone marrow failure causing anaemia (low red cells/haemaglobin), neutropenia (low white cells) and thrombocytopenia (low platelets)
  - Chronic lymphocytic leukaemia (CLL)
    - Rare in children
    - Has more differentiated cells and associated with:
      - Enlarged lymph nodes
      - Hepatosplenomegaly
      - Shortness of breath
      - Fatigue
    - May be asymptomatic and found on routine full blood count (FBC)
  - Acute myeloid leukaemia (AML)
    - More common in adults
    - Rapid progression and can be fatal if untreated
  - Chronic myeloid leukaemia (CML)
    - More common in adults
    - May be asymptomatic
    - Many patients have enlarged spleen and raised white cell count associated with the presence of Philadelphia chromosome
  - Rare types include hairy cell leukaemia (involving B cells with hair-like cytoplasmic projections) and myeloproliferative disorders (e.g. polycythaemia vera, essential thrombocythemia), a group of disorders involving bone marrow failure that can develop into acute leukaemia

Symptoms

- Recurrent infections, fever (low levels of 'normal' white cells)
- Abnormal or excessive bruising or bleeding (low platelets)
- Fatigue, breathlessness, dizziness, palpitations (anaemia)
- Bone and joint pain (especially in children with ALL)
- Muscle weakness
- Night sweats
- Central nervous system involvement – headaches, convulsions, fits, coma

Examination

- Pale
- Enlarged lymph nodes (lymphadenopathy)
- Enlarged spleen (splenomegaly)
- Enlarged liver (hepatomegaly)
- Gum hypertrophy, stomatitis
- Bruising – purpura (purple-coloured spots) or petechiae (pinpoint, round spots on the skin)
- Fever

Investigations

- Blood tests
  - Full blood count – anaemia, low or high white cells (depending on type) and low platelets
  - Blood film – immature white cells (blasts) may be seen
  - Urate – hyperuricaemia may be found
  - U&E – signs of renal failure may be seen
  - Genetic testing – Philadelphia chromosome (secondary care)
- Bone marrow or lymph node biopsy
  - Cytogenetic analysis and immunophenotyping – indicates which cell type is present
- Lumbar puncture
  - If CNS involvement suspected – immature (blast) cells may be seen
- Infection screening
  - May include blood cultures
- Chest X-ray
  - Widened mediastinum suggesting mediastinal mass (enlarged mediastinal nodes)

Management

- The prognosis has improved, with most children with ALL surviving
- The chronic leukaemias generally progress slowly, and treatment improves and prolongs survival for most
- Treatment is usually managed by haematologists or oncologists, dependent on type and presentation but may include:
  - Blood and/or platelet transfusion
  - Allopurinol (for hyperuricemia)
  - Chemotherapy – involving multi – drug regimens that may need to be taken for years
  - Radiotherapy – helps lymphadenopathy and splenomegaly
  - Bone marrow (stem cell) transplant may be curative but comes with significant risks
  - Immunoglobulin transfusions if recurrent infections

4.26

Soft Tissue Sarcoma

Soft tissue sarcomas are rare malignant tumours found in a range of soft (connective) tissues usually causing a painless lump. Although they are rare, they are an important part of the differential diagnosis for a soft tissue mass.

There are more than 50 different types of sarcoma based on what type of connective tissue is affected, with leiomyosarcoma being the most common, followed closely by fibrosarcoma and liposarcoma. The cause may remain uncertain for most people.

Tissue Type	Sarcoma
Smooth muscle	Leiomyosarcoma
Skeletal muscle	Rhabdomyosarcoma
Fat	Liposarcoma
Cartilage	Chondrosarcoma
Fibrous tissue	Fibrosarcoma
Cells around joints and tendons	Synovial sarcoma

History

- Leiomyosarcoma and liposarcomas are more common in older people usually >50 years old
- Men and women are affected equally
- Rhabdomyosarcoma more commonly affects children
- Synovial sarcoma tends to affect young adults
- There is an association with rare genetic syndromes (e.g. neurofibromatosis and retinoblastoma)
- Risk factors identified include:
  - Radiotherapy – sarcomas may arise four to ten years after treatment (e.g. angiosarcoma)
  - Infection (e.g. Epstein – Barr virus and Herpes virus 8/Kaposi's sarcoma)
  - HIV infection – due to increased risk of Kaposi's sarcoma
  - Lymphoedema – associated with angiosarcoma
  - Toxins and pesticides (e.g. benzenes and vinyl chloride, which are used in manufacturing)

Symptoms

- A painless lump that is continuously growing
- Can occur anywhere but more common in the lower limb
- Neuropathic pain – due to compression of nerves by a soft tissue mass
- Rash of Kaposi's sarcoma may be found – purplish macular or papular lesions on the skin or in the mouth
- Systemic features – weight loss, fatigue and anorexia are signs of advanced disease
- Gastrointestinal (GI) symptoms include GI bleeding and acute abdominal pain – may be seen with GI stromal tumours

Examination

- A soft tissue mass usually more than five cm
- Usually located deep to fascia and is less apparent on muscle contracture
- Fixed or immobile
- May have regrown following a previous soft tissue mass excision
- Oedema may be a feature in upper limb tumours
- Lymphadenopathy (disease or swelling of lymph nodes) – may be a sign of metastatic disease

Investigations

- Ultrasound
  - Used to identify more superficial masses and identify nature (e.g. cystic)
- MRI
  - Is the preferred modality for imaging
  - May show a mass with variable enhancement and central necrosis
- Core biopsy
  - Is undertaken to enable grading and tissue typing of the sarcoma
- CT scan
  - Used for staging (from stage I to IV) based on size and spread to lymph nodes or distant sites (e.g. lung metastases)
- Chest X-ray
  - May be used to identify lung metastases
- Blood tests
  - Full blood count – clotting if any suspicion of GI bleeding
  - HIV test – may be positive in AIDS related Kaposi's sarcoma

Management

All patients with suspected sarcoma should be managed in a specialist centre with multidisciplinary care usually involving surgery and support from oncologists.

SURGERY

- Wide excision with clearly negative margins
- This may involve limb amputation in some cases

RADIOTHERAPY

- Often used as an adjuvant therapy (i.e. following surgery to reduce recurrence)

CHEMOTHERAPY

- Therapeutic – prior to surgery to reduce the tumour size and reduce metastases
- Palliative – in widespread, metastatic disease for symptom control and to prolong life

4.27

Systemic Conditions: Shorts

Acromegaly

Acromegaly describes excessive secretion of growth hormone in adults causing bones and tissues to grow. In childhood this is called 'gigantism.' This is most commonly caused by a secretory tumour of the pituitary gland.

Symptoms include enlargement of hands and feet, prominence of jaw, orbit and frontal ridges of the face, fatigue, headache, loss of libido, carpal tunnel syndrome, skin tags and sweating. Pituitary tumours can disrupt the optic chasm, causing a loss of peripheral vision. It is associated with an increased risk of osteoarthritis, metabolic disorders, cardiomyopathy and bowel cancer.

Diagnosis is based on blood tests (including raised IGf1 and an abnormal glucose tolerance test) and an MRI to identify tumours.

Treatment, if caused by a pituitary adenoma, depends on its size and impact and may include medication, radiotherapy or surgical excision.

Anti-phospholipid Antibody Syndrome

Anti-phospholipid antibody syndrome is an autoimmune condition that can cause blood clots. It is associated with the presence of antiphospholipid antibodies (e.g. anticardiolipin antibodies and lupus anticoagulant) which make the blood more likely to clot.

Blood clots (thrombosis) may be arterial (causing strokes, heart attacks and transient ischaemic attacks) or venous (causing deep vein thrombosis or pulmonary embolisms). Recurrent miscarriages may be seen (usually in the second/third trimester) as well as low platelets (thrombocytopaenia) in up to half of patients. Diagnosis is based on the presence of autoantibodies with treatment focussing on reducing the risk of blood clots using anticoagulants.

Charcot Marie Tooth Syndrome/Disease

Charcot Marie Tooth syndrome/disease is a genetically inherited disease that is the most common heritable cause of peripheral neuropathy in the UK. It occurs when the genes that are involved in making neurons and the myelin sheath are defective.

It presents in puberty with clumsiness, weakness (usually of the ankles) and foot drop (causing a high stepping gait). Pes cavus and distal atrophy of the arm and leg muscles may be seen with an inverted champagne bottle appearance on the legs.

Investigations include nerve conduction studies and genetic testing. Treatment includes physiotherapy, occupational therapy and surgery (nerve release), with most patients having mild disability and a normal lifespan.

Chronic Fatigue Syndrome (CFS)/Myalgic Encephalomyelitis (ME)

Chronic fatigue syndrome is classified as a neurological illness defined by the presence of severe, disabling fatigue. Diagnosis is based on the presence of debilitating fatigue, post-exertion malaise, unrefreshing sleep (+/- sleep disturbance) and cognitive difficulties ('brain fog') for a minimum of three months that impact on the individual's ability to engage in work, school, social and personal activities and that is not explained by another condition.

There may be additional features of autonomic dysfunction (i.e. dizziness, palpitations, fainting that may be worse on standing), nausea, muscle twitches and jerks, food and drink intolerances, hypersensitivity (sound, light, touch, taste, smell, temperature) and widespread pain (myalgia, arthralgia, headaches).

Diagnosis is made by specialist teams, and management is holistic and multidisciplinary including counselling and supportive care, energy management strategies, flare up management, psychological therapies, and individualised programmes of physical activity/exercise.

Compartment Syndrome

Compartment syndrome relates to increased pressure within a closed osteofascial compartment due to trauma, prolonged immobilisation, bleeding or infection. The resulting reduction in circulation can cause ischaemia and necrosis if left untreated.

The majority of compartment syndromes occur after fractures and can affect any number of compartments in the upper and lower limbs but most commonly the anterior tibial compartment of the leg.

A recent history of trauma or fracture, burns, blood clots, infections or a limb within a plaster cast or splint are risks for developing compartment syndrome. Symptoms include paraesthesia, swelling and tenderness with pain that worsens, despite immobilisation. It is also aggravated with passive stretching of the relevant muscles. Pallor, loss of pulse, paralysis and reduced temperature are late signs. Treatment involves removal of any splints or dressing and, in some cases, surgery to relieve the compression (fasciotomy). Diagnosis includes measuring of compartment pressures and Doppler ultrasound.

Chronic exertional compartment syndrome is a cause of exertional leg pain, most commonly in athletes, relating to raised intra-compartmental pressure. Characteristic pain and muscle tightness relating to activity with raised compartment pressures is found after exercise alongside muscle herniation and abnormal gait (pronation). Fasciotomy remains the definitive treatment, but conservative approaches including activity modification and reduced intensity of training may be useful.

Complex Regional Pain Syndrome (CRPS)

Previously known as Sudeck's atrophy, CRPS is a chronic regional pain syndrome characterised by a combination of autonomic and inflammatory features. Its precise cause is uncertain, but it is often seen following an injury (e.g. fracture or surgery to a limb) and can cause life altering disability.

Diagnosis is based on presence of key clinical symptoms that include:

- Pain – with allodynia and/or hyperalgesia
- Vasomotor changes – change in skin colour and temperature
- Sudomotor changes – localised oedema and sweating
- Motor changes – reduced range of movement, weakness, tremor and spasm
- Trophic (soft tissue) changes due to disrupted nerve supply including:
  - Hair – thicker or thinner
  - Skin – thin, shiny, clammy
  - Nails – brittle, thickened

Treatment includes a multidisciplinary approach including physiotherapy, psychology and may include bisphosphonates, neuropathic medication, sympathetic blocks and TENs.

Guillain-Barre Syndrome

Guillain – Barre syndrome describes a group of conditions characterised by inflammation and damage to peripheral nerves after an infection.

These include:

- Acute inflammatory demyelinating polyneuropathy (AIDP) – the most common type
- Acute motor axonal neuropathy (AMAN) – only affects motor nerves
- Acute motor sensory axonal neuropathy (AMSAN) – rare variant affecting both motor and sensory nerves
- Miller Fisher syndrome – ophthalmoplegia (paralysis of eye muscles), ataxia (with balance, coordination and speech difficulties) and areflexia (absence of deep tendon reflexes)

They most commonly occur following an influenza-like illness or gastroenteritis, and patients can present with back and/or leg pain with progressive, symmetrical muscle weakness that usually starts in the legs before affecting the arms. It is associated with paraesthesia in the hands and feet that occurs before developing a flaccid paralysis with hyporeflexia that usually recovers within four weeks.

A significant proportion of patients can develop respiratory muscle weakness that can be fatal. Other symptoms include slurred speech, facial weakness, visual, speech and swallowing difficulties.

Investigation includes nerve conduction studies (may show evidence of demyelination), lumbar puncture (elevated protein but normal cell count), liver function tests and spirometry. Treatment includes supportive respiratory management (including ventilation), haemodynamic support, plasma exchange and immunoglobulin therapy.

Muscular Dystrophy

Muscular dystrophy is a group of inherited conditions causing progressive muscle weakness and wasting, with Duchenne muscular dystrophy (DMD) being the most common and rapidly progressive form. It is associated with marked disability from a young age and, although life expectancy has improved, it remains a life limiting condition.

Features included delayed motor milestones, imbalance in lower limb strength, gait abnormalities (including toe walking), falls, calf hypertrophy, reduced muscle tone and tendon reflexes (but normal sensation) hyperactivity, intellectual disability, bladder and bowel incontinence, arrhythmia, respiratory compromise and Gower's sign (due to weakness of hip and knee extensors and ankle dorsiflexors).

Blood tests can show a creatinine kinase (CK) up to 50-100 higher than normal range. Further tests may include muscle biopsies and genetic testing (Xp21 mutation may be found in DMD).

Management will include multidisciplinary care focussed on maintaining and supporting mobility, corticosteroids (can delay progression), ACE inhibitors (reduce cardiac complications), surgery (tendon release), genetic counselling, family and psychological support

Myasthenia Gravis

Myasthenia gravis (MG) is an auto-immune condition with antibodies (IgG) formed against acetylcholine receptors in the post-synaptic membrane of the neuromuscular junction in skeletal muscle. This can cause weakness, usually with slowly increasing fatigue in muscles usually around the eyes and face as well as the muscles used for speech, chewing and swallowing (bulbar muscles).

Symptoms include muscle weakness that characteristically increases with exercise and is eased with rest. It is associated with double vision (diplopia), drooping eyelids (ptosis), difficulties with chewing food, nasal sounding speech, loss of facial muscles (causing a flattened smile and difficulty making facial expressions), shoulder or hip girdle weakness and, more rarely, difficulty breathing.

There are genetic links and links to changes in the thymus gland (part of the lymphatic system). Diagnosis includes looking for auto-antibodies, lung function tests, EMG, nerve stimulation tests and CT chest (looking for thymoma or thymic dysplasia found in many patients with MG).

Management includes immunosuppressive drugs (including steroids), cholinesterase inhibitors, thymectomy (for patients with thymoma) and plasmapheresis or IV immunoglobulins. Myasthenia crisis is an acute inability to swallow and difficulty breathing (triggered by infection, aspiration, surgery, trauma and some medications) that may need mechanical ventilation.

Myositis (Polymyositis/Dermatomyositis)

Myositis is the name for a group of rare conditions leading to progressive muscle weakness and pain caused by autoimmune-mediated muscle and skin damage. Features include:

- Progressive symmetrical muscle weakness and inflammation (myositis) – usually affecting the shoulder and pelvic girdle muscles
- Arthralgia and/or myalgia
- Difficulty swallowing and speaking caused by muscle weakness
- Respiratory difficulties – due to respiratory muscle weakness and lung fibrosis
- Skin changes – in dermatomyositis there is a purplish rash (mostly on the hands and face), redness of nails and red papules over the knuckles (Gottron's papules)
- There is an association of up to half of patients with dermatomyositis having a malignancy – usually gastric or ovarian

The differential diagnosis includes polymyalgia rheumatica (PMR). The key differences between the two are that PMR does not characteristically cause weakness of muscles or a rise in CK, whereas polymyositis and myositis do

Investigations include:

- Muscle biopsies – showing inflammation and necrosis in muscle
- Blood tests – raised creatinine kinase (CK), positive antinuclear antibodies (ANA) and positive anti-Jo1 and anti-Mi2 (ENA)
- EMG – shows fibrillation potentials

Management includes rest during flares and treatment of any associated tumours (ovarian or gastric). Medications used include steroids, azathioprine or methotrexate

Paraneoplastic Syndromes

Paraneoplastic syndromes are a collection of syndromes occasionally seen in patients with advanced cancer, most commonly lung, ovarian, lymphatic or breast cancer. The symptoms tend to evolve over days to weeks and may be the first symptoms encountered in a previously undiagnosed cancer.

They are not a direct result of the tumour but thought to be caused by factors including:

- Hormones secreted by tumours (e.g. hypercalcaemia caused by parathyroid hormone (PTH) secretion or Cushing's syndrome from adrenocorticotrophin hormone (ACTH) or corticotropin releasing factor (CRF) secretion)
- Tumour-related inflammation (e.g. dermatomyositis, polymyositis)
- Autoimmune responses from cells fighting the tumour cells mistakenly targeting cells in the body including those in the nervous system (e.g. antibody mediated peripheral neuropathy, Lambert Eaton myasthenic syndrome, cortical cerebellar degeneration and polymyopathy)

Other manifestations include skin changes (e.g. acanthosis nigricans and pemphigus) and hypertrophic osteoarthropathy (arthritis, periostitis and finger clubbing seen with some lung cancers).

Treatment focusses on managing the original cancer and use of immunosuppressants including corticosteroids, immunoglobulins and plasmapheresis as well as supportive care including speech and physical therapy.

Prostate Cancer

Prostate cancer is the most common cancer in men. The risk of developing it increases with age, and it mostly impacts men over the age of 50.

Investigation is prompted by the presence of lower urinary tract symptoms including difficulty starting or stopping urination (hesitancy and terminal dribbling), a weaker stream of urine, needing to pass urine during the night (nocturia) and retention of urine. Late stage/metastatic features include fatigue, weight loss, bone pain and enlarged lymph nodes.

Diagnosis of prostate cancer is suspected if these symptoms occur alongside changes in the prostate on examination (an irregularly/craggy enlarged prostate) and a rise in the prostate specific antigen (PSA). It should be considered in men when presenting with hypercalcaemia, bony pain or pathological fractures as a possible presentation of metastatic cancer.

PSA should not be tested if the patient has ejaculated or had vigorous exercise in past 48 hours nor should it be screened for in the presence of a UTI or if they have had a prostate biopsy within the last six weeks. Treatment depends on stage and spread of cancer and may involve surgery, radiotherapy or hormone therapy.

Raynaud's Phenomenon

Raynaud's phenomenon is caused by exaggerated vasospasm in the digits causing pain and well demarcated colour change, often in response to cold. The vasospasm causes ischaemia with characteristic colour changes of the digits turning white, then blue (deoxygenation) then red as they re-perfuse. The last stage is often accompanied by pain and a throbbing sensation.

In the vast majority of patients, it is primary (idiopathic), but care should be taken to screen for secondary causes such as connective tissue diseases as it is found in around half of patients with SLE, dermatomyositis or polymyositis. It is also associated with atherosclerosis and hypothyroidism.

Treatment of primary Raynaud's includes preventing the peripheries from getting cold (using warm gloves and/or socks in cold weather), smoking cessation, where relevant, and medication such as calcium channel blockers.

Sarcoidosis

Sarcoidosis is a multi-system inflammatory disorder of unknown origin involving formation of granulomas (focal areas of inflammation) in multiple organs where they can cause fibrosis and permanent damage.

This generally affects people in their 20s and 30s and may be asymptomatic. When symptomatic it can cause features including fatigue, weight loss and night sweats. It commonly affects the lungs (causing breathlessness, cough, wheeze) and may cause lymphadenopathy as well as arthritis and myopathy. Virtually any organ can be affected.

Initial investigations may include chest X-ray, blood tests (serum ACE, FBC, U&Es, LFTs) ECG and a CT scan of the chest.

Treatment may be conservative, as many resolve spontaneously or, if symptomatic, may include analgesia, steroids and TNF inhibitors (e.g. etanercept, adalimumab)

Scleroderma

Scleroderma is a group of connective tissue diseases that are divided into two main types: systemic sclerosis (a multi-system disease) and localised scleroderma (sometimes called morphoea), which only affects the skin. Scleroderma is a rare condition driven by a combination of microvascular changes, immune dysregulation and fibrosis. It generally affects women in their 40 and 50s and can co-exist with SLE, myositis or inflammatory arthritis.

Systemic sclerosis has multiple subtypes and has a widespread impact on the body with a significant increase in mortality, generally with cardiorespiratory complications.

Signs and symptoms include:

- Skin – tightening and thickening of the skin due to an accumulation of scar tissue giving it a characteristic shiny appearance. This is most often seen in the fingers with ulceration of the tips of fingers and/or toes. This can contribute to loss of movement and muscle atrophy
- Bones – osteolysis (resorption of bone) occurring most commonly in the tips of phalanges
- Raynaud's phenomenon can manifest before the development of other symptoms
- Generalised symptoms such as fatigue, weight loss, arthralgia
- Depression
- Respiratory symptoms – shortness of breath on exertion and a chronic cough caused by pulmonary fibrosis and pulmonary hypertension
- Cardiac complications – congestive cardiac failure (late-stage symptom)
- Renal failure – associated with rapidly increasing hypertension
- Gastrointestinal – oesophageal stricture and/or immobility, small bowel malabsorption

The designation 'CREST syndrome' has been used to describe a subtype of patients with:

- **C**alcinosis – deposits of calcium in skin (associated with digital ulcers)
- **R**aynaud's phenomenon – vasospasm causing pain and colour change in fingers
- **E**sophageal hypomotility – causes heartburn and problems with swallowing
- **S**clerodactyly – thickening and swelling of fingers or toes
- **T**elangiectasia – non-blanching red spots on skin

Investigations are similar to other connective tissue diseases, with blood tests including ANA (raised titre) and ENA (anti-Scl-70, anticentromere and antinucleolus antibodies found), FBC (showing anemia and elevated ESR). X-rays[1] may show calcium deposits in the fingers and resorption of bone in distal phalanges.[2]

Treatment includes DMARDs and management of individual complications (e.g. Raynaud's disease and gastrointestinal reflux).

Shingles

Shingles is an acute, self-limiting viral infection caused by the herpes zoster virus (HSV). Infection involves reactivation of the virus, which lies dormant in the ganglia of dorsal and cranial nerves from when it would have first manifested itself as chicken pox, usually caught in childhood. In adults, the virus tends to be reactivated as we age (normally over 50 years old) especially if there is a reduction in immunity (e.g. with HIV infection, malignancies, chemotherapy or use of long-term corticosteroids).

The virus causes inflammation (initially ganglionitis) that accounts for the early symptoms of pain and parasthesia lasting for two to three days followed by the virus being carried down the nerve to the skin where it causes local inflammation and eruption of vesicles in the dermatomal distribution of the nerve affected. This usually affects only one dermatome on one side of the body.

Shingles is less infectious than chicken pox but, if transmitted, can cause chicken pox in someone who has not had it before. It is non-infectious once the lesions have crusted over.

[1]Rutckowska, U. (2021). Imaging in diagnosis of systemic sclerosis. *Journal of Clinical Medicine, 10*(2), 248.

[2]Siao-Pin, S., Damian, L. O., Muntean, L. M. Rednic, S. (2016). Acroosteolysis in systemic sclerosis: an insight into hypoxia-related pathogenesis. *Experimental and Therapeutic Medicine, 12*(5), 3459-3463.

Treatment aims to reduce the severity and consequences of infection rather than eradicating the virus and is most effective if initiated early. It includes antivirals (e.g. aciclovir) with analgesia.

Complications include post-herpetic neuralgia and bacterial superinfection. In patients who are immunocompromised, infection can become widely disseminated with organ and neurological involvement with significant mortality. Shingles affecting the ophthalmic branch of the trigeminal nerve with involvement of the eye requires specialist (ophthalmology) advice due to risks of permanent visual impairment and vision loss if untreated.

A live vaccine is widely used for those over 50 years old to reduce the incidence of shingles and its complications.

Systemic Vasculitis

The term 'vasculitis' describes a group of autoimmune conditions characterised by inflammation of blood vessels that can cause problems in the organs or tissues they supply. They can affect any organ in the body and can exist on their own or related to another condition. Vasculitis can be categorised according to the size of vessels affected:

Large
- Giant cell arteritis (GCA)
- Takayasu's arteritis

Medium
- Polyarteritis nodosa (PAN) – also caused by hepatitis B
- Kawasaki disease – an acute vasculitis affecting mostly children

Small
- Anti-neutrophil cytoplasmic antibody (ANCA) associated vasculitis including:
  - Granulomatosis with polyangiitis GPA (Wegener's granulomatosis)
  - Microscopic polyangiitis (MPA)
  - Eosinophilic granulomatosis with polyangiitis (Churg-Strauss syndrome)
- Immune complex-associated
- Anti-glomerular basement membrane-associated
- Bechet's syndrome

Symptoms will vary according to which type of vasculitis and which organ is affected
- Systemic features – malaise, fever and weight loss alongside arthralgia, myalgia and headaches
- Skin changes – purpura (red or purple discoloured spots on the skin), ulcers, livedo reticularis (pink-blue mottling of skin – although this can be physiological response to cold) as well as nail infarcts and digital gangrene
- Renal changes – causing hypertension, glomerulonephritis (inflammation and damage to the glomeruli) and ultimately renal failure
- Respiratory changes – usually seen in small vessel vasculitis causing cough, blood in sputum (pulmonary haemorrhage), wheeze and breathlessness
- ENT – includes nosebleeds and nasal crusting, loss of hearing and sinus problems
- Episcleritis and/or scleritis – inflammation in and around the whites of the eye is a feature with visual loss associated more with large vessel vasculitis (e.g. GCA)
- Neurological changes – fits, confusion, altered mood and psychosis as well as motor and sensory deficits and stroke
- Gastrointestinal – mouth ulcers, diarrhoea, malabsorption and abdominal pain due to infarction of blood vessels to the gut with medium vessel involvement
- Cardiovascular – Takayasu's arteritis (a type of vasculitis predominantly affecting the aorta and its branches) causing systemic features (malaise, fatigue, fever, weight loss), limb claudication, angina, myocardial infarction and/or heart failure

Blood tests may show raised ESR, CRP and a positive ANCA. Raised creatinine and protein and/or blood on urinalysis is suggestive of renal failure.

Management includes the use of steroids and immunosuppressants to reduce inflammation, push symptoms into remission and reduce the chance of recurrence. Severe vasculitis is a medical emergency requiring same day admission to hospital to avoid end organ damage (e.g. renal failure).

Peripheral Vascular Disease

Signs of acute arterial ischaemia
- Pulseless
- Paraesthesia
- Pale
- Paralysis
- Perishingly cold
- Pain – on squeezing muscle

Signs of chronic arterial insufficiency
- Loss of hair
- Diminished pedal pulses
- Arterial ulcers
- Severe pain - usually over pressure points
- An absence of skin signs suggesting venous disease (e.g. lipodermatosclerosis)
- Often exists in the presence of known cardiovascular disease (hypercholesterolaemia, hypertension, heart disease)

Signs of chronic venous insufficiency
- Lipodermatosclerosis – pigmentation caused by haemosiderin deposition (product of blood breaking down once it comes out of vessels) – this can progress to cause thickening underneath the skin and narrowing of the distal lower limb (inverted champagne bottle appearance)
- Venous ulcers
  - Usually above the medial malleolus
  - Less painful than arterial ulcers
  - Sign of severe venous disease
- Varicose eczema

DIAGNOSTICS

5.1

Imaging

5.1.1 IR(ME)R Guidelines and Regulations

The Ionising Radiation (Medical Exposure) Regulations [IR(ME)R] are designed to protect patients from the risk of harm when being exposed to the radiation used in X-rays, nuclear scans and treatments such as radiotherapy. In the United Kingdom (UK), they are enforced by the Care Quality Commission, with the employer taking ultimate responsibility.

X-rays are a naturally occurring form of radiation, but exposure to high dose or repeated X-rays can cause changes in our DNA that may lead to cancer. The amount of damage is related to how much exposure there has been and for how long. This is quantified using the internationally recognised unit millisieverts (mSv). Background radiation (the natural radiation that is present in the environment at a particular location) is two to three mSv/year in the UK. Typically, one mSv is associated with a one in 20,000 chance of inducing cancer.

The principles of radiation exposure aim to expose the individual to the minimum dose of radiation required for the task. The amount of radiation and risks from common imaging techniques can be expressed as follows:

Procedure	Radiation Dose (mSv)	Equivalent of Background Radiation for...	Lifetime Additional Risk of Fatal Cancer Per Exam
Hand/Foot X-ray	0.001	<1.5 days	1 in a few million
DEXA Scan	0.001	<1.5 days	1 in a few million
Chest X-ray	0.02	Three days	1 in a million
Thoracic Spine X-ray	0.7	Four months	1 in 30,000
Lumbar Spine X-ray	1.5	Six months	1 in 15,000
CT Abdomen and Pelvis	10	4.5 years	1 in 2000

Statistics taken from Public Health England guidance on patient dose information. (2008). Available at https://www.gov.uk/government/publications/medical-radiation-patient-doses/patient-dose-information-guidance

5.1.2 X-Rays

X-rays are used to produce images of structures within the body, particularly bones. They are a form of naturally occurring radiation similar to light rays but of a higher energy that allows them to pass through the body.

Images are created by placing the patient (or part of the patient) between an X-ray emitter and an X-ray detector (or radiographic film). X-rays are absorbed to varying degrees by different tissues in the body (i.e. they easily pass through air-filled cavities like the lungs and bowel as well as soft tissues like muscle and fat but are almost completely absorbed by harder tissues such as bone). The rays that pass through easily turn the radiographic film black, whereas those that are absorbed or partially absorbed will leave the film white or shades of grey, giving us a picture of internal structures.

Advantages

- X-rays are cheap (much cheaper than computed tomography and magnetic resonance imaging)
- Does not take long to do
- Widely available – in hospitals and community settings and portable X-ray units
- Non-invasive
- No significant contraindications (apart from abdominal or pelvic imaging in pregnancy)
- Can identify fractures or dislocations, bony asymmetry and deformity, and congenital anomalies of the joints and spine like scoliosis, spina bifida and vertebral deformities
- Can identify degenerative changes (osteoarthritis) in the form of joint space narrowing, marginal osteophytes and bony sclerosis
- Bone tumours (benign and malignant) may be identifiable in the form of lytic (black) or sclerotic (white) lesions
- X-rays have a screening role (e.g. mammograms that can identify more radiopaque masses and calcification within the breast tissue that might suggest a tumour)
- They can also be used therapeutically:
    - Fluoroscopic guided interventions using real-time X-rays to guide interventions such as spinal epidural injections and medial branch block denervations
    - Radiotherapy – using a much higher dose of radiation to destroy cancerous cells by disrupting their DNA

Limitations

- Poor visualisation of soft tissue structures
- Factors like obesity and excessive bowel gases may obscure some abnormalities or make the interpretation of X-rays difficult
- X-rays are a source of radiation to the patient, with increased risk when used on children

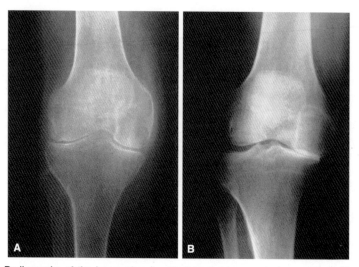

Fig 5.1.2.1 Radiographs of the knees showing the two most common forms of arthritis. (A) Severe rheumatoid arthritis with almost complete loss of joint space (B) Typical osteoarthritis with near-total loss of joint space in one compartment and a normal joint space in the other. From Goldman, L., Ausiello, D. (2004). *Cecil textbook of medicine* (22nd ed.). Philadelphia: WB Saunders.

5.1.3   Computed Tomography

Computed tomography (CT) works by using X-rays fired in a narrow beam that is quickly rotated around the patient's body toward digital X-ray receptors. This generates a series of X-ray images that are then fed into a computer to create cross-sectional images known as 'tomographic' images. These images can be collated into three-dimensional pictures that can help with diagnosis and with planning procedures and interventions. CT images will contain more information than standard X-rays.

Advantages

- Excellent depiction of bone anatomy and changes seen in a range of bone pathologies (e.g. complex bone fractures, severely eroded joints or bone tumours). These are often seen on CT before they are visible on X-rays
- More widely available and accessible than MRI
- Cheaper than MRI
- Does not take long to do
- Can be used safely in patients with metallic implants, shells, and magnetic fixation devices and used when an MRI scan may be contraindicated
- Can be used to detect calcification in soft tissues, including muscles and tendons
- CT has certain organ-specific uses, including:
  - Detecting possible tumours or pathologies within the abdomen
  - Identifying various types of cardiac disease
  - Locating injuries, tumours, clots leading to stroke or signs of haemorrhage in the head
  - Identifying tumours, pulmonary embolisms (blood clots), excess fluid and other conditions such as emphysema or infection in the lungs

Limitations

- High risk of radiation exposure – a standard CT delivers a significant amount of radiation dose to the patient (almost 100 times that of a chest X-ray)
- Not as good as MRI at defining soft tissues
- Artefacts from metallic fixation devices or shells may badly affect the quality of the image and can obscure some anatomical and pathological findings
- As it uses X-rays, precautions are taken to avoid abdominal or pelvic CT scans in pregnant women and are avoided in children, if possible

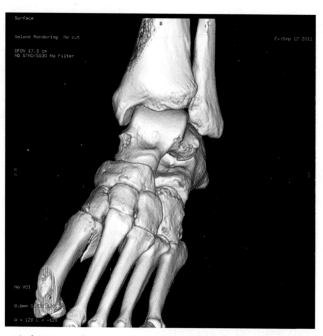

Fig 5.1.3.2 Computed tomography scan three-dimensional reconstruction demonstrating Lisfranc injury with fracture at the base of the first and second metatarsal. From Rynders, S. D., Hart, J. A. (2022). *Orthopaedics for physician assistants* (2nd ed.). Philadelphia: Elsevier.

5.1.4   Ultrasound

Ultrasound (US) works by using a transducer that produces high-frequency sound waves at far higher frequencies than those detectable by the human ear. The US probe is placed on the skin, with the application of a gel for better transmission of the sound waves. The sound waves pass into the body, where they are then reflected off organs and tissues and detected by the US transducer and transformed into a real-time image on the screen. The probe is manipulated to identify relevant anatomy and get more information about the structures using different angles and planes.

The different tissues of the body reflect the sound waves differently, allowing for discrimination between tissues. Bone and fat reflect sound very well (hyperechoic), creating a bright signal seen as white on the screen, whereas sound waves pass through cartilage and muscle more easily (hypoechoic), creating a darker signal, seen as grey regions on the screen. Fluid and fluid-filled structures, like blood vessels, do not reflect the sound waves at all (anechoic) and appear as a black signal on the screen.

Advantages

- Cheap
- Non-invasive (in most musculoskeletal applications)
- Dynamic assessment of structures – joints and tissues can be moved, and observation of pathological changes can be made in real time. Patients are able to provide feedback during the assessment, allowing functional assessment
- Portable – US machines can be moved around easily within clinic settings or pitch-side, allowing for 'point of care ultrasound' (POCUS)
- The ability to discriminate between soft tissues means it can be helpful to guide interventions (e.g. aspiration and injection of bursae and joint spaces)
- No ionising radiation or contrast dyes are used
- Can be used to:
  - Assess the presence of synovitis in suspected inflammatory arthritis
  - Identify soft tissue trauma and damage (e.g. muscle injuries and tendinopathies)
  - Discern the nature of soft tissue masses (if fluid-filled or solid)
  - Detect effusions within joints and bursae and enable aspiration
  - Identify nerve changes (e.g. identification of Morton's neuroma)
- May be used in acute or emergency care settings as a 'focused assessment with sonography for trauma' to identify free fluid in the abdomen as a sign of damage to internal abdominal organs and vessels and pericardial effusions

Limitations

- Obese patients – imaging of deeper structures is limited in patients with large amounts of subcutaneous fat or muscle
- Artefact – any angulation of the probe away from 90° to the target creates a loss of reflected sound waves (anisotropy) and reduced signal creating a falsely hypoechoic signal. Very hyperechoic structures like bone can also create a 'shadow,' reducing accurate visualisation of the structures behind them

- Diagnostic US is very operator dependent and is only as good as the person holding the probe. Whilst images can be captured and stored, the real-time visualisation of structures means it is hard for another clinician to be able to interpret them after the examination
- The standard of the images is dependent on the quality of the equipment used. Low-quality images can compromise their ability to be effective diagnostic tools

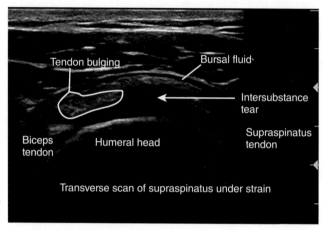

Fig 5.1.4.3 Example of a transverse ultrasound image obtained during dynamic ultrasound imaging demonstrating impingement of the supraspinatus musculotendinous unit. From Waldman, S. (2021). *Physical diagnosis of pain: An atlas of signs and symptoms* (4th ed.). Philadelphia: Elsevier.

5.1.5 Dual Energy X-Ray Absorptiometry

Also known as a bone density scan, a Dual Energy X-ray Absorptiometry (DEXA) scan involves passing low-dose X-rays through selected regions of bone to assess how much radiation passes through as a measure of bone density. This uses small amounts of radiation, less than the equivalent of two days of normal background radiation.

There are different types of bone density scans. Usually, they involve X-rays of the hip and lumbar spine. The is because these areas tend to be vulnerable to osteoporotic fractures, and assessment of these regions can help predict the likelihood of future fractures. When X-rays cannot be done on the hip or spine, then bone density can be tested on peripheral bones (e.g. the radius).

Results are expressed as the number of standard deviations (SD) between:
- The individual being tested and a healthy young adult – the T score
- The individual being tested and someone of the same age – the Z score

The higher the standard difference, the lower the bone mineral density. The T score is needed for diagnosis, according to the World Health Organization, whereas the Z score is used more to give a clinician an idea of risk compared to an age-matched population.

Interpreting T Scores

- Above -1 SD is normal (i.e. between 0 and -1)
- Between -1 and -2.5 SD is defined as mildly reduced bone mineral density compared with peak bone mass (osteopenia)
- At or below -2.5 SD (T score) is diagnostic of osteoporosis

Advantages

- Cheap
- Non-invasive
- Widely available
- Good reproducibility and standardisation
    - Allows repeated assessment to quantify response to treatment

Limitations

- Accuracy may be limited in certain groups:
    - Those with significant degenerative changes
    - Previous spinal surgery
    - Very obese patients
    - Patients taking corticosteroids

5.1.6   Magnetic Resonance Imaging

Magnetic resonance imaging (MRI) works by placing the body in a very strong magnetic field that causes the hydrogen ions found in cells throughout the body to align with the magnetic field. Their direction is then altered by applying a radiofrequency pulse which, when turned off, allows the ions to then realign with the magnetic field and release a signal that is picked up by the MRI sensors. The signal strength varies depending on what tissue the hydrogen ions are in (bone, fat and muscle), allowing for subsequent discrimination between them. Contrast agents like gadolinium can be given during the scan to speed up how quickly the hydrogen ions realign, giving a brighter signal. MRI has a wide range of uses in musculoskeletal medicine and neurology and is often the diagnostic medium of choice due to its superior views of soft tissues.

The machine can be adjusted to suppress or enhance certain signals, which can be useful in providing information in a range of clinical presentations. The two basic types of MRI are T1-weighted and T2-weighted images (often referred to as T1 and T2 images), which refers to different timings of the radiofrequency pulse sequences. T1 images highlight fat tissue within the body, so it appears bright, whilst fluids appear dark. T2 images highlight fat and water within the body, so both are highlighted on the scan.

- Vascular structures (e.g. blood vessels or highly vascular tissues like tumours) can be further enhanced by the use of gadolinium in T2 images. Fat can also be 'suppressed' to help differentiate boundaries between fat and soft tissue or bone marrow tumours
- Short tau inversion recovery (STIR) sequences can be used to better enhance oedema in tissues (e.g. around fractures in bone or inflammation in joints) by manipulating T2 images to not just suppress but completely remove the high signal from fat.

Advantages

- MRI does not use ionising radiation like CT or X-rays (this is particularly helpful if repeated imaging is required)
- Superior visualisation of soft tissues compared to regular X-rays and CT
- Can be used to investigate:
  - Rotator cuff injury (tendinopathy and/or tear)
  - Avascular necrosis
  - Biceps tendon injury (tendinopathy and/or tear)
  - Inflammatory processes
  - Tumours
  - Muscle atrophy or denervation
  - Fracture

Limitations

- It tends to be more expensive than CT or X-ray imaging
- It takes longer to gather the images
- If the subject moves during the scan, it can reduce the quality and value of resultant images, known as 'movement artefact'
- Because of the strong magnetic field, patients must remove any external metalwork (piercings, rings, belts and keys). It is contraindicated for anyone with metalwork in their body, including pacemakers, nerve stimulators, implantable cardioverter-defibrillators, loop recorders, insulin pumps, cochlear implants, deep brain stimulators and capsules from capsule

endoscopy. Some metallic implants are compatible with MRI (e.g. hip replacements), but this needs to be checked
- Contrast agents can cause problems for people with significant renal failure
- The scans can be very noisy, with patients normally requiring ear defenders. This can be very disturbing for some patients
- Being placed in a narrow tube can cause claustrophobia, anxiety and distress among patients
- Whilst there is little evidence of harm to a foetus, it is generally avoided during the first trimester of pregnancy, especially when contrast agents may be used

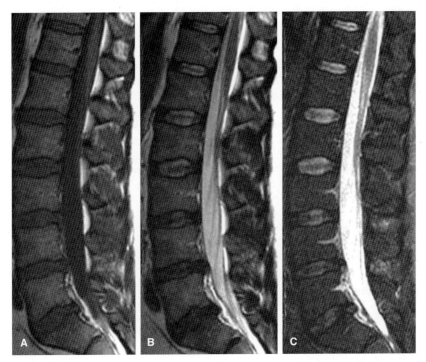

Fig 5.1.6.4 MRI sequences. The images through the lumbar spine demonstrate the different appearances obtained with different techniques. (A) Sagittal T1-weighted image (B) T2-weighted image (C) Short tau inversion recovery (STIR) sequence. From Winn, H. R. (2022). *Youmans & Winn neurological surgery* (8th ed.). Philadelphia: Elsevier.

5.1.7   Radioisotope Bone Scans

A radioisotope bone scan is also known as a radionuclide scan, bone scintigraphy or nuclear medicine scan. It is designed to pick up increased metabolic activity within bones and joints by using radioisotopes, such as 99 mTc (phosphate molecules labelled with the radioactive isotope of technetium), that are injected intravenously and absorbed into bone. The amount of tracer absorbed by bones is proportionate to blood flow and osteoblastic activity. Areas of increased uptake are detectable as the radioactive tracer gives off gamma rays as it decays. These show up as 'hot spots' on special scanners called a gamma camera.

Advantages

- The sensitivity of the scan is high if it involves osteoblastic activity and can identify pathologies earlier than other imaging modalities
- Is useful as a 'survey' technique to assess large areas of the body for pathology (e.g. bone metastases)
- Bone scans are useful for investigating a wide range of pathologies, including:
  - Malignancies: osteoblastic primary and secondary bone cancers
  - Infection: osteomyelitis, discitis and septic arthritis
  - Vascular pathologies: avascular necrosis or bone infarction
  - Metabolic disease: Paget's disease, osteomalacia
  - Benign tumours (e.g. osteoid osteoma)
  - Inflammatory disease: inflammatory arthropathies
  - Fractures: degree of uptake reduces with time in a healing fracture so it can identify new or old fractures (e.g. vertebral fracture)
  - Identification of pars defects (when used with SPECT)

Limitations

- Because absorption is increased in any regions with increased osteoblastic activity, it is not specific to any single pathology and may require other imaging to support a diagnosis
- Two-dimensional images give poor spatial resolution
- High dose of radiation
- They are contraindicated in pregnancy
- They are avoided in breastfeeding
- Radioisotopes can cause an allergic reaction
- They are not as useful in pathologies with a predominantly osteoclastic process, resulting in lytic lesions (e.g. multiple myeloma) that are unlikely to concentrate the tracer
- It can be hard to distinguish pathological change from a physiological healing process if there has been trauma or surgery to the region of interest within the previous six to 12 months

5.1.8 Positron Emission Tomography

Positron emission tomography (PET) scans use radioisotopes that are injected into the bloodstream to detect areas of the body with increased metabolic activity. They are most commonly used in the assessment and detection of cancers but may also be used in the assessment of epilepsy and dementia and for planning cardiac surgery (coronary artery bypass grafts).

PET scans usually involve the use of a radioactive labelled sugar which, once introduced to the bloodstream, will follow the increased blood flow to tissues and cells that are more metabolically active (e.g. cancer). These radioisotopes produce positrons as they decay. These positrons react with electrons in the body and produce photons that are then picked up by the PET scanner to create three-dimensional images.

5.1.9   Single Photon Emission Computed Tomography

Single photon emission computed tomography (SPECT) scans involve injecting radioisotopes into the bloodstream that emit gamma rays, which are detected using a gamma camera. This is different from a PET scan as the radioactive tracer remains in the blood rather than being absorbed by tissues. They are used to help with conditions characterised by increased blood flow in certain regions of the body. For example, in epilepsy, they can show increased blood flow to certain areas of the brain, and in cardiac conditions, they can pick up changes in the blood supply to the heart tissue. In musculoskeletal health, they are used to better identify less obvious fractures, bone infections and bone tumours or metastases, where they are valuable in clarifying if a lesion is aggressive or not. They can also be used to identify changes in complex regional pain syndrome where there may be increased blood flow thought to relate to abnormal sympathetic activity.

They are often used in combination with a standard CT scan (when it is called a SPECT-CT scan), or standard radioisotope bone scans to gain more information and improve the ability to detect pathologies.

Nerve Conduction Studies and Electromyography

Nerve conduction studies (NCS) and electromyography (EMG) can help locate and characterise problems in peripheral nerves and muscles by measuring their electrical activity and, in the case of motor nerves, the electrical activity in the muscles they supply.

NCS use electrodes attached to the skin to generate a signal that is detected by electrodes distal to the source of stimulation. EMG activity can be measured in a whole muscle using surface electrodes or a smaller area of muscle using needle electrodes inserted into the muscle during activity or at rest.

There are two main components measured:

- The propagated nerve action potential (NAP) – the electrical signal as it runs down the nerve
- A compound muscle action potential (CMAP) – the collective electrical activity of a muscle in response to the action potentials

They assess for features including:

- The speed of the action potential along a nerve (conduction velocity)
- The size of the response of the muscle (size of the CMAP)
- The time it takes for the muscle to respond to the arrival of the action potential (aka the 'latency') - most affected by demyelinating processes
- If there is any variation in the muscle response between stimulation points along the nerve (known as a conduction block)
- Sensory NAP (SNAP) - changes may indicate axonal loss
- F-waves - unique to motor nerves, these measure the part of the electrical impulse that travels back towards the nerve root identifying conditions such as Guillain-Barre disease

Advantages

- Helps identify and characterise the nature of nerve or muscle pathology, identifying demyelination, axonal loss or both
- Informs prognosis and the likelihood of recovery in nerve injury
- Monitors disease progression

Limitations

- They only measure medium to large motor and sensory nerves (e.g. motor fibres and sensory fibres for vibration and joint position sense). Activity in smaller unmyelinated fibres (involved in pain and temperature sensation) is not picked up accurately with these studies

- Physiological variation and activity, including spontaneous fibrillation in muscles, can confuse the interpretation
- Accuracy in the placement of electrodes and their stability, limb position and temperature can affect the accuracy
- It is important that the right equipment and settings are used
- The results require interpretation by an experienced clinician (often a neurologist) in combination with the clinical picture

Summary of Blood Tests

All reference ranges quoted here relate to adults unless otherwise specified. Please be aware that values may vary between laboratories, in certain populations and are prone to change so should be used as a guide only.

Test	Normal Range	Purpose/Indication	Interpretation
Alanine amino-transferase (ALT)	5–35 IU/L	Useful predominantly to identify and monitor liver disease as it is found in cells of liver but also in heart, kidney and skeletal muscle (anything causing damage to these organs will cause it to be released into bloodstream)	Increased Mildly: • Myositis • Pancreatitis • Myocardial infarction • Infectious mononucleosis (EBV) • Shock • Injury to liver/heart/kidney/muscle Moderately: • Cirrhosis • Malignancy • Obstructive jaundice • Hepatotoxic drugs • Severe burns • Significantly raised: • Hepatitis • Hepatic necrosis • Hepatic ischaemia
Albumin (Alb)	35–50 g/L	Main protein in blood. Helps to maintain osmotic pressure in blood. Transports blood constituents such as fatty acids, hormones, enzymes and other substances	Increased: • Dehydration Decreased: • Acute/inflammatory illness • Urinary protein loss • Advanced liver disease • Gastrointestinal loss • Severe malnutrition

Continued on following page

Test	Normal Range	Purpose/Indication	Interpretation
Alkaline phosphatase (ALP)	30–130 IU/L	Used to detect and monitor diseases including of liver and bone It is seen in active osteoblasts, so increases in childhood, puberty and in healing fractures It is also produced by the placenta and in membranes of bile ducts in liver It can also be raised after a recent meal	Increased: • Liver disease. If so, expect a rise in gamma-glutamyl transpeptidase (GGT) (as well as AST/ALT) • Bone and other diseases, including cancer (primary/secondary), Paget's disease, hyperparathyroidism, renal failure, thyrotoxicosis, rheumatoid arthritis (RA), osteomalacia/rickets and Crohn's/ulcerative colitis • Puberty (up to 650 U/L) • Pregnancy (up to 400 U/L) • Transient hyperphosphatasaemia of childhood (up to 30 000 U/L for up to 3/12) • Familial benign hyperphosphatasaemia Decreased: • Malnutrition • Milk-alkali syndrome • Pernicious anaemia • Vitamin C deficiency (scurvy)
Anti-nuclear antibodies (ANA)	Result is described as a titre	Screening for SLE (positive in 95% of cases)	<1:40=negative 1:40 or 1:80=borderline >1:160=consistent with autoimmune disease
Anti-cyclic citrullinated peptide (Anti-CCP)	Positive or negative	Is a type of autoantibody that targets a protein (citrullinated protein) that is found in some people's joints Useful to help diagnose RA Better specificity than rheumatoid factor	+ in 60%-70% of people who get RA, needs interpretation in context but can indicate: • Risk of developing RA in a healthy person • Better than rheumatoid factor at predicting those in early stages of arthritis who will develop RA In those who are RA +ve, anti-CCP predicts an increased chance of erosive disease
Anti-DNA antibodies	Result is described as a titre	Positive in 60%–80% of SLE also present in low titres in RA, autoimmune hepatitis and other immune disorders	<1:20 or 1:40 equivocal >1:80 supports a diagnosis of SLE

Test	Normal Range	Purpose/Indication	Interpretation
Aspartate transaminase (AST)	5–35 IU/L	Enzyme found in heart, liver, pancreas, skeletal muscle, kidney and red blood cells Damage to any of these organs causes a release of this enzyme into bloodstream	Increased: <ul><li>Liver disease</li><li>Myocardial Infarction (increases 6–12 h post-MI, peaking at 24–36 h)</li><li>Congestive cardiac failure</li><li>Trauma</li><li>Muscular dystrophy</li><li>Dermatomyositis</li><li>Haemolysis</li><li>Renal infarction</li><li>Acute pancreatitis</li><li>After surgery/IM injections</li><li>Hypothyroidism</li></ul> Decreased: <ul><li>Severe/end-stage liver disease (no further enzyme to release)</li></ul>
Basophils	0.0–0.10 ×10/L	Smallest group of white cells Circulate in bloodstream and migrate into tissues becoming mast cells Significant role in immediate hypersensitivity reactions (including anaphylaxis)	Increased: <ul><li>Viral infections</li><li>Urticaria</li><li>Post-splenectomy</li><li>Hypothyroidism</li><li>Ulcerative colitis</li><li>Systemic mastocytosis</li><li>Malignancy</li><li>Myeloproliferative disorders:<ul><li>Chronic myeloid leukaemia</li><li>Myelofibrosis</li><li>Polycythaemia rubra vera</li></ul></li><li>Haemolysis</li></ul>
Bilirubin	3–17 μmol/L	Breakdown product of red cells Normally metabolised by liver into a water-soluble form and excreted via kidneys	Increased: <ul><li>Haemolysis</li><li>Gilberts disease (impaired conjugation)</li><li>Jaundice</li><li>Physiological</li><li>Breastfeeding</li><li>Haemolytic disease of newborns</li></ul>
Ca 15-3	Reference range may be supplied with report or reported as 'normal' or 'raised'	Tumour marker	Found in breast cancer (also raised in other benign and malignant conditions)
Ca 19-9	< 40 kU/L	Tumour marker	Found in pancreatic cancer (and other gastrointestinal (GI) malignancies)

Continued on following page

Test	Normal Range	Purpose/Indication	Interpretation
Ca 125	Age related reference ranges supplied with report or reported as 'normal' or 'raised'	Tumour marker	Found in ovarian cancer. Also lung, pancreas, colon and uterine cancer (also raised in endometriosis, PID, cirrhosis and pregnancy) NICE recommend pelvic ultrasound in females with Ca 125 >35 kU/L alongside symptoms (pelvic mass, abdominal pain/ bloating and increased urinary frequency)
Calcium (corrected)	2.12–2.60 mmol/L	Essential mineral used in formation of bone and teeth, muscle contraction, normal functioning of a number of enzymes, blood clotting and normal heart rhythm	Hypercalcaemia • Primary hyperparathyroidism • Malignancy (myeloma, breast, lung, kidney, thyroid, prostate, ovary or colon) • Chronic renal failure
Carcino embryonic antigen (CEA)	Age related reference ranges supplied with report	Tumour marker	Found in colorectal, pancreatic, breast, lung, small intestine, stomach and ovarian cancer
Cholesterol	<5 mmol/L	Has a role in cell membranes and as a precursor of steroid hormones and bile salts. It is found in certain foods and synthesised in liver and is associated with cardiovascular disease (and gallstone production)	Primary hyperlipidaemia • Predominantly genetically inherited Secondary hyperlipidaemia • Hypothyroidism • Obesity • Steroids • Diabetes • Alcohol • Biliary obstruction • Drugs (beta-blockers/ thiazide diuretics)
Complement (C3 and C4)	Reference range may be supplied with report	Proteins within complement cascade that are involved in cell lysis, marking cells for destruction (opsonisation) and clearance of immune complexes	Increased: • Bacterial infection • Inflammatory conditions (RA, spondyloarthropathies) Decreased: • SLE • Inherited syndromes (hereditary hypocomplementemic syndrome)
C-reactive protein (CRP)	<5 mg/L	Acute phase protein Made in liver stimulated by action of cytokines (IL1/6 and TNF) Increases within 4–6 h of onset of inflammation, doubling every 8 h, but has a short half-life (4–7 h)	Increased: • Inflammation • Autoimmune disease • Malignancy • Tissue injury • Obesity • Infection. Bacterial infections will cause a greater rise in CRP (150–350 mg/L) compared to a viral infection

Test	Normal Range	Purpose/Indication	Interpretation
Creatinine (Cr)	70–100 μmol/L	Breakdown product from muscle and protein metabolism and influenced by diet (meat) Excreted by the kidneys	Steadily increases with age as a measure of deteriorating glomerular filtration rate. Anything that increases creatinine or reduces the kidneys' ability to clear it will increase it. Used to monitor renal disease/diabetic renal disease/transplants and monitoring nephrotoxic drugs (including NSAIDs)
Creatinine kinase (CK)	Males 5–190 U/L Females 5–165 U/L	CK is found mostly in heart muscle, skeletal muscle and brain and can be used as a marker of damage to cells in these structures Levels tend to rise at around 6 h after injury and reach a peak at 18 h before returning to normal	Increased: • Myocardial infarction • Myopathies, including myositis • Vigorous exercise • Cardioversion • Chronic alcoholism Surgery and repeated IM injections
Estimated glomerular filtration rate (eGFR in mL/min/1.73m^2)	Chronic kidney disease: stage 1: (normal) >90 stage 2: 60–89 stage 3a: 45–59 stage 3b: 30–44 stage 4: 15–29 stage 5: <15 (severe)	Uses rate of glomerular filtration as a means to assess kidney function It is measured in millilitres per minute/1.73m^2	Decreases with: • Age • Renal disease • Diabetes • Hypertension • Medication e.g. NSAIDs, ACE inhibitors, diuretics and others
Eosinophils	0.004–0.4 ×10^9/L	Pro-inflammatory cells with a significant role in allergies, parasitic infections and some cancers	Increased: • Allergy • Drug effects • Parasitic infections • Tuberculosis • Malignancies (lymphoma, Hodgkin's, ovarian)
Erythrocyte sedimentation rate (ESR)	Men <10 Women <15	Non-specific measure of disease (including inflammation)	Increased: • Inflammation (infection, RA) • Malignancy • Myocardial infarction • Anaemia (and macrocytosis) • Age • Female gender • Pregnancy Decreased: • Polycythaemia • Microcytosis • Sickle-cell anaemia
Extractable nuclear antigens (ENA)	Anti Ro, anti La, RNP, Scl 70, Jo 1, Mi2	Assessed in conjunction with ANA, it is possible to extract some of nuclear antigens and test patient's serum to see if they have antibodies against them. This can add information to aid diagnosis but is not diagnostic on its own	Found in: • Sjögren's disease • SLE • Polymyositis • RA • Diffuse scleroderma • CREST

Continued on following page

Test	Normal Range	Purpose/Indication	Interpretation
Folate (aka Vitamin B9)	0.36– 1.44 µmol/L	A dietary vitamin found in liver and dark green leafy vegetables). It is important for red cell synthesis and a cause of anaemia when low	Low in: • Alcohol misuse • Pregnancy • Malabsorptive disorders
Gamma-glutamyl transpeptidase (GGT)	*Males* 25–195 u/L *Females* 7–33 u/L	Liver enzyme found in all liver cells. Useful to differentiate between bone and liver causes of a raised ALP (raised GGT linked with liver disease)	Increased: • Excessive alcohol use (but can be normal in chronic alcoholism) • Cholestatic disorders • Medication (e.g. anticonvuslants)
Glucose (fasting)	3.5–5.5 mmol/L	One of the body's fuel sources From the building blocks of carbohydrates found in bread, fruit, rice and vegetables	Has been used to diagnose diabetes (if fasting levels >7.0 mmol/L or 2 h post – prandial levels are >11.1 mmol/L)
Glycosylated haemoglobin (HbA1c)	Normal: <42 mmol/ mol (6%)	Is used to diagnose diabetes and as a measure of longer-term blood sugar control (over the previous three months). It measures glycosylation of haemoglobin, which is affected by blood glucose concentration	Prediabetes: 42 to 47 mmol/mol (6.0% − 6.4%) Diabetes: 48 mmol/mol + (6.5% +)
Haemoglobin (Hb)	*Men* 130–180 g/L *Women* 115–160 g/L	Measure of main component in red cells responsible for gas transfer. Increased or decreased levels can indicate disease and guide treatment Anaemia can be classified according to size of red cells, which changes characteristically with different types of anaemia This is described as mean cell volume (MCV) and described as being normal-sized (normocytic), larger (microcytic) or smaller (microcytic) than normal	Increased (polycythaemia): • Primary • Polycythaemia rubra vera • Secondary • Chronic respiratory disease • Congenital heart disease • High altitude Decreased (anaemia): • Microcytic (MCV<75 fL) ◦ Iron deficiency anaemia (bleeding, cancer, menses, malabsorption, pregnancy) ◦ Anaemia of chronic disease ◦ Rarely thalassaemia, sideroblastic anaemia, hyperthyroidism • Normocytic (MCV 76–96 fL) ◦ If alongside pancytopaenia may indicate bone marrow failure ◦ Normal or reduced reticulocytes: chronic inflammatory disease, hypothyroidism, chronic kidney disease, liver disease, haemochromatosis ◦ Raised reticulocytes: haemolytic anaemia, bleeding • Macrocytic (MCV >6 fL) ◦ Megaloblastic: B12/folate deficiency ◦ Non-megaloblastic: alcohol misuse, liver disease, hypothyroidism (severe), reticulocytosis, drugs (e.g. azathioprine)

Test	Normal Range	Purpose/Indication	Interpretation
High-density lipoprotein (HDL)	>1.0 mmol/L	Lipids (cholesterol, phospholipids and triglycerides) need to be linked with proteins in complexes (called lipoproteins) to enable transport around the body Lipoproteins vary in size. The smaller the size, the higher the density of lipids, from very low-density lipoprotein [VLDL] to high-density [HDL]). HDL is anti-atherogenic (i.e. its concentration is *inversely* related to risk of cardiovascular disease [possibly because it has a role in transporting cholesterol from tissues to the liver]	Decreased: • Smoking • Obesity (visceral fat especially) • Very low-fat diets • The presence of high triglycerides (that promote transfer of cholesterol from HDL to VLDL) • Metabolic syndrome (as a risk factor) • Genetic inherited (e.g. familial hypoalphalipoproteinaemia)
HLA B-27 (human leucocyte antigen)	Positive or negative	Human leucocyte antigens are proteins found on the surface of white blood cells. Their role is to help identify differences between our own healthy tissues and foreign/dangerous substances. HLA B27 causes white cells to attack our own healthy cells in error (termed 'autoimmune disease')	Found in 7%–10% in general (healthy) population but seen in: • Ankylosing spondylitis (95%–98%) • Reiter's disease (90%) • Arthropathies related to Crohn's/UC (70%) • Juvenile idiopathic arthritis • Anterior uveitis
Human chorionic gonadotrophin (HCG IU/L)	• Non-pregnant females <5 • Male <2	Hormone produced by placental cells in pregnancy and tumours, including testicular tumours, choriocarcinoma, hydatiform mole and trophoblastic disease	Peaks of up to 200,000 at around 10 to 12 weeks of pregnancy
Lactate dehydrogenase (LDH)	100–250 U/L	Enzyme found in liver, myocardium, skeletal muscle and red blood cells	Increased: • Lymphoma • Myocardial infarction • Tumours (germ cell) • Megaloblastic anaemia (low B12/folate) • Liver disease (especially hepatitis) • Skeletal muscle damage
Low-density lipoprotein (LDL)	<2.5 mmol/L	A lipid storage molecule Accounts for two-thirds to four-fifths of serum cholesterol Mostly stores cholesterol (very little triglyceride) and is the main transport mechanism of cholesterol out of the liver LDL interacts with HDL and passes cholesterol to HDL. These relatively 'empty' particles are atherogenic (increased lipid deposition in arteries) associated with vascular disease and are often raised alongside triglycerides even in normal total cholesterol	Increased: • Familial hypercholesterolaemia • Diet (e.g. trans fats, vegetable oil) • Hypothyroidism • Medication: thiazide diuretics, beta-blockers, steroids, contraceptives • Renal disease • Diabetes

Continued on following page

Test	Normal Range	Purpose/Indication	Interpretation
Lymphocytes	1.0–4.5 ×10⁹/L	Important immune cells (T and B cells), part of adaptive immune response, involved in production of antibodies and identifying infected cells	Increased: • Viral infections (EBV, Hepatitis, CMV) • Chronic lymphocytic leukaemia (CLL) Decreased: • Viral illness (!) • Pancytopaenia • Hodgkin's lymphoma • Congestive cardiac failure • AIDs • Steroid therapy
Mean corpuscular volume (MCV)	76–96 fL	Indicator of red blood cell disease Helpful in identifying different causes of anaemia	Macrocytosis (increased size >98 fL) • B12/folate deficiency • Reticulocytosis • Alcoholism • Liver disease • Myeloma • Hypothyroidism • COPD • Myelodysplasia • Cytotoxic drugs (e.g. hydroxyurea) Microcytosis (microcytic anaemia) • Iron deficiency • Thalassaemia trait

Monocytes	0.2–0.8 × 10⁹/L	Multiple roles in adaptive immune system (replenishing macrophage stores) respond to infection, inflammation and cancers	Increased:
			• rarely in isolation but can be seen in
			  ◦ Chronic myeloid leukaemia
			  ◦ Infections (e.g. TB)
			  ◦ Polycythaemia rubra vera

Test	Normal Range	Purpose/Indication	Interpretation
Neutrophils	$2.0–7.5 \times 10^9$/L	They are the most abundant cells of the immune response, designed to travel in the blood-stream to fight infection. Neutropenia (low neutrophils) is considered mild when $<2 \times 10^9$, but if below 0.5×10^9, there is a significantly increased risk of spontaneous infection (much more so when below 0.2×10^9)	Increased: (neutrophilia) • Infection • Injury • Inflammation • Malignancy • Drugs (steroids, heparin, adrenaline) • Haemorrhage • Metabolic disorders Decreased: (neutropenia) • Viral infection • Typhoid • Sepsis • B12/folate deficiency • Aplastic anaemia • Malignancy (haematological or bone marrow) • Immune-mediated (e.g. post viral, SLE) • Hypertension • Thyrotoxicosis • Medication: chemotherapy but also phenothiazines, carbamazepine, chlorpromazine, thiazides, sulphonamides, indomethacin
Parathyroid hormone (PTH)	1.0–6.0 pmol/L	Hormone produced by parathyroid glands that act on kidneys and bones to increase calcium as part of bone metabolism	Increased (alongside elevated calcium) • Primary hyperparathyroidism (adenoma 85%; hyperplasia 15%) • Lithium therapy • Familial benign hypocalciuric hypercalcaemia Increased (without raised calcium) • Renal failure (secondary hyperparathyroidism) • Vitamin D deficiency
Phosphate	Adults 0.80–1.50 mmol/L	Used in cases of hypercalcaemia and in renal failure to help identify cause	Increased: • Sample error (haemolysed sample) • Renal failure • Increased intake (IV therapy and vitamin D excess) • Hypoparathyroidism Decreased: • Hypercalcaemia (associated with hyperparathyroidism/malignancy) • Alcoholism • Antacids (aluminium containing), nutritional recovery • Post-diabetic acidosis

Continued on following page

Test	Normal Range	Purpose/Indication	Interpretation
Plasma viscosity (PV)	1.50–1.72 mPa/s	An alternative to ESR in many labs	Increased: • Inflammation/infection • RA • Malignancy • Myocardial infarction • Anaemia • Macrocytosis Decreased: • Polycythaemia • Microcytosis • Sickle-cell anaemia
Platelets (Plt)	150–400 x 10⁹/L	Contribute to formation of blood clots; hence low platelets increases the risk of bleeding 0–20 × 10⁹/L = severe and potentially life-threatening and requires action (referral to haematology) Increased platelets are increasingly seen as a risk marker for cancer, so important to think of this if noted on FBC	Increased (thrombocytosis): • Blood loss • Surgery • Trauma • Infection • Inflammation • Malignancy • Myeloproliferative disorders • Polycythaemia • Thrombocythaemia Decreased (thrombocytopaenia): • Infection (often marked but transient) • Medication: salicylates, sulphonamides, antibiotics • Alcohol/liver disease • Idiopathic thrombocytopenic purpura • Leukaemia • Bone marrow infiltration (myeloma/malignancy) • Pregnancy
Potassium (K)	3.5–5.3 IU/L	Is most abundant cation (+ charged ion) in body, and changes in this can affect cellular membrane excitability and impact function of nerves and muscles (cardiac muscle in particular)	Increased: • Haemolysis of sample • Renal failure • Diabetic ketoacidosis • Addison's disease • Mineralocorticoid deficiency Decreased: • Medication: diuretics, salbutamol, insulin • Vomiting, diarrhoea • Inadequate intake (alcoholism/anorexia)
Prostate-specific antigen (PSA)	age 40-49 <2.5 µg/L age 50-59 <3.5 µg/L age 60-69 <4.5 µg/L age 70-79 + <6.5 µg/L	A screening test for prostate cancer. Should always be assessed in context with symptoms and examination	Increased: • Prostate cancer • Benign prostatic hypertrophy • Urine/prostate infection • Ejaculation • Post prostate biopsy

Test	Normal Range	Purpose/Indication	Interpretation
Reticulocyte count	20–100 × 10⁹/L	Immature blood cells used to identify conditions that affect red blood cells	Increased: • Chronic or acute blood loss (increased turnover) • Haemolytic anaemia • Bone marrow infiltration Decreased: • Aplastic anaemia (autoimmune condition where body does not produce enough red blood cells)
Rheumatoid factor (RhF)	Reported as positive or negative	RhF is an antibody present in autoimmune conditions as well as being present in normal population from 2%–10% (rises with age)	Associated with: • RA (80% of cases) • Sjögren's (90%) • SLE (30%) • Other connective tissue disorders, infection • Malignancy
Sodium (Na)	135–145 mmol/L	One of the essential minerals Affects water distribution in body and is involved in nerve conduction Originates in diet and is excreted via urine and sweat Changes will often relate to diseases affecting fluid/electrolyte balance in body When decreased, needs to be assessed in context of plasma osmolality (measure of balance between electrolytes and solutes) and water (solvent)	Decreased (hyponatraemia) with: • Raised osmolality ○ Hyperglycaemia • Normal osmolality ○ Hyperlipidaemia ○ Hyperproteinaemia • Decreased osmolality with: ○ Hypovolaemia: caused by diuretics, diarrhoea/vomiting, Addison's disease, oedema (cirrhosis, cardiac failure, nephrotic syndrome) ○ Euvolaemia: caused by increased water intake, drugs, hypothyroidism, renal insufficiency
Thyroid autoantibodies	These include • Anti-TPO • Anti-thyroglobulin antibodies • Thyroid-stimulating antibody (also known as TS antibody or TSH receptor antibody)	Presence of thyroid autoantibodies indicates autoimmune thyroid disease but may be seen in 10% of population who have normal thyroid function (euthyroid) but may progress to thyroid disease	Anti-TPO and anti-thyroglobulin antibodies present in: • Hashimoto's thyroiditis • Primary hypothyroidism (seen in 90% of cases) • Autoimmune disease: these are found in presence of other autoimmune conditions such as diabetes and pernicious anaemia Thyroid-stimulating antibody • Seen in Grave's disease (autoimmune thyrotoxicosis)

Continued on following page

Test	Normal Range	Purpose/Indication	Interpretation
Thyroid-stimulating hormone (TSH)	0.5–4.2 mU/L	Main marker used to identify thyroid dysfunction	Increased: • Primary hypothyroidism • Hashimoto's thyroiditis • Subacute thyroiditis • Ectopic TSH from tumours (e.g. lung, breast cancer) • Medication: lithium, metoclopramide, clomiphene, domperidone, amiodarone, contrast medium Decreased: • Hyperthyroidism: usually TSH is <0.03 in clinical thyrotoxicosis • Subclinical hyperthyroidism • Patients on excessive T4 or T3 therapy • Medication: steroids, L-dopa, bromocriptine, heparin • Non-thyroidal illness
Thyroxine (T4) T4 is produced in much greater quantities than T3	70–140 mmol/L	T4 is effectively a 'pre-hormone' that gets converted into active form T3 in tissues	Increased: • Hyperthyroidism • T4 therapy • Medication: amiodarone, NSAIDs, steroids, iodine, heparin, Hashimoto's thyroiditis (less common) • Subacute thyroiditis Decreased • Hypothyroidism • Hypopituitarism • Hashimoto's thyroiditis • Medication: T3, phenytoin, lithium, carbamazepine
Tri-iodothyronine (T3)	1.2–3.0 nmol/L	T3 is active hormone, 80% of which comes from conversion of T4, and the rest is made directly in thyroid gland It affects a wide range of organs and systems, including temperature regulation, basal metabolic rate and nerve and bone health	Increased: • Hyperthyroidism • T3 therapy • Subacute thyroiditis • Hashimoto's thyroiditis Decreased: • Hypothyroidism • T4 therapy (although it is generally normal) • Medication: amiodarone, steroids, propranolol, lithium, iodine • Hypopituitarism

Test	Normal Range	Purpose/Indication	Interpretation

Triglycerides (fasting)	0.5–2.3 mmol/L	A type of lipid with a significant link to morbidity. Of note, a triglyceride above 10.0 mmol/L indicates a risk of acute pancreatitis and requires immediate treatment	Increased:
			Primary
			  • Familial (either combined with other raised lipids or in isolation)
			Secondary
			  • Obesity
			  • Alcohol
			  • Diabetes
			  • Hypothyroidism
			  • Liver disease
			  • Nephrotic syndrome
			  • Pancreatitis
			  • Pregnancy
			  • Medication: oestrogen, oral contraceptive pill, beta-blockers, steroids, thiazides

Urea (Ur)	2.5–6.7 mmol/L	A breakdown product of protein used as a measure of renal function. It is also made in the liver, so affected by liver disease	Increased: • Renal impairment (but less reliable than creatinine) • High protein diet (can skew results) • Catabolic states such as acute illness • Infection • Dehydration (increased reabsorption) • GI bleeding (increased cell breakdown) • Prostatic hypertrophy (outflow obstruction) • Medication: steroids, diuretics Decreased: • loss of albumin in dialysis • Liver disease • Malnutrition • In a normal pregnancy
Urate	*Men* 210–480 μmol/L *Women* 150–390 μmol/L	Used to primarily to identify gout	Increased: • Gout • High purine diet (meat, shellfish) • Alcohol • Renal insufficiency • Medication: diuretics, chemotherapy, salicylates • Metabolic syndrome • Pregnancy • Hypothyroidism • Malignancies (leukaemia/lymphoma especially)

Continued on following page

Test	Normal Range	Purpose/Indication	Interpretation
Vitamin B12	>170 pmol/L	Is a dietary vitamin found in meat and animal proteins It is involved in manufacture of blood cells	Increased: • B12 supplementation • Leukaemia, myeloproliferative disorders • Liver disease Decreased: • Vegetarian diet • Medication: oral contraceptive pill, metformin, methotrexate, colchicine, anticonvulsants • Pregnancy • Pernicious anaemia • Malabsorption, including past gastrectomy/ileectomy • Folate deficiency
Vitamin D	<25 nmol/L: deficient 25–50 nmol/L: insufficient >50 nmol/L: sufficient	Regulates calcium and phosphate absorption. Implicated in bone metabolic disorders (secondary hyperparathyroidism/rickets/osteomalacia) and as a potential cause of myalgia/fatigue	Decreased: Due to reduced intake of vitamin D • Lack of sunlight • Lack of dietary vitamin D • Fat malabsorption (vitamin D is fat soluble, e.g. coeliac disease) Due to reduced liver production of 25 (OH) D3 • Deficiency of 1αhydroxylase (hereditary or in renal failure) • Medication: carbamazepine, phenytoin (increased degradation) • Nephrotic syndrome Due to reduced renal production of calcitriol • Deficiency of 1αhydroxylase • Suppression of 1αhydroxylase (PTH deficiency in hypoparathyroidism or end organ resistance seen in pseudohypoparathyroidism) Increased: • Excessive intake: supplements or prescribed • Increased calcitriol production (hyperparathyroidism) • Production by sarcoidosis, sarcomas and lymphomas

Pain Medications

Amitriptyline

[A-mee-trip'ti-leen]

Amitriptyline is a tricyclic antidepressant that was developed in the early 1960s to treat major depressive orders. More recently, it has also been used at low doses to treat neuropathic pain and is often prescribed as a first or second line treatment for these conditions. Amitriptyline also has sedative qualities that may be beneficial for some but can cause confusion and increase risk of falls in others, particularly the elderly.

Class of Medication

Tricyclic antidepressant

Mechanism of Action

Amitriptyline inhibits the reuptake of serotonin and noradrenaline at presynaptic membranes, thereby increasing their availability at postsynaptic receptor sites. By maintaining higher levels of these neurotransmitters in the synaptic cleft, it achieves its antidepressant effect by improving mood and sense of well-being. However, the mechanism by which it works for pain is likely to differ, as analgesia is achieved at much lower doses than those needed to treat depression.

Amitriptyline also blocks other receptors including adrenergic, muscarinic, histamine and dopamine receptors. Its antimuscarinic properties account for many of its adverse effects (most notably dry mouth and eyes, urinary retention, tachycardia, confusion and cognitive dysfunction), and its antihistamine effect causes drowsiness and sedation. This limits its therapeutic usefulness as newer tricyclic medications are more effective and have fewer adverse effects, although its sedative qualities are often utilised to encourage sleep and reduce the need for additional sleeping medication.

Prescribed For

- Depression
- Neuropathic pain
- Migraine prophylaxis
- Chronic tension-type headache prophylaxis
- Emotional lability in multiple sclerosis
- Abdominal pain

Adverse Effects

- Dry mouth
- Constipation
- Urinary retention

- Bowel obstruction
- Dilated pupil
- Blurred vision
- Arrythmia and ECG changes (prolonged QT/QRS durations)
- Decreased sweating
- Impaired concentration
- Confusion
- Attention deficit
- Memory impairment
- Fatigue

Contraindications

- Arrhythmias
- Heart block
- Following myocardial infarction
- During manic phase of bipolar disorder

Cautions

- Cardiovascular disease
- Chronic constipation
- Diabetes
- History of bipolar disorder
- History of psychosis
- Hyperthyroidism
- Increased intra-ocular pressure
- Patients at risk of suicide
- Pheochromocytoma
- Prostatic hypertrophy
- Pyloric stenosis
- Angle-closure glaucoma
- Urinary retention

Adult Dosage

Neuropathic Pain

Initial dose: 10–25 mg taken at night
Titration: increased by 10–25 mg every three to seven days in one to two divided doses
Usual dose: 25–75 mg daily, taken at night
Maximum dose: 100 mg per dose. Doses above 100 mg should be used with caution

Notes on Dosage and Administration

- Doses above 75 mg should be used with caution in the elderly and those with cardiovascular disease
- Patients should be slowly titrated to the dose that provides adequate analgesia with tolerable adverse side effects
- Amitriptyline is currently not recommended for major depressive disorders due to the increased risk of fatality in overdose

- The analgesic and anti-depressive effect is normally seen after two to four weeks of dosing
- Although individual responses vary, adverse effects are generally mild and usually decrease within two weeks
- Although amitriptyline is often effective in treating neuropathic pain, it does not work for most people. It is estimated that around one in four people will benefit from taking it (Moore et al, 2015)

Driving and Skilled Tasks
- Amitriptyline is a sedative drug and can impair general attention and concentration. Patients should be cautioned about their ability to drive or operate machinery. Drinking alcohol while taking amitriptyline can potentiate adverse effects

Treatment Cessation
- After long-term use, suddenly stopping the medication may produce withdrawal symptoms such as headache, malaise, insomnia and irritability. The dose should be gradually reduced over four weeks. If withdrawal symptoms emerge, a longer period may be necessary

Aspirin

[As'pe-rin]

Aspirin is also known as acetylsalicylic acid and is used to treat mild to moderate pain, fever and inflammation. It also suppresses normal platelet function and is widely used prophylactically to reduce the risk of heart attacks, ischaemic stroke and blood clots. Although readily available, aspirin should be used with caution as it can irritate the stomach and cause gastrointestinal ulceration and haemorrhage. It can provoke sensitivity reactions such as asthma attacks and bronchospasm.

Class of Medication

- Non-opioid analgesic
- Anti-platelet
- Antipyretic

Mechanism of Action

Aspirin irreversibly inhibits the activity of cyclooxygenase (COX), an enzyme which is responsible for the formation of prostaglandin, a potent inflammatory mediator. By inhibiting COX, the conversion of arachidonic acid (which is released during irritation or injury) into prostaglandin is prevented, thereby reducing inflammation, pain and swelling. It also counteracts fever through the vasodilation of peripheral vessels, allowing the dissipation of excess heat.

In addition, aspirin's inhibition of COX reduces the production of the pro-aggregatory factor thromboxane from arachidonic acid, reducing platelet aggregation. This occurs at low doses and prevents the formation of blood clots, reducing the risk of heart attacks or strokes.

Prostaglandins are produced throughout the body and play key roles in protecting the stomach mucosa, maintaining kidney function and platelet aggregation. As a result, long-term use of aspirin can cause gastrointestinal bleeding, gastrointestinal ulceration and haemorrhage, as well as hypersensitivity reactions (such as bronchospasm) and exacerbate asthma.

Prescribed For

- Mild to moderate pain
- Pyrexia
- Acute migraine
- Cardiovascular disease
- Secondary prevention of deep-vein thrombosis
- Secondary prevention of pulmonary embolism
- Management of unstable angina and non-ST-segment elevation myocardial infarction
- Management of ST-segment elevation myocardial infarction
- Transient ischaemic attack
- Ischaemic stroke

- Atrial fibrillation
- Following coronary bypass surgery
- Prevention of pre-eclampsia in women at moderate or high risk

Adverse Effects

- Asthmatic attack
- Bronchospasm
- Dyspepsia
- Haemorrhage

Contraindications

- Active peptic ulceration
- Bleeding disorders
- Children under 16 years (risk of Reye's syndrome)
- Previous history of hypersensitivity to aspirin or any other NSAID
- Haemophilia
- Previous peptic ulceration
- Severe cardiac failure

Cautions

- Allergic disease
- Anaemia
- Asthma
- Dehydration
- Elderly
- G6PD deficiency
- Hypertension
- May mask symptoms of infection
- Avoid during fever or viral infection in children
- Thyrotoxicosis

Adult Dosage

Mild-To-Moderate Pain and Pyrexia

Dose: 300–900 mg every four to six hours as required
Maximum: 4 g per day

Acute Migraine

Dose: 900 mg for one dose – taken as soon as migraine symptoms develop

Cardiovascular Disease (Secondary Prevention)

Dose: 75 mg daily

Notes on Dosage and Administration

- Aspirin should not be given to children under 16 years of age due to the risk of developing Reye's syndrome, a rare but life threatening brain and liver disorder
- Take with or just after food to slow gastrointestinal absorption and minimise gastric irritation

Driving and Skilled Tasks

Has no reported influence.

Treatment Cessation

Aspirin should not be stopped abruptly after long-term use as it may trigger a rebound effect with an increased risk of cardiovascular events after discontinuation. Patients wishing to stop taking aspirin should be advised to speak to their doctor or consultant.

Baclofen

(bak-loe·fen)

Baclofen is a skeletal muscle relaxant and antispasmodic that acts on the central nervous system to reduce severe spasticity resulting from a number of disorders, including multiple sclerosis, spinal cord injury, motor neurone disease, cerebral palsy and stroke.

Class of Medication

- Central-acting skeletal muscle relaxant
- Antispasmodic
- Gamma-aminobutyric acid (GABA) agonist

Mechanism of Action

Baclofen is structurally similar to the inhibitory neurotransmitter GABA. Although its exact mechanism of action is unknown, it is thought to stimulate GABA receptors in the central nervous system and inhibit the release of excitatory neurotransmitters. This depresses reflex transmission and increases descending pain inhibitory effects.

Prescribed For

- Muscle spasm in palliative care
- Chronic severe spasticity
- Hiccups (due to gastric distention in palliative care)

Adverse Effects

- Confusion
- Constipation
- Depression
- Diarrhoea
- Dizziness
- Drowsiness
- Dry mouth
- Euphoric mood
- Fatigue
- Gastrointestinal disorder
- Hallucination
- Headache
- Hyperhidrosis
- Hypotension

- Muscle weakness
- Myalgia
- Nausea
- Paraesthesia
- Respiratory depression
- Skin reactions
- Sleep disorders
- Urinary disorders
- Vision disorders
- Vomiting

Contraindications

- Active peptic ulceration

Cautions

- Drowsiness may affect performance of skilled tasks (e.g. driving)
- It also enhances the effects of alcohol

Adult Dosage

Pain Of Muscle Spasm In Palliative Care

Dose: 5–10 mg three times a day

Severe Chronic Spasticity Resulting From Disorders Such As Multiple Sclerosis Or Traumatic Partial Section Of The Spinal Cord

Dose: Initially 5 mg three times a day, gradually increased up to 60 mg daily in divided doses
Maximum dose: 100 mg per day

Notes on Dosage and Administration

- Benefits may occur after one to three hours, but it may take several weeks for the full benefits to be felt
- There is an important distinction between centrally mediated spasticity and more peripherally driven muscle spasm. Baclofen's use in muscle spasm for longer term musculoskeletal pain conditions characterised by muscle spasm (including back pain and fibromyalgia) is controversial, and there is little evidence to support its long-term use

Driving and Skilled Tasks

Patients should avoid driving and hazardous tasks until they know how baclofen affects them. It can cause drowsiness, decreased alertness and blurred vision.
Alcohol enhances its effects.

Treatment Cessation

Avoid abrupt withdrawal as it risks creating a hyperactive state. It may also exacerbate spasticity and precipitate autonomic dysfunction, including hyperthermia, psychiatric reactions and convulsions. To minimise risk, the dose should be gradually reduced over at least one to two weeks.

6.4

Buprenorphine

(byoo·pruh·naw·feen)

Buprenorphine is a semi-synthetic opioid used to treat moderate-to-severe pain arising from surgery, serious injury or cancer. It is also a partial opioid agonist, and its mechanism of action suggests an important role in managing opioid dependence. However, its use in managing pain is prone to the same pitfalls and cautions as any other opioid with risks of significant side effects, tolerance, dependence, withdrawal and addiction.

Class of Medication

Opioid receptor partial agonist

Mechanism of Action

Buprenorphine is a partial agonist with a high affinity for the mu opioid receptor. This means that it will preferentially bind to the mu receptor and block the effect of other opioids like heroine or morphine, even when they are present. However, when bound to the opioid receptor, it will only elicit a partial response, no matter how much of the drug is administered. This reduces the risk of overdose and respiratory depression and makes buprenorphine an important medication in opiate misuse and detoxication regimes.

Opioid drugs work by activating specific opioid receptors (mu, kappa and delta) located in the central nervous system, gastrointestinal system and peripheral tissue. Its widespread effects include analgesia, sedation, anxiolysis, euphoria, respiratory depression and gastrointestinal system smooth muscle contraction.

Opioids exert their analgesic effect in two ways:
- In the presynaptic nociceptive neurone, it reduces the influx of calcium, which in turn reduces neurotransmitter release. As a consequence, there is reduced nociceptive transmission to the postsynaptic neurone
- In the postsynaptic neurone, it increases the efflux of potassium from the neurone. This results in hyperpolarisation of the nociceptive neurone and reduces the nociceptive signal passing up to the spinal cord to the brain

The net result is a significant decrease in nociceptive transmission.

Prescribed For

- Moderate-to-severe pain not responsive to other opioids or non-opioids
- Treatment of opioid dependence
- Treatment of chronic cancer pain
- Premedication and intraoperative analgesia

Adverse Effects

For All Opioids

- Arrhythmias
- Confusion
- Constipation
- Dizziness
- Drowsiness
- Dry mouth
- Euphoric mood
- Flushing
- Hallucination
- Headache
- Hyperhidrosis
- Hypotension (with high doses)
- Miosis
- Nausea (more common on initiation)
- Palpitations
- Respiratory depression (with high doses)
- Skin reactions
- Urinary retention
- Vertigo
- Visual impairment
- Vomiting (more common on initiation)
- Withdrawal syndrome

For Buprenorphine (Patches)

- Appetite decreased
- Weakness, lack of energy or strength
- Breathlessness
- Abdominal pains
- Oedema
- Sleep disorders

Contraindications

FOR ALL OPIOIDS

- Acute respiratory depression
- Comatose patients
- Head injury (opioid analgesics interfere with pupillary responses vital for neurological assessment)
- Increased intracranial pressure (opioid analgesics interfere with pupillary responses vital for neurological assessment)
- Risk of paralytic ileus

For Buprenorphine (Patches)

- Not to be worn in MRI scan (contain metals)
- History of keloid or hypertrophic scar formation

Cautions

FOR ALL OPIOIDS

- Adrenocortical insufficiency (reduced dose is recommended)
- Asthma (avoid during an acute attack)
- Central sleep apnoea
- Convulsive disorders
- Current or history of mental health disorder
- Current or history of substance use disorder
- Debilitated patients (reduced dose is recommended)
- Diseases of the biliary tract
- Elderly (reduced dose is recommended)
- Hypotension
- Hypothyroidism (reduced dose is recommended)
- Impaired respiratory function (avoid in chronic obstructive pulmonary disease)
- Inflammatory bowel disorders
- Myasthenia gravis
- Obstructive bowel disorders
- Prostatic hypertrophy (in adults)
- Shock
- Urethral stenosis

Cautions

For Buprenorphine

- Impaired consciousness

Adult Dosage

Transdermal Application Of Patches In Moderate, Non-Cancer Pain Not Responding To Non-Opioid Analgesics

Initial dose: 5 micrograms/hour using 7 day patches.

Dose adjustments: Dose is adjusted at intervals of at least 3 days (72 hours) using a patch on the next strength usually up to no more than a maximum dose of one 20 mcg/hr (7 day) patch.

In Patients Who Have Already Been Receiving Strong Opioid Analgesics

Initial dose: Should be based on the previous 24 hours opioid requirements. For chronic non-cancer pain, usual maximum one 35 micrograms/hour patch, seek specialist advice if further dose increases required.

Dose adjustments: Analgesic effect should not be evaluated until the system has been worn for 24 hours (to allow for gradual increase in plasma-buprenorphine concentration). If necessary, the dose should be adjusted at intervals of at least three days (72 hours) using a patch of the next strength or a combination of two patches applied in different places (applied at the same time to avoid confusion). A maximum of two patches can be used at any one time.

Notes on Dosage and Administration

- Buprenorphine comes as transdermal patches (available as 72-hourly, 96-hourly and seven-day patches), tablets and injections (usually only administered in-hospital)
- Opiates are at their most effective when used for short – medium term ($<$12 weeks) or intermittent use
- Do not use other opioids within 24 hours of patch removal as they have a long duration of action
- Dependence/addiction is associated with prolonged use (longer than three months) of opioids for non-malignant pain
- Guidelines do not recommend opioids for chronic primary pain, including chronic lower back pain and fibromyalgia
- There is an increased risk in individuals with current or history of substance use disorder or mental health disorders
- When using patches, patients and carers should be advised to:
  - Not exceed the prescribed dose
  - Follow the correct frequency of patch application, avoid touching the adhesive side of patches, and wash hands after application
  - Not cut patches and avoid exposure of area of skin where patch is sited to heat, including via hot water, as it accelerates drug release and shortens duration of action
  - Ensure that old patches are removed before applying a new one
  - Follow instructions for safe storage and properly dispose of used patches or those which are not needed

Driving and Skilled Tasks

Drowsiness may affect performance of skilled tasks (e.g. driving); effects of alcohol can be enhanced. Driving at the start of therapy with opioid analgesics, and following dose changes, should be avoided.

Treatment Cessation

Avoid abrupt withdrawal after long-term treatment. They should be withdrawn gradually to avoid withdrawal symptoms, following the guidelines of reduction, by no more than 10% every two to four weeks.

6.5

Celecoxib

(cel-e-cox-ib)

Celecoxib is a non-steroidal anti-inflammatory drug (NSAID). However, unlike ibuprofen or naproxen, it is selective in which enzyme it inhibits. As a result, celecoxib is associated with a decreased risk of stomach ulceration and gastrointestinal bleeding with long-term use (>120 days) but has a greater risk of cardiovascular and renal events when compared to those of traditional NSAIDs.

Class of Medication

- Non-steroidal anti-inflammatory drug
- Selective cyclooxygenase-2 (COX-2) inhibitor

Mechanism of Action

Celecoxib selectively inhibits COX-2, which is responsible for the production of prostaglandins involved in pain and inflammatory pathways. Most traditional NSAIDs are non-selective and inhibit both COX isoforms (COX-1 and COX-2). Because COX-1 is thought to play a pivotal role in protecting the stomach lining (mucosa), medications that do not inhibit COX-1 but selectively target COX-2 are thought to lower the risk of stomach upsets, ulceration and bleeding with long-term use. However, they appear to be associated with a higher risk of thrombotic events.

Prescribed For

- Pain and inflammation in osteoarthritis
- Pain and inflammation in rheumatoid arthritis
- Ankylosing spondylitis

Adverse Effects

- Angina pectoris
- Benign prostatic hyperplasia
- Cough
- Diarrhoea
- Dizziness
- Dysphagia
- Dyspnoea
- Fluid retention
- Gastrointestinal discomfort
- Gastrointestinal disorders
- Headache

- Hypersensitivity
- Hypertension
- Increased risk of infection
- Influenza-like illness
- Injury
- Insomnia
- Irritable bowel syndrome
- Joint disorders
- Muscle tone increased
- Myocardial infarction
- Nausea
- Nephrolithiasis
- Oedema
- Skin reactions
- Vomiting
- Weight increase

Contraindications

- Active gastrointestinal bleeding
- Active gastrointestinal ulceration
- Cerebrovascular disease
- Inflammatory bowel disease
- Ischaemic heart disease
- Mild to severe heart failure
- Peripheral arterial disease

Cautions

- Allergic disorders
- Cardiac impairment
- Coagulation defects
- Connective-tissue disorders
- Dehydration (risk of renal impairment)
- Elderly (risk of serious side effects and fatalities)
- History of cardiac failure
- History of gastrointestinal disorders
- Hypertension
- Left ventricular dysfunction
- May mask symptoms of infection
- Oedema
- Risk factors for cardiovascular events

Adult Dosage

Pain and Inflammation in Osteoarthritis

Initial dose: 200 mg daily in one to two divided doses
Titration: increased if necessary to 200 mg twice daily. Discontinue if no improvement after two weeks
Maximum dose: 400 mg

Pain and Inflammation In Rheumatoid Arthritis

Initial dose: 100 mg twice daily
Titration: increased if necessary to 200 mg twice daily. Discontinue if no improvement after
  two weeks
Maximum dose: 400 mg

Ankylosing Spondylitis

Initial dose: 200 mg daily in one to two divided doses
Titration: increased if necessary to 400 mg daily in one to two divided doses. Discontinue if
  no improvement after two weeks
Maximum dose: 400 mg

Notes on Dosage and Administration

- Recent research suggests that selective COX-2 inhibitors may be associated with higher
  risks of thrombotic events (especially myocardial infarction and stroke) than those associ-
  ated with non-selective NSAIDs
- Celecoxib should be used with caution with patients at greater risk of cardiovascular events
- The risks associated with celecoxib may increase with dose and duration of exposure.
  Therefore, the shortest duration and lowest effective dose should be used
- Advise patients to take the medication with food to decrease absorption rates and adverse
  effects

Driving and Skilled Tasks

Some patients may experience dizziness, vertigo or somnolence while taking celecoxib and should
be advised to avoid driving or operating machinery.

Treatment Cessation

With short-term use, the medication can be discontinued as soon as it is no longer required.
Following sustained, long-term use, there are no firm guidelines, but some prescribers may reduce
the dose slowly over a few days before complete discontinuation.

Codeine Phosphate

(kow·deen fos ·feit)

Codeine is an opioid that is used to treat mild-to-moderate pain and is often used as a second-line treatment when non-opioid analgesics such as aspirin, ibuprofen or paracetamol are insufficient. Codeine affects gut motility, which can cause constipation, although this can have a therapeutic benefit when used to manage acute diarrhoea.

Class of Medication

Weak opioid agonist

Mechanism of Action

Codeine is a prodrug, which means that it must be converted via metabolic processes in the liver before it becomes an active pharmacological agent. Codeine is converted to morphine by Cytochrome P450 2D6, a metabolising enzyme. Approximately 5–10% of the population are poor or non-metabolisers of codeine and so get very little pain relief. Conversely, 0.5–2% of the population can rapidly metabolise codeine and, as such, risk overdose.

Once metabolised into morphine, codeine produces its analgesic effect by activating descending inhibitory pathways via opioid receptors located in the central nervous system.

Prescribed For

- Mild-to-moderate pain
- Acute diarrhoea

Adverse Effects

- Arrhythmias
- Confusion
- Constipation
- Dizziness
- Drowsiness
- Dry mouth
- Euphoric mood
- Flushing
- Hallucination
- Headache
- Hyperhidrosis
- Hypotension (with high doses)
- Miosis

- Nausea (more common on initiation)
- Palpitations
- Respiratory depression (with high doses)
- Skin reactions
- Urinary retention
- Vertigo
- Visual impairment
- Vomiting (more common on initiation)
- Withdrawal syndrome

Contraindications

For All Opioids

- Acute respiratory depression
- Comatose patients
- Head injury (opioid analgesics interfere with pupillary responses vital for neurological assessment)
- Increased intracranial pressure (opioid analgesics interfere with pupillary responses vital for neurological assessment)
- Risk of paralytic ileus

For Codeine

- Acute ulcerative colitis
- Antibiotic-associated colitis
- Children under 18 years who undergo the removal of tonsils or adenoids for the treatment of obstructive sleep apnoea
- Conditions where abdominal distension develops
- Conditions where inhibition of peristalsis should be avoided
- Known ultra-rapid codeine metabolisers

Cautions

For All Opioids

- Adrenocortical insufficiency
- Asthma (avoid during an acute attack)
- Central sleep apnoea
- Convulsive disorders
- Current or history of mental health disorder
- Current or history of substance use disorder
- Debilitated patients (reduced dose is recommended)
- Diseases of the biliary tract
- Elderly (reduced dose is recommended)
- Hypotension
- Hypothyroidism (reduced dose is recommended)
- Impaired respiratory function (avoid in chronic obstructive pulmonary disease)
- Inflammatory bowel disorders
- Myasthenia gravis
- Obstructive bowel disorders

- Prostatic hypertrophy
- Shock
- Uethral stenosis

Adult Doses

Mild-to-Moderate Pain

Dose: 30–60 mg every four hours if required
Maximum dose: 240 mg daily

Acute Diarrhoea

Dose: 30 mg three to four times a day
Usual dose: 15–60 mg three to four times a day
Maximum dose: 240 mg daily

Notes on Dosage and Administration

- Codeine is often combined with non-opioids drugs such as paracetamol (co-codamol) to provide an additive effect
- Dependence and addiction are associated with prolonged use of opioids for non-malignant pain (longer than three months)
- Guidelines do not recommend opioid use for chronic primary pain, including chronic lower back pain and fibromyalgia
- There is an increased risk in individuals with current or history of substance use disorder or mental health disorders

Driving and Skilled Tasks

Drowsiness may affect performance of skilled tasks. Driving at the start of therapy with opioid analgesics, and following dose changes, should be avoided. Opioids enhance the effects of alcohol

Treatment Cessation

Avoid abrupt withdrawal after long-term treatment

Opioids should be reduced gradually to avoid withdrawal symptoms. Guidelines suggest reducing the dose by no more than 10% every two to four weeks

Diazepam

(dai·a·zuh·pam)

Diazepam is the best-known and most commonly prescribed benzodiazepine. It is used to reduce feelings of anxiety, restlessness and agitation and can also induce sedation and promote drowsiness to overcome insomnia. It also acts as a muscle relaxant and is used to relieve muscle spasm. However, it bears significant risks and needs to be used with caution. It is important that patients be aware of the risks, which include dependency with repeated use, drowsiness, impaired judgement and loss of motivation.

Class of Medication

Benzodiazepine

Mechanism of Action

Diazepam works by binding to GABA-A receptor on chloride ion channels, which leads to an increase in the frequency at which the channels opens. The increased conductance of chloride ions leads to hyperpolarisation of the neuronal membrane and reduced excitability of the neuron.

In the limbic system, which is involved in behavioural, emotional and fight and flight responses, this leads to a reduction in anxiety, while in the spinal cord and motor neurons its binding to GABA-A receptors is responsible for its muscle relaxant effect.

It also binds to receptors in the cortex, thalamus and cerebellum, which mediates its sedative, amnestic (loss of memory) and anticonvulsant effects.

Prescribed For

- Sedation
- Skeletal muscle relaxation – including in conditions characterised by muscle spasticity such as stroke and spinal cord injury
- Reducing anxiety
- Reducing/stopping seizures

Adverse Effects

- Drowsiness
- Lethargy
- Fatigue
- Impaired motor coordination
- Dizziness
- Vertigo
- Slurred speech

- Blurry vision
- Mood swings
- Euphoria
- Hostile or erratic behaviour
- Dependence and addiction
- Withdrawal
- Sleep disorders
- Suicidal ideation
- Tremor

Contraindications

- Acute pulmonary insufficiency
- Marked neuromuscular respiratory weakness
- Not for use alone to treat chronic psychosis
- Depression (or anxiety associated with depression)
- Obsessional states
- Phobic states
- Sleep apnoea syndromes
- Stable myasthenia gravis

Cautions

- Avoid prolonged use and abrupt withdrawal – risk of dependence is significantly reduced by short-term use (ideally no more than two to four weeks)
- Avoid in debilitated patients (or reduce dose)
- Caution in elderly (reduce dose)
- Avoid in people with a history of alcohol or drug dependence or abuse
- Caution with those with personality disorder (within the fearful group—dependent, avoidant, obsessive-compulsive) as may increase risk of dependence

Adult Dosage

Muscle Spasm

Dose: 2–15 mg daily in divided doses, then increased if necessary to 60 mg daily (20 mg three times a day), adjusted according to response; the dose is only increased in conditions of known spasticity

Anxiety

Dose: 2 mg three times a day, then increased if necessary to 15–30 mg daily in divided doses, for debilitated patients, use elderly dose.
For the elderly: 1 mg three times a day, then increased if necessary to 7.5–15 mg daily in divided doses

Insomnia

Dose: 5–15 mg daily, to be taken at bedtime

Notes on Dosage and Administration
- Avoid prolonged use (>4 weeks) to reduce the risk of dependency

■ When diazepam and other benzodiazepines are taken with opioids they can increase CNS depressant effects, increasing the risk of sedation, respiratory depression, coma and death

■ Diazepam has an onset within one to two hours with a half-life of over 30 hours (this increases by as much as three times in elderly patients or those with kidney problems) so is considered a long-acting medication

Driving and Skilled Tasks

Diazepam may cause drowsiness, impair judgement and increase reaction time, and so affects ability to drive or perform skilled tasks.

The hangover effects of a night dose may impair performance the following day.

Diazepam enhances the effect of alcohol.

Treatment Cessation

Diazepam should not be stopped abruptly following long-term use as withdrawal can cause seizures, confusion, depression, sweating and diarrhoea. A slow taper of 1–2 mg every three to seven days is recommended, depending on how long the patient has been on the medication.

Diclofenac

[dik-lo-fen-ak]

Diclofenac is a non-steroidal anti-inflammatory drug (NSAID) used to relieve pain and inflammation caused by musculoskeletal disorders, rheumatic disease, postoperative pain and gout. Although diclofenac is widely used throughout the world, it has a greater cardiovascular health risk compared with those of other non-steroidal anti-inflammatory drugs – even at low doses.

Class of Medication

Non-steroidal anti-inflammatory drug

Mechanism of Action

Prostaglandins are produced in response to injury or infection and play a key role in generating the inflammatory response. Diclofenac works by inhibiting cyclooxygenase (COX), an enzyme responsible for prostaglandin synthesis. As a result, less prostaglandin is produced, leading to a reduction in inflammation and pain.

Prostaglandin receptors are found throughout the body and have a number of roles including:
- Maintaining the gastric mucosa
- Preventing thrombus formation
- Constricting and dilating the blood vessels
- Regulating the contraction of smooth muscle tissue

By inhibiting prostaglandin formation, NSAIDs impact on these other functions, giving rise to some of their adverse effects.

Prescribed For

- Pain and inflammation in musculoskeletal disorders
- Pain and inflammation in rheumatic disease, including juvenile idiopathic arthritis
- Acute gout
- Postoperative pain

Adverse Effects

With Oral Use

- Appetite decreased
- Diarrhoea
- Dizziness
- Gastrointestinal discomfort
- Gastrointestinal disorders

- Headache
- Nausea
- Rash (discontinue)
- Vertigo
- Vomiting

With Topical Use

- Conjunctivitis
- Muscle tone increased
- Rash (discontinue)
- Sensation abnormal
- Skin ulcer

Contraindications

- Previous history of hypersensitivity to diclofenac or any other NSAID
- Active gastrointestinal bleeding
- Active gastrointestinal ulceration
- Avoid suppositories in proctitis
- Cerebrovascular disease
- History of gastrointestinal bleeding or perforation related to previous NSAID therapy
- History of recurrent gastrointestinal haemorrhage or ulceration (two or more distinct episodes)
- Ischaemic heart disease
- Mild to severe heart failure
- Peripheral arterial disease

Cautions

With Systemic Use

- Allergic disorders
- Cardiac impairment (NSAIDs may impair renal function)
- Coagulation defects
- Connective-tissue disorders
- Dehydration (risk of renal impairment)
- Elderly (risk of serious side effects and fatalities)
- History of cardiac failure
- History of gastrointestinal disorders (e.g. ulcerative colitis, Crohn's disease)
- Hypertension
- May mask symptoms of infection
- Oedema
- Risk factors for cardiovascular events

With Topical Use

- Avoid contact with eyes
- Avoid contact with inflamed or broken skin
- Avoid contact with mucous membranes
- Not for use with occlusive dressings
- Topical application of large amounts can result in systemic effects, including hypersensitivity and asthma (renal disease has also been reported)

Adult Dosage

Pain and Inflammation in Musculoskeletal Disorders, Pain and Inflammation in Rheumatic Disease Including Juvenile Idiopathic Arthritis, Acute Gout, Postoperative Pain

Dose: 75–150 mg daily in two to three divided doses

Relief of Pain in Musculoskeletal Conditions, Adjunctive Treatment in Knee or Hand Osteoarthritis

Using gel containing diclofenac sodium 1%, applied to the skin.

Dose: Apply three to four times a day

Therapy should be reviewed after 14 days (or after 28 days for osteoarthritis).

Notes on Dosage and Administration

- Diclofenac carries a higher risk of upper gastrointestinal bleeding compared with those associated with paracetamol and ibuprofen – although the risk is similar to that associated with naproxen
- It has a higher cardiovascular risk and should only be initiated after careful consideration for patients with significant risk factors for cardiovascular events (e.g. hypertension, hyperlipidaemia, diabetes mellitus, smoking)
- A number of patients historically prescribed diclofenac find it beneficial for treating pain and inflammation. They need to be made aware of the risks involved with continued use and weigh up the improved quality of life against the potential side effects

Driving and Skilled Tasks

Diclofenac generally has no adverse effects on the ability to drive and use machinery. However, patients who experience visual disturbances, dizziness, vertigo, somnolence, central nervous system disturbances, drowsiness or fatigue while taking NSAIDs should refrain from driving or operating machinery.

Treatment Cessation

Generally, there is no need to taper doses when stopping the medication after short-term use. However, patients who have been taking NSAIDs for long periods should not stop abruptly as it may increase their risk of heart attack or stroke. They should speak to their GP about slowly tapering the dose down.

6.9

Dihydrocodeine

(dai·hai·druh·kow·deen)

Dihydrocodeine is a semi-synthetic derivative of codeine with the same analgesic properties. Dihydrocodeine is sometimes used as an alternative to codeine and has a stronger analgesic action and a greater euphoric effect. Consequently, there is a greater risk of dependence and substance abuse, which needs to be taken into consideration when prescribing.

Class of Medication

Weak opioid

Mechanism of Action

Dihydrocodeine is metabolised into dihydromorphine in the liver and produces its analgesic effect by activating descending inhibitory pathways via opioid receptors located in the central nervous system.

Dihydrocodeine is structurally related to codeine. However, unlike codeine, which needs to be metabolised into morphine by a specific enzyme (CYP2D6), dihydrocodeine is not dependent on this pathway to produce its analgesic effect. Therefore, patients who are identified as poor or ultra-rapid metabolisers of codeine might find that dihydrocodeine provides more effective pain relief.

Prescribed For

- Moderate to severe pain
- Chronic severe pain

Adverse Effects

For All Opioids

- Arrhythmias
- Confusion
- Constipation
- Dizziness
- Drowsiness
- Dry mouth
- Euphoric mood
- Flushing
- Hallucination
- Headache
- Hyperhidrosis

- Hypotension (with high doses)
- Miosis
- Nausea (more common on initiation)
- Palpitations
- Respiratory depression (with high doses)
- Skin reactions
- Urinary retention
- Vertigo
- Visual impairment
- Vomiting (more common on initiation)
- Withdrawal syndrome

For Dihydrocodeine

- Dysuria
- Mood altered

Contraindications

For All Opioids

- Acute respiratory depression
- Comatose patients
- Head injury (opioid analgesics interfere with pupillary responses vital for neurological assessment)
- Increased intracranial pressure (opioid analgesics interfere with pupillary responses vital for neurological assessment)
- Risk of paralytic ileus

Cautions

For All Opioids

- Adrenocortical insufficiency
- Asthma (avoid during an acute attack)
- Central sleep apnoea
- Convulsive disorders
- Current or history of mental health disorder
- Current or history of substance use disorder
- Debilitated patients (reduced dose is recommended)
- Diseases of the biliary tract
- Elderly (reduced dose is recommended)
- Hypotension
- Hypothyroidism (reduced dose is recommended)
- Impaired respiratory function (avoid in chronic obstructive pulmonary disease)
- Inflammatory bowel disorders
- Myasthenia gravis
- Obstructive bowel disorders
- Prostatic hypertrophy
- Shock
- Uethral stenosis

For Dihydrocodeine

- Pancreatitis
- Severe cor pulmonale (right-sided heart failure normally caused by pulmonary hypertension)

Adult Dosages

Moderate to Severe Pain

Dose: 30–60 mg every four hours if required

Chronic Severe Pain

Dose: 60–120 mg every 12 hours

DF118 Forte®
Dose: 40–80 mg three times a day
Maximum dose: 240 mg per day

Notes on Dosage and Administration
- Dihydrocodeine is often combined with non-opioids drugs such as paracetamol (co-dydramol) to provide an additive effect
- Dependence and addiction are associated with prolonged use of opioids for non-malignant pain (longer than three months)
- Guidelines do not recommend opioid use for chronic primary pain, including chronic lower back pain and fibromyalgia
- There is an increased risk in individuals with current or history of substance use disorder or mental health disorders

Driving and Skilled Tasks
- Drowsiness may affect performance of skilled tasks
- Driving at the start of therapy with opioid analgesics, and following dose changes, should be avoided
- Opioids enhance the effects of alcohol

Treatment Cessation
- Avoid abrupt withdrawal after long-term treatment
- Opioids should be withdrawn gradually to avoid withdrawal symptoms
- Guidelines suggest reducing the dose no more than 10% every two to four weeks

Duloxetine

(du-lox-er-teen)

Duloxetine belongs to a class of drugs called serotonin and noradrenaline reuptake inhibitors (SNRIs), which are mainly used to treat depression but also have a role in treating anxiety, chronic primary pain and the pain associated with diabetic neuropathy.

Class of Medication

Serotonin and noradrenaline reuptake inhibitor.

Mechanism of Action

Duloxetine inhibits the reuptake of serotonin and noradrenaline by neurons within the central nervous system. These neurotransmitters have a number of important functions, including the regulation of sleep, mood, attention and memory. Low levels of serotonin can cause anxiety, suicidal thoughts and depression, while low levels of noradrenaline can lead to a loss of concentration and depression. By preventing serotonin and noradrenaline being reabsorbed back into the neurons, the availability of these neurotransmitters is maintained.

Prescribed For

- Major depressive disorder
- Generalised anxiety disorder
- Diabetic neuropathy
- Moderate to severe stress urinary incontinence

Adverse Effects

- Anxiety
- Appetite creased
- Constipation
- Diarrhoea
- Dizziness
- Drowsiness
- Dry mouth
- Fall
- Fatigue
- Flushing
- Gastrointestinal discomfort
- Gastrointestinal disorders
- Headache

- Muscle complaints
- Nausea
- Pain
- Palpitations
- Paraesthesia
- Sexual dysfunction
- Skin reactions
- Sleep disorders
- Sweat changes
- Tinnitus
- Tremor
- Urinary disorders
- Vision disorders
- Vomiting
- Weight changes
- Yawning

Cautions

- Bleeding disorders
- Cardiac disease
- Elderly
- History of mania
- History of seizures
- Hypertension
- Increased intra-ocular pressure
- Susceptibility to angle-closure glaucoma

Adult Dosage

Major Depressive Disorder

Dose: 60 mg once daily

Generalised Anxiety Disorder

Initial dose: 30 mg once daily
Titration: increased 60 mg once daily
Maximum dose: 120 mg per day

Diabetic Neuropathy

Initial dose: 60 mg once daily
Discontinue if inadequate response after two months. Review treatment at least every three months
Maximum dose: 120 mg per day, administered in divided doses

Notes on Dosage and Administration

Serotonin syndrome, a potentially life-threatening condition caused by high levels of serotonin, may occur with duloxetine treatment – particularly with concomitant use of other medications that inhibit the uptake of serotonin or prevent it from being broken down. These include amitriptyline, tramadol and other anti-depressants.

Driving and Skilled Tasks
Duloxetine may be associated with sedation and dizziness. Patients should be informed that if they experience these symptoms, especially when starting treatment, they need to avoid potentially hazardous tasks such as driving or operating machinery.

Treatment Cessation
The dose should be reduced over at least one to two weeks. Abrupt withdrawal or marked reduction of the dose can lead to nausea, vomiting, headache, anxiety, dizziness, paraesthesia, sleep disturbances and tremor. The risk of withdrawal symptoms is dependent on the duration and dose of therapy and the rate of dose reduction.

Etoricoxib

(E-tor-e-cox-ib)

Etoricoxib is a selective cyclooxygenase-2 (COX-2) inhibitor with a lower risk of gastrointestinal toxicity compared to traditional non-steroidal anti-inflammatory drugs. It is used to treat pain and inflammation in a number of long-term conditions including osteoarthritis and ankylosing spondylitis.

Class of Medication

Non-steroidal anti-inflammatory drug

Mechanism of Action

Etoricoxib selectively inhibits COX-2, which is responsible for the production of prostaglandins involved in pain and inflammatory pathways. Most traditional NSAIDs are non-selective and inhibit both COX isoforms (COX-1 and COX-2). Because COX-1 is thought to play a pivotal role in protecting the stomach lining (mucosa), medications that do not inhibit COX-1 but selectively target COX-2 are thought to lower the risk of stomach upsets, ulceration and bleeding with long-term use.

Prescribed For

- Pain and inflammation in osteoarthritis
- Pain and inflammation in rheumatoid arthritis
- Pain and inflammation in ankylosing spondylitis
- Acute gout

Adverse Effects

- Arrhythmias
- Asthenia
- Bronchospasm
- Constipation
- Diarrhoea
- Dizziness
- Fluid retention
- Gastrointestinal discomfort
- Gastrointestinal disorders
- Headache
- Hypertension
- Increased risk of infection
- Influenza like illness

- Nausea
- Oedema
- Oral ulceration
- Palpitations
- Skin reactions
- Vomiting

Contraindications

- Previous history of hypersensitivity to etoricoxib or any other NSAID
- Active gastrointestinal bleeding
- Active gastrointestinal ulceration
- Cerebrovascular disease
- Inflammatory bowel disease
- Ischaemic heart disease
- Mild to severe heart failure
- Peripheral arterial disease
- Uncontrolled hypertension (persistently above 140/90 mmHg)

Cautions

- Allergic disorders
- Cardiac impairment
- Coagulation defects
- Connective-tissue disorders
- Dehydration (risk of renal impairment)
- History of cardiac failure
- History of gastrointestinal disorders
- Hypertension
- Left ventricular dysfunction
- May mask symptoms of infection
- Oedema
- Risk factors for cardiovascular events

Adult Dosage

Pain and Inflammation in Osteoarthritis

Initial dose: 30 mg once daily
Titration: increased if necessary to 60 mg once daily
Maximum dose: 60 mg daily

Pain and Inflammation in Rheumatoid Arthritis and Ankylosing Spondylitis

Initial dose: 60 mg once daily
Titration: increased if necessary to 90 mg once daily
Maximum dose: 90 mg daily

Acute Gout

Dose: 120 mg once daily for a maximum of eight days

Notes on Dosage and Administration

- Research suggests that selective COX-2 inhibitors may be associated with a higher risk of thrombotic events (especially myocardial infarction and stroke) than those associated with non-selective NSAIDs
- Etoricoxib should be used with caution in patients at greater risk of cardiovascular events
- The risk associated with etoricoxib may increase with dose and duration of exposure. Therefore, the shortest duration and lowest effective dose should be used
- Advise patients to take the medication with food to decrease absorption rates and adverse effects

Driving and Skilled Tasks

Some patients experience dizziness, vertigo or somnolence while taking etoricoxib and should be advised to avoid driving or operating machinery.

Treatment Cessation

With short-term use, the medication can be stopped as soon as it is no longer required.

Fentanyl

(fen·tuh·nil)

Fentanyl is a synthetic opioid that acts as a potent analgesic with approximately 80–100 times the strength of morphine at equivalent doses. It is usually reserved for treating severe pain arising from surgery, injury or cancer. Fentanyl has the same mechanism of action as that of other opioids; however, due to its potency, it is also highly addictive.

Class of Medication

- Strong opioid analgesic

Mechanism of Action

Fentanyl works by activating specific opioid receptors (mu, kappa and delta) located in the central nervous system, gastrointestinal system and peripheral tissue. Its widespread effects include analgesia, sedation, anxiolysis, euphoria, respiratory depression and gastrointestinal system smooth muscle contraction

Fentanyl exerts its analgesic effect in two ways:
- In the presynaptic nociceptive neurone, it reduces the influx of calcium, which in turn reduces neurotransmitter release. As a consequence, there is reduced nociceptive transmission to the postsynaptic neuron
- In the postsynaptic neurone, it increases the efflux of potassium from the neuron. This results in hyperpolarisation of the nociceptive neuron and reduces the nociceptive signal passing up to the spinal cord to the brain

The net result is a significant decrease in nociceptive transmission

Prescribed For

- Chronic intractable pain not currently treated with a strong opioid analgesic (not opiate-naïve patients)
- Analgesia and enhancement of anaesthesia during operation
- Breakthrough pain in patients receiving opioid therapy for chronic cancer pain

Adverse Effects

For All Opioids

- Arrhythmias
- Confusion
- Constipation
- Dizziness

- Drowsiness
- Dry mouth
- Euphoric mood
- Flushing
- Hallucination
- Headache
- Hyperhidrosis
- Hypotension (with high doses)
- Miosis
- Nausea (more common on initiation)
- Palpitations
- Respiratory depression (with high doses)
- Skin reactions
- Urinary retention
- Vertigo
- Visual impairment
- Vomiting (more common on initiation)
- Withdrawal syndrome

For Fentanyl (Patches)

- Anxiety
- Decreased appetite
- Weakness, loss of energy
- Depression
- Shortness of breath
- Diarrhoea
- Abdominal pains
- Hypertension
- Sleep disturbance
- Muscle pains
- Oedema
- Abnormal sensation
- Altered temperature sensation.
- Tremor

Contraindications

For All Opioids

- Acute respiratory depression
- Comatose patients
- Head injury (opioid analgesics interfere with pupillary responses vital for neurological assessment)
- Increased intracranial pressure (opioid analgesics interfere with pupillary responses vital for neurological assessment)
- Risk of paralytic ileus

For Fentanyl (Patches)

- Do not use in opioid naive patients

Cautions

For All Opioids

- Adrenocortical insufficiency (reduced dose is recommended)
- Asthma (avoid during an acute attack)
- Central sleep apnoea
- Convulsive disorders
- Current or history of mental health disorder
- Current or history of substance use disorder
- Debilitated patients (reduced dose is recommended)
- Diseases of the biliary tract
- Elderly (reduced dose is recommended)
- Hypotension
- Hypothyroidism (reduced dose is recommended)
- Impaired respiratory function (avoid in chronic obstructive pulmonary disease)
- Inflammatory bowel disorders
- Myasthenia gravis
- Obstructive bowel disorders
- Prostatic hypertrophy (in adults)
- Shock
- Urethral stenosis

Adult Dosage

Chronic Intractable Pain Not Currently Treated With A Strong Opioid Analgesic (Not Opioid Naive Patients)

Initial dose: 12 micrograms/hour every 72 hours or 25 micrograms every 72 hours when starting
Titration: Evaluation of the analgesic effect should not be made before the patch has been worn for 24 hours (to allow for the gradual increase in plasma-fentanyl concentration). Previous analgesic therapy should be phased out gradually from time of first patch application. Dose should be adjusted at 72-hour intervals in steps of 12–25 micrograms/hour if necessary. After a dose increase, the patch should be worn through two 72-hour applications before any further increase in dose

Notes on Dosage and Administration

- Fentanyl comes as transdermal patches, nasal spray, tablets and lozenge
- Serious harm, including fatalities, has been reported with the use of fentanyl patches, and there is considerable risk of respiratory depression linked with its use
- Patients and carers should be advised to:
  - Not exceed the prescribed dose
  - Follow the correct frequency of patch application, avoid touching the adhesive side of patches, and wash hands after application

- Not cut patches and avoid exposure to heat, including via hot water, as it accelerates drug release and shortens duration of action
- Ensure that old patches are removed before applying a new one
- Follow instructions for safe storage and properly dispose of used patches or those which are not needed
- Dependence/addiction is associated with prolonged use (longer than 3 months) of opioids for non-malignant pain
- Guidelines do not recommend use for chronic primary pain, including chronic lower back pain and fibromyalgia
- There is an increased risk in individuals with current or history of substance use disorder or mental health disorders

Driving and Skilled Tasks
Driving or performing skilled tasks at the start of therapy with opioid analgesics, and following dose changes, should be avoided as fentanyl may impair mental and/or physical abilities. Patients are advised to not drive or perform hazardous tasks until they know how the medication will affect them.

Treatment Cessation
Avoid abrupt withdrawal after long-term treatment. They should be withdrawn gradually to avoid withdrawal symptoms following guidelines of reduction by no more than 10% every two to four weeks.

Gabapentin

[ga-ba-pen-tin]

Gabapentin is used in conjunction with other anticonvulsants to control certain types of seizures in patients with epilepsy. It has also been shown to provide good levels of pain relief in people with postherpetic neuralgia and peripheral diabetic neuropathy. Although it is widely prescribed for other types of neuropathic pain, there is little evidence of its effectiveness in these conditions (Wiffen et al., 2017).

Class of Medication

- Anti-epileptic

Mechanism of Action

The mechanism by which gabapentin relieves nerve pain and lowers the risk of seizures is unclear. It is thought that gabapentin exerts it anti-nociceptive activity by binding to specific voltage-gated calcium channels, which inhibits neurotransmitter release and reduces synaptic transmission. This reduction in neuronal excitability is what provides gabapentin with its anti-nociceptive and anticonvulsant effects.

Prescribed For

- Peripheral neuropathic pain
- Adjunctive treatment of focal seizures with or without secondary generalisation
- Monotherapy for focal seizures with or without secondary generalisation
- Menopausal symptoms in women with breast cancer
- Oscillopsia in multiple sclerosis
- Spasticity in multiple sclerosis

Adverse Effects

- Anxiety
- Abnormal appetite
- Arthralgia
- Asthenia
- Abnormal behaviour
- Confusion
- Constipation
- Cough
- Depression
- Diarrhoea

- Dizziness
- Drowsiness
- Dry mouth
- Dysarthria
- Dyspnoea
- Emotional lability
- Flatulence
- Abnormal gait
- Gastrointestinal discomfort
- Headache
- Hypertension
- Increased risk of infection
- Insomnia
- Leucopoenia
- Malaise
- Movement disorders
- Muscle complaints
- Nausea
- Nystagmus
- Oedema pain
- Abnormal reflexes
- Seizure (in children)
- Sensation abnormal
- Sexual dysfunction
- Skin reactions
- Abnormal thinking
- Tooth disorder
- Tremor
- Vasodilation
- Vertigo
- Visual impairment
- Vomiting

Cautions

- Diabetes mellitus
- Elderly
- High doses of oral solution in adolescents and adults with low body-weight
- History of substance abuse
- Mixed seizures (including absences)
- Respiratory depression

Adult Dosage

Neuropathic Pain

Initial dose: 300 mg once daily on day 1, then 300 mg twice daily on day 2, then 300 mg three times a day on day 3

Alternatively, initially 300 mg three times a day on day 1

Titration: Increased in steps of 300 mg every two to three days in three divided doses, adjusted according to response

Maximum: 3.6 g per day

Notes on Dosage and Administration

Gabapentin has recently been reclassified as a Class C, schedule 3 controlled drug in the UK as it has abuse potential. It can induce feelings of euphoria, intense relaxation and calmness, especially if conventional dosages are not followed. The reclassification is intended to prevent people from stockpiling prescriptions and makes getting repeat prescriptions more difficult.

Driving and Skilled Tasks

Gabapentin acts on the central nervous system and may cause drowsiness, dizziness or other related symptoms; especially at the beginning of treatment or after an increase in dose. These may only occur to a mild or moderate degree but can be dangerous in patients driving or operating machinery.

Treatment Cessation

Gabapentin should not be stopped suddenly as patients could develop significant and serious withdrawal effects, including heightened anxiety, heart palpitations, sweating, confusion and agitation. It is possible to prevent withdrawal seizures and other symptoms by gradually reducing the dose of gabapentin. The rate of reduction will be dependent on the current dosage, length of time on the medication and patient's beliefs and expectations.

6.14

Ibuprofen

(eye-byoo'proe-fen)

Ibuprofen is the most commonly used and prescribed non-steroidal anti-inflammatory drug (NSAID). It has prominent analgesic and antipyretic properties and has fewer side-effects than those associated with other NSAIDs - especially at low doses. However, its anti-inflammatory effects are weaker than other non-selective NSAIDs.

Class of Medication

- NSAID

Mechanism of Action

Prostaglandins are produced in response to injury or infection and play a key role in generating the inflammatory response. Ibuprofen works by inhibiting cyclooxygenase (COX), an enzyme responsible for prostaglandin synthesis. As a result, less prostaglandin is produced, leading to a reduction in inflammation and pain.

Prostaglandin receptors are found throughout the body and have a number of roles including:
- Maintaining the gastric mucosa
- Preventing thrombus formation
- Constricting and dilating blood vessels
- Regulating the contraction of smooth muscle tissue

By inhibiting prostaglandin formation, NSAIDs impact on these other functions, giving rise to some of their adverse effects.

Prescribed For

- Pain and inflammation in rheumatic disease and other musculoskeletal disorders
- Mild-to-moderate pain including dysmenorrhoea
- Migraine
- Dental pain
- Headache
- Fever
- Symptoms of colds and influenza
- Neuralgia
- Pyrexia with discomfort for more than three days

Adverse Effects

Side-effects are uncommon but include:
- Gastrointestinal discomfort
- Hypersensitivity
- Rash (discontinue)
- Skin reactions

Contraindications

- Contraindicated in patients with a history of hypersensitivity to aspirin or any other NSAID
- Active gastrointestinal bleeding
- Active gastrointestinal ulceration
- History of gastrointestinal bleeding or perforation related to previous NSAID therapy
- History of recurrent gastrointestinal haemorrhage (two or more distinct episodes)
- History of recurrent gastrointestinal ulceration (two or more distinct episodes)
- Severe heart failure
- Varicella infection

Cautions

- Allergic disorders
- Cardiac impairment
- Cerebrovascular disease
- Coagulation defects
- Connective-tissue disorders
- Dehydration (risk of renal impairment)
- Elderly (risk of serious side-effects and fatalities)
- Heart failure
- History of gastrointestinal disorders (e.g. ulcerative colitis, Crohn's disease)
- Ischaemic heart disease
- May mask symptoms of infection
- Peripheral arterial disease
- Risk factors for cardiovascular events
- Uncontrolled hypertension

Adult Dosage

Pain and Inflammation in Rheumatic Disease and Other Musculoskeletal Disorders

Mild-to-Moderate Pain Including Dysmenorrhoea

Postoperative Analgesia

Dental Pain

Initial dose: 300–400 mg three to four times a day
Titration: Increased if necessary up to 600 mg four times a day
Maintenance: 200–400 mg three times a day, may be adequate
Maximum dose: 2.4 g

Modified-release medicines

Initial dose: 1.6 g once daily, taken in the early evening

Titration: Increased if necessary to 2.4 g daily in two divided doses. Dose to be increased only in severe cases

Max dose: 2.4 g

Acute Migraine

Initial dose: 400–600 mg in one dose. To be taken as soon as migraine symptoms develop

Notes on Dosage and Administration

- Although the analgesic effect of ibuprofen should occur soon after taking the medication, the anti-inflammatory effect may take up to three weeks to occur
- If an appropriate response is not achieved within a week for analgesia and within three weeks for inflammation, another NSAID should be trialled
- Ibuprofen should be taken with food to minimise gastrointestinal side effects

Driving and Skilled Tasks

Ibuprofen generally has no adverse effects on the ability to drive and use machinery. However, at high doses side-effects such as fatigue, somnolence, vertigo and visual disturbances may be experienced. In these cases, the ability to drive or operate machinery may be impaired in individual cases. This effect is potentiated by simultaneous consumption of alcohol

Treatment Cessation

Generally, there is no need to taper doses when stopping the medication. However, patients who have been taking NSAIDs for long periods should not stop taking them suddenly as the abrupt cut off may increase their risk of heart attack or stroke. They should speak to their GP about slowly tapering the dose down

Meloxicam

(mel-ox'-e-cam)

Meloxicam is a non-steroidal anti-inflammatory drug (NSAID) used to relieve pain caused by osteoarthritis, rheumatoid arthritis and various other musculoskeletal conditions (especially in children who cannot tolerate other NSAIDs). It is longer acting than most other NSAIDs and is often considered a favourable option for those who require once-daily dosing. Meloxicam is a preferential COX-2 inhibitor, especially at low doses, but whether it reduces the risk of adverse gastrointestinal effects remains debatable.

Class of Medication

- NSAID

Mechanism of Action

Meloxicam preferentially inhibits cyclooxygenase-2 (COX-2), which is responsible for the production of prostaglandins involved in pain and inflammatory pathways. Most traditional NSAIDs are non-selective and inhibit both COX isoforms (COX-1 and COX-2). Because COX-1 is thought to play a pivotal role in protecting the stomach lining (mucosa), medications that selectively target COX-2 are thought to lower the risk of stomach upsets, ulceration and bleeding with long-term use.

Prescribed For

- Exacerbation of osteoarthritis (short-term)
- Pain and inflammation in rheumatic disease and ankylosing spondylitis
- Relief of pain and inflammation in juvenile idiopathic arthritis and other musculoskeletal disorders in children intolerant to other NSAIDs

Adverse Effects

- Constipation
- Diarrhoea
- Gastrointestinal discomfort
- Gastrointestinal disorders
- Headache
- Nausea
- Vomiting

Contraindications

- Contraindicated in patients with a history of hypersensitivity to aspirin or any other NSAID
- Active gastrointestinal bleeding or ulceration
- Following coronary artery bypass graft surgery
- History of gastrointestinal bleeding or perforation related to previous NSAID therapy
- History of recurrent gastrointestinal haemorrhage or ulceration (two or more distinct episodes)
- Severe heart failure

Cautions

- Allergic disorders
- Cardiac impairment
- Cerebrovascular disease
- Coagulation defects
- Connective-tissue disorders
- Dehydration (risk of renal impairment)
- Elderly (risk of serious side-effects and fatalities)
- Heart failure
- History of gastrointestinal disorders (e.g., ulcerative colitis, Crohn's disease)
- Ischaemic heart disease
- May mask symptoms of infection
- Peripheral arterial disease
- Risk factors for cardiovascular events
- Uncontrolled hypertension

Adult Dosage

Exacerbation of Osteoarthritis (Short-Term)

Initial dose: 7.5 mg once daily
Titration: Increased if necessary, up to 15 mg once daily
Maximum dose: 15 mg daily

Pain and Inflammation in Rheumatic Disease
Ankylosing Spondylitis

Initial dose: 15 mg once daily
Titration: Reduced to 7.5 mg once daily if required
Maximum dose: 15 mg daily. In elderly, maximum 7.5 mg once daily

Notes on Dosage and Administration
The main advantage of prescribing meloxicam over other NSAIDs is that it has a long duration of action, so it only needs to be taken once a day.

Driving and Skilled Tasks
Meloxicam is likely to have no or negligible influence on the ability to drive or operate machinery.

Treatment Cessation
Patients who have been taking NSAIDs for long periods should not stop taking them suddenly as the abrupt cut off may increase their risk of heart attack or stroke. They should speak to their GP about slowly tapering the dose down.

6.16

Morphine Sulphate

(maw·feen sul-fayt)

Morphine is an opiate alkaloid derived from the opium poppy (Papaver somniferum) and produced synthetically as a potent analgesic used for managing moderate to severe pain.

It has historically been prescribed for acute and chronic pain. However, as with all opioids, its role in managing long-term, persistent pain is currently being reviewed and debated. Its therapeutic benefits are often limited due to tolerance, withdrawal, risk of abuse, extensive side effect profile and risk to long-term health.

Class of Medication

- Opiate (μ receptor agonist)

Mechanism of Action

Opioid drugs work by activating specific opioid receptors (mu, kappa and delta) located in the central nervous system, gastrointestinal system and peripheral tissue. Its widespread effects include analgesia, sedation, anxiolysis, euphoria, respiratory depression and gastrointestinal system smooth muscle contraction.

Opioids exert their analgesic effect in two ways:

- In the presynaptic nociceptive neurone, it reduces the influx of calcium, which in turn reduces neurotransmitter release. As a consequence, there is reduced nociceptive transmission to the postsynaptic neurone
- In the postsynaptic neuron it increases the efflux of potassium from the neuron. This results in hyperpolarisation of the nociceptive neuron and reduces the nociceptive signal passing up to the spinal cord to the brain

The net result is a significant decrease in nociceptive transmission.

Prescribed For

- Acute and chronic pain
- Pain relief in palliative care
- Myocardial infarction (pain relief)
- Breathlessness in palliative care

Adverse Effects

For All Opioids

- Arrhythmias
- Confusion

- Constipation
- Dizziness
- Drowsiness
- Dry mouth
- Euphoric mood
- Flushing
- Hallucination
- Headache
- Hyperhidrosis
- Hypotension (with high doses)
- Miosis
- Nausea (more common on initiation)
- Palpitations
- Respiratory depression (with high doses)
- Skin reactions
- Urinary retention
- Vertigo
- Visual impairment
- Vomiting (more common on initiation)
- Withdrawal syndrome

For Morphine

- Appetite decreased
- Asthenic conditions
- Gastrointestinal discomfort
- Insomnia
- Neuromuscular dysfunction

Contraindications

For All Opioids

- Acute respiratory depression
- Comatose patients
- Head injury (opioid analgesics interfere with pupillary responses vital for neurological assessment)
- Increased intracranial pressure (opioid analgesics interfere with pupillary responses vital for neurological assessment)
- Risk of paralytic ileus

For Morphine

- Acute abdomen
- Delayed gastric emptying
- Heart failure secondary to chronic lung disease
- Phaeochromocytoma

Cautions

For All Opioids

- Adrenocortical insufficiency (reduced dose is recommended)
- Asthma (avoid during an acute attack)
- Central sleep apnoea
- Convulsive disorders
- Current or history of mental health disorder
- Current or history of substance use disorder
- Debilitated patients (reduced dose is recommended)
- Diseases of the biliary tract
- Elderly (reduced dose is recommended)
- Hypotension
- Hypothyroidism (reduced dose is recommended)
- Impaired respiratory function (avoid in chronic obstructive pulmonary disease)
- Inflammatory bowel disorders
- Myasthenia gravis
- Obstructive bowel disorders
- Prostatic hypertrophy (in adults)
- Shock
- Urethral stenosis

For Morphine

- Cardiac arrhythmias
- Pancreatitis
- Severe cor pulmonale

Adult Dosage

Acute Pain

Initial dose: 10 mg every four hours, adjusted according to response

For the elderly
Initial dose: 5 mg every four hours, adjusted according to response

Chronic Pain

Initial dose: 5–10 mg every four hours, adjusted according to response

Pain (with Modified-Release 12-Hourly Preparations)

Dose: Every 12 hours, dose adjusted according to daily morphine requirements, dosage requirements should be reviewed if the brand is altered

Pain (with Modified-Release 24-Hourly Preparations)

Dose: Every 24 hours, dose adjusted according to daily morphine requirements, dosage requirements should be reviewed if the brand is altered

Notes on Dosage and Administration

- Opiates are at their most effective with short to medium term (<12 weeks) or intermittent use
- Evidence is lacking that they benefit most people with long-term pain
- 80% of people will experience at least one side effect
- Significant increase in risks when above 120 mg daily equivalent morphine
- Patients need a clear plan as well as an understanding of expectations
- The affinity of opioids for the different receptors, and their rate of metabolism, will vary between patients, hence the variation in clinical effectiveness

Driving and Skilled Tasks

Morphine may modify the patient's reactions to a varying extent depending on the dosage and susceptibility. Drowsiness may affect performance of skilled tasks (e.g. driving). Driving at the start of therapy with opioid analgesics, and following dose changes, should be avoided. If affected, patients should not drive or operate machinery. Opioids also enhance the effects of alcohol.

Treatment Cessation

- Avoid abrupt withdrawal after long-term treatment
- Opioids should be withdrawn gradually to avoid abstinence symptoms
- Follow guidelines by reducing no more than 10% every two to four weeks

6.17

Naproxen

(na-prox'en)

Naproxen is a non-steroidal anti-inflammatory (NSAID) medication used to relieve pain and inflammation caused by musculoskeletal disorders, rheumatic disease, migraine and gout. Although its mechanism of action is similar to that of ibuprofen, naproxen is longer acting and so only needs to be administered twice a day. This may make it a better option for treating chronic inflammatory conditions and those requiring an easier dosing regimen.

Class of Medication

- NSAID

Mechanism of Action

Prostaglandins are produced in response to injury or infection and play a key role in generating the inflammatory response. Naproxen works by inhibiting cyclooxygenase (COX), an enzyme responsible for prostaglandin synthesis. As a result, less prostaglandin is produced, leading to a reduction in inflammation and pain.

Prostaglandin receptors are found throughout the body and have a number of roles including:
- Maintaining the gastric mucosa
- Preventing thrombus formation
- Constricting and dilating blood vessels
- Regulating the contraction of smooth muscle tissue

By inhibiting prostaglandin formation, NSAIDs impact these other functions, giving rise to some of their adverse effects.

Prescribed For

- Pain and inflammation in rheumatic disease
- Pain and inflammation in musculoskeletal disorders
- Dysmenorrhoea
- Acute gout
- Acute migraine

Adverse Effects

- Confusion
- Dizziness
- Drowsiness
- Headache
- Disturbances

- Tinnitus
- Fatigue
- Visual disturbance
- Rash
- Pruritis
- Purpura

Contraindications

- Contraindicated in patients with a history of hypersensitivity to aspirin or any other NSAID
- Active gastrointestinal bleeding or ulceration
- History of gastrointestinal bleeding or perforation related to previous NSAID therapy
- History of recurrent gastrointestinal haemorrhage or ulceration (two or more distinct episodes)
- Severe heart failure

Cautions

- Allergic disorders
- Cardiac impairment
- Cerebrovascular disease
- Coagulation defects
- Connective-tissue disorders
- Dehydration (risk of renal impairment)
- Elderly (risk of serious side-effects and fatalities)
- Heart failure
- History of gastrointestinal disorders (e.g., ulcerative colitis, crohn's disease)
- Ischaemic heart disease
- May mask symptoms of infection
- Peripheral arterial disease
- Risk factors for cardiovascular events
- Uncontrolled hypertension

Adult Dosage

Pain and Inflammation in Rheumatic Disease

Initial dose: 0.5–1 g daily in one to two divided doses

Pain and Inflammation in Musculoskeletal Disorders
Dysmenorrhoea

Initial dose: 500 mg, then 250 mg every six to eight hours as required
Maximum dose: 1.25 g daily after the first day

Acute Gout

Dose: 750 mg, then 250 mg every eight hours until attack has passed

Acute Migraine

Dose: 500 mg for one dose, to be taken in combination with sumatriptan as soon as migraine symptoms develop

Notes on Dosage and Administration
- Although the analgesic effect of naproxen should occur soon after taking the medication the anti-inflammatory effect may take up to three weeks
- If an appropriate response is not achieved within a week for analgesia and within three weeks for inflammation, another NSAID should be trialled
- Naproxen should be taken with food to minimise gastrointestinal side effects

Driving and Skilled Tasks
Naproxen generally has no adverse effects on the ability to drive and use machinery. However, at high doses undesirable effects such as dizziness, drowsiness, fatigue and visual disturbances are possible after taking NSAIDs. If affected, patients should not drive or operate machinery.

Treatment Cessation
Generally, there is no need to taper doses when stopping naproxen. However, patients who have been taking NSAIDs for long periods should not stop taking them suddenly as the abrupt cut off may increase their risk of heart attack or stroke. They should speak to their GP about slowly tapering the dose down.

Oxycodone

(ok·see·kow·down)

Oxycodone is a semi-synthetic opioid that acts on mu, kappa and delta receptors. It is a potent analgesic with twice the strength of morphine at equivalent oral doses (10 mg oxycodone = 20 mg morphine). Oxycodone has the same mechanism of action as those of other opioids but with potentially fewer side effects. Its clinical efficacy is similar to that of morphine.

Class of Medication

- Strong opioid

Mechanism of Action

Like other opioid drugs, oxycodone works by activating specific opioid receptors (mu, kappa and delta), located in the central nervous system, gastrointestinal system and peripheral tissue. Its widespread effects include analgesia, sedation, anxiolysis, euphoria, respiratory depression and gastrointestinal system smooth muscle contraction.

Opioids exert their analgesic effect in two ways:
- In the presynaptic nociceptive neuron it reduces the influx of calcium, which in turn reduces neurotransmitter release. As a consequence, there is reduced nociceptive transmission to the postsynaptic neuron
- In the postsynaptic neurone, it increases the efflux of potassium from the neuron. This results in hyperpolarisation of the nociceptive neuron and reduces the nociceptive signal passing up to the spinal cord to the brain.

The net result is a significant decrease in nociceptive transmission.

Prescribed For

- Severe pain
- Postoperative pain
- Moderate to severe pain in palliative care

Adverse Effects

For All Opioids:

- Arrhythmias
- Confusion
- Constipation
- Dizziness
- Drowsiness

- Dry mouth
- Euphoric mood
- Flushing
- Hallucination
- Headache
- Hyperhidrosis
- Hypotension (with high doses)
- Miosis
- Nausea (more common on initiation)
- Palpitations
- Respiratory depression (with high doses)
- Skin reactions
- Urinary retention
- Vertigo
- Visual impairment
- Vomiting (more common on initiation)
- Withdrawal syndrome

For Oxycodone:

- Anxiety
- Bronchospasm
- Depression
- Diarrhoea
- Dyspnoea
- Gastrointestinal discomfort
- Hiccups
- Mood altered
- Tremor

Contraindications

For All Opioids:

- Acute respiratory depression
- Comatose patients
- Head injury (opioid analgesics interfere with pupillary responses vital for neurological assessment)
- Increased intracranial pressure (opioid analgesics interfere with pupillary responses vital for neurological assessment)
- Risk of paralytic ileus

For Oxycodone:

- Acute abdomen
- Chronic constipation
- Cor pulmonale
- Delayed gastric emptying

Cautions

For All Opioids:

- Adrenocortical insufficiency (reduced dose is recommended)
- Asthma (avoid during an acute attack)
- Central sleep apnoea
- Convulsive disorders
- Current or history of mental health disorder
- Current or history of substance use disorder
- Debilitated patients (reduced dose is recommended)
- Diseases of the biliary tract
- Elderly (reduced dose is recommended)
- Hypotension
- Hypothyroidism (reduced dose is recommended)
- Impaired respiratory function (avoid in chronic obstructive pulmonary disease)
- Inflammatory bowel disorders
- Myasthenia gravis
- Obstructive bowel disorders
- Prostatic hypertrophy (in adults)
- Shock
- Urethral stenosis

For Oxycodone:

- Pancreatitis
- Toxic psychosis

Adult Dosage

Severe Pain/Postoperative Pain

Immediate release medicines
Initial dose: 5 mg every four to six hours
Titration: Dose to be increased if necessary according to the severity of pain. Some patients may require higher doses than the maximum daily dose
Max dose: 400 mg per day

Modified (slow) release medicines:
Initial dose: 10 mg every 12 hours
Titration: Dose to be increased if necessary according to the severity of pain. Some patients may require higher doses than the maximum daily dose
Max dose: 200 mg every 12 hours

For Onexila XL®
Initial dose: 10 mg every 24 hours
Titration: Dose to be increased if necessary according to the severity of pain. Some patients may require higher doses than the maximum daily dose
Max dose: 400 mg per day

Notes on Dosage and Administration

- Oxycodone comes in an immediate-release preparation, with peak plasma levels at one hour following ingestion, although its analgesic effect starts within 15 minutes. The modified-release preparation acts about an hour after ingestion, reaching peak plasma levels at three hours
- Oxycodone is a prodrug (like codeine and tramadol) and is metabolised by cytochrome P450 enzymes in the liver. As a result, some people cannot completely metabolise it and receive no benefit and at the other end of the scale are ultra-metabolisers who are at increased risk of toxicity and overdose

Driving and Skilled Tasks

Drowsiness may affect the performance of skilled tasks (e.g. driving); the effects of alcohol are enhanced. Driving at the start of therapy with opioid analgesics, and following dose changes, should be avoided.

Treatment Cessation

- Avoid abrupt withdrawal after long-term treatment
- Opioids should be withdrawn gradually to avoid withdrawal symptoms
- Follow guidelines by reducing no more than 10% every two to four weeks

Paracetamol

(par-ra-cet-a-mol)

Paracetamol is widely used as a first line analgesic for a range of pain conditions and to reduce fever. It has a similar mechanism of action to that of non-steroidal anti-inflammation drugs, but has, at best, weak anti-inflammatory properties. Paracetamol is often combined with other pain medications (codeine, ibuprofen, tramadol, etc.) as it may offer better analgesia than either drug alone. Paracetamol is generally safe to use at prescribed doses and has very few side-effects, though it can cause liver damage if taken in overdose.

Class of Medication

- Non-opioid analgesic

Mechanism of Action

The mechanism of action of paracetamol is still not clear, but it is thought to act on a number of pain pathways. It inhibits cyclooxygenase (COX), an enzyme responsible for prostaglandin synthesis. This reduction in prostaglandin production increases pain thresholds in the brain and spinal cord, leading to his analgesic and anti-pyretic effects.

It is thought that paracetamol inhibits COX within the central nervous system, rather than at the site of injured or inflamed tissue, which explains its lack of anti-inflammatory activity. It also preferentially inhibits COX-2 and therefore does not have the same detrimental effect on gastrointestinal mucosa or anti-platelet activity as those of COX-1 inhibition.

Paracetamol reduces fever by reducing prostaglandin production in the thermoregulatory region of the thalamus – an area of the brain that regulates body temperature.

Paracetamol also activates descending serotonergic pathways that interact with nociceptors in the dorsal horn to increase the pain thresholds.

Prescribed For

- Mild-to-moderate pain
- Pyrexia
- Acute migraine

Adverse Effects

General side effects are rare. Liver damage and, less frequently, renal damage occurs following overdose.

Cautions

- Body-weight under 50 kg – increased risk of toxicity even at therapeutic doses
- Chronic alcohol consumption
- Chronic dehydration
- Chronic malnutrition
- Long-term use (especially in those who are malnourished)
- Co-administration of enzyme-inducing anti-epileptic medications may increase toxicity – doses should be reduced
- Adult doses
- Mild-to-moderate pain
- Pyrexia

Adult Dosage

Mild-to-Moderate Pain

Pyrexia

Dose: 0.5–1 g every four to six hours; maximum 4 g per day

Acute Migraine

Dose: 1 g for one dose. To be taken as soon as migraine symptoms develop

Notes on Dosage and Administration

- Due to its easy and widespread availability many people are not aware of the maximum dose (4 g a day) and may regularly exceed it
- Even a small increase over the maximum dose may increase the risk of liver toxicity in people who regularly drink more than the recommended amount of alcohol

Driving and Skilled Tasks

Paracetamol does not affect driving or skilled tasks

Treatment Cessation

Paracetamol can be stopped immediately

Pregabalin

(Pre-ga-ba-lin)

Pregabalin is primarily an anticonvulsant drug but is increasingly being prescribed for peripheral and central neuropathic pain. Pregabalin is effective in treating postherpetic neuralgia, painful diabetic neuralgia and mixed or unclassified post-traumatic neuropathic pain. Significant variability is observed in people's response to pregabalin, with some deriving substantial or moderate benefits, while others have no benefits or discontinue treatment (Derry et al., 2019).

Class of Medication

- Anti-epileptic

Mechanism of Action

The mechanism by which pregabalin relieves nerve pain and lowers the risk of seizures is not fully understood. It is thought that pregabalin exerts its effect by binding to specific voltage-gated calcium channels, thereby inhibiting neurotransmitter release in the central nervous system. This prevents synaptic transmission and reduces neuronal excitability which provides its anti-nociceptive, anticonvulsant and anxiolytic effects.

Prescribed For

- Peripheral and central neuropathic pain
- Adjunctive therapy for focal seizures with or without secondary generalisation
- Generalised anxiety disorder

Adverse Effects

- Abdominal distension
- Appetite abnormal
- Asthenia
- Cervical spasm
- Concentration impaired
- Confusion
- Constipation
- Diarrhoea
- Dizziness
- Drowsiness
- Dry mouth
- Feeling abnormal
- Gait abnormal

- Gastrointestinal disorders
- Headache
- Increased risk of infection
- Joint disorders
- Memory loss
- Mood altered
- Movement disorders
- Muscle complaints
- Nausea
- Oedema
- Pain
- Sensation abnormal
- Sexual dysfunction
- Sleep disorders
- Speech impairment
- Vertigo
- Vision disorders
- Vomiting
- Weight changes

Cautions

- Conditions that may precipitate encephalopathy
- Elderly
- History of substance abuse
- Severe congestive heart failure
- Respiratory depression

The following patients may be at higher risk of experiencing severe respiratory depression, and dose adjustment may be necessary:
- Patients with compromised respiratory function
- Respiratory or neurological disease
- Renal impairment
- Concomitant use of central nervous system depressants
- Elderly

Adult Dosage

Peripheral and Central Neuropathic Pain

Initial dose: 150 mg daily in two to three divided doses

Titration: increased if necessary to 300 mg daily in two to three divided doses; dose to be increased after three to seven days, then increased if necessary up to 600 mg daily in two to three divided doses; dose to be increased after seven days

Adjunctive Therapy For Focal Seizures with or without Secondary Generalisation

Initial dose: 25 mg twice daily

Titration: increased in steps of 50 mg daily. Dose to be increased at seven-day intervals, increased to 300 mg daily in two to three divided doses for seven days, then increased if necessary up to 600 mg daily in two to three divided doses

Generalised Anxiety Disorder

Initial dose: 150 mg daily in two to three divided doses

Titration: increased in steps of 150 mg daily if required, dose to be increased at seven-day intervals, increased if necessary; up to 600 mg daily in two to three divided doses

Notes on Dosage and Administration

Along with gabapentin, pregabalin has recently been reclassified as a Class C, schedule 3 controlled drug in the UK as it has abuse potential. It can induce feelings of euphoria, intense relaxation and calmness, especially if conventional dosages are not followed. The reclassification is intended to prevent people from stockpiling prescriptions and makes getting inappropriate repeat prescriptions more difficult.

Driving and Skilled Tasks

Pregabalin may cause dizziness and somnolence and therefore may influence the ability to drive or use machinery. Patients are advised not to drive, operate complex machinery or engage in other potentially hazardous activities until it is known whether it affects their ability to perform these activities.

Treatment Cessation

Pregabalin should not be stopped suddenly as patients may develop significant and serious withdrawal effects including heightened anxiety, heart palpitations, sweating, confusion and agitation. It is possible to prevent withdrawal seizures and other symptoms by gradually reducing the dose of pregabalin. The rate of reduction will be dependent on the current dosage, length of time on the medication and patient's beliefs and expectations.

6.21

Tramadol

(tra·muh·dol)

Tramadol is a centrally acting analgesic used to treat moderate to moderately severe pain. It is structurally similar to codeine and morphine, but it does not have the same potency as those of some other opioids and is therefore considered to have a lower potential for abuse.

Class of Medication

- Weak opioid

Mechanism of Action

Tramadol has two separate modes of action that contribute independently to its overall analgesic effect. Tramadol is metabolised in the liver to form O-desmethyltramadol (M1), which acts on μ opioid receptors and provides the primary analgesic effect. This is the same receptor that morphine binds to, but it has a lower affinity to the receptor; thus, its efficacy is only about a tenth of that of morphine. It is worth noting that about 7% of the population does not have the enzyme required to convert tramadol into its active metabolite and so will not receive any analgesic benefit. Tramadol also acts as a serotonin and noradrenaline reuptake inhibitor and therefore maintains the availability of these neurotransmitters in the central nervous system.

Prescribed For

- Moderate-to-severe pain
- Postoperative pain

Adult Dosage

Moderate to Severe Pain (By Mouth Using Immediate Release Medicines)

Dose: Initially 100 mg, then 50–100 mg every four to six hours
Maximum dose: 400 mg in 24 hours

Moderate to Severe Pain (with Modified-Release 12-Hourly Preparations)

Dose: 50–100 mg twice daily, increased if necessary to 150–200 mg twice daily. Doses exceeding the usual maximum dose are not generally required
Maximum dose: 400 mg in 24 hours

Moderate-to_severe Pain (with Modified-Release 24-Hourly Preparations)

Initial dose: 100–150 mg once daily, increased if necessary up to 400 mg once daily
Maximum dose: 400 mg in 24 hours

Adverse Effects

For All Opioids

- Arrhythmias
- Confusion
- Constipation
- Dizziness
- Drowsiness
- Dry mouth
- Euphoric mood
- Flushing
- Hallucination
- Headache
- Hyperhidrosis
- Hypotension (with high doses)
- Miosis
- Nausea (more common on initiation)
- Palpitations
- Respiratory depression (with high doses)
- Skin reactions
- Urinary retention
- Vertigo
- Visual impairment
- Vomiting (more common on initiation)
- Withdrawal syndrome

For Tramadol

- Fatigue

Contraindications

For All Opioids

- Acute respiratory depression
- Comatose patients
- Head injury (opioid analgesics interfere with pupillary responses vital for neurological assessment)
- Increased intracranial pressure (opioid analgesics interfere with pupillary responses vital for neurological assessment)
- Risk of paralytic ileus

For Tramadol

- Acute intoxication with alcohol, analgesics (including opioids) or hypnotics
- Compromised respiratory function (in children)
- Not suitable for narcotic withdrawal treatment
- Uncontrolled epilepsy

Cautions

For All Opioids

- Adrenocortical insufficiency
- Asthma (avoid during an acute attack)
- Central sleep apnoea
- Convulsive disorders
- Current or history of mental health disorder
- Current or history of substance use disorder
- Debilitated patients (reduced dose is recommended)
- Diseases of the biliary tract
- Elderly (reduced dose is recommended)
- Hypotension
- Hypothyroidism (reduced dose is recommended)
- Impaired respiratory function (avoid in chronic obstructive pulmonary disease)
- Inflammatory bowel disorders
- Myasthenia gravis
- Obstructive bowel disorders
- Prostatic hypertrophy
- Shock
- Urethral stenosis

For Tramadol

- Excessive bronchial secretions
- History of epilepsy – use tramadol only if compelling reasons
- Impaired consciousness
- Not suitable as a substitute in opioid-dependent patients
- Postoperative use (in children)
- Susceptibility to seizures – use tramadol only if compelling reasons
- Variation in metabolism

Notes on Dosage and Administration

- Tramadol reduces the seizure threshold, so care must be taken when using it in patients with epilepsy and in those with drug or alcohol dependence/addiction
- There is also an increased seizure risk in patients taking tramadol within the recommended dosage ranges
- A risk of serotonin syndrome is associated with the use of tramadol. The risk is increased if it is taken in conjunction with selective serotonin reuptake inhibitors, tricyclic antidepressants, monoamine oxidase inhibitors and triptans (used to treat migraines and cluster headaches). This leads to increased serotonin levels in the central nervous system, which produces a spectrum of cognitive, autonomic, neuromuscular and somatic symptoms (i.e. confusion, agitation, sweating, tachycardia, hyperreflexia and incoordination). In some instances, it can be fatal

■ Not everyone metabolises tramadol at the same rate. Poor metabolisers experience better pain relief than that experienced by intermediate metabolisers, who may experience insufficient relief. Ultra-rapid metabolisers are more likely to experience adverse effects from tramadol because of the more rapid release of M1

Driving and Skilled Tasks
Even when taken according to instructions, tramadol may cause effects such as drowsiness and dizziness and may impair the reactions of drivers and machine operators. This is increased if used in conjunction with alcohol and other psychotropic substances. When prescribing tramadol, patients should be warned of the potential cognitive function impairment. They should not drive until they know how the medication affects them.

Treatment Cessation
Avoid abrupt withdrawal after long-term treatment. Opioids should be reduced gradually to avoid withdrawal symptoms. Guidelines suggest reducing by no more than 10% every two to four weeks.

APPENDICES

Acronyms and Abbreviations

A&E	accident and emergency
AAA	abdominal aortic aneurysm
Ab	antibody
ABG	arterial blood gas
ABI	acquired brain injury/ankle-brachial index
ACE	angiotensin-converting enzyme
ACEI	angiotensin-converting enzyme (ACE) inhibitor
ACL	anterior cruciate ligament
ACT	activated clotting time/airway clearance technique/acceptance commitment therapy
ACTH	adrenocorticotrophic hormone
ADH	anti-diuretic hormone
ADL	activities of daily living
ADR	adverse drug reaction
AE	air entry
AEA	above elbow amputation
AF	atrial fibrillation
AFO	ankle-foot orthosis
Ag	antigen
AGN	acute glomerulonephritis
AI	aortic insufficiency
AIDS	acquired immunodeficiency syndrome
AJ	ankle jerk
AKA	above-knee amputation
AL	acute leukaemia
ALD	alcoholic liver disease
ALI	acute lung injury/acute limb ischaemia
ALP	alkaline phosphatase
ALS	amyotrophic lateral sclerosis
AMI	acute myocardial infarction
AML	acute myeloid leukaemia
AN	antenatal
ANA	antinuclear antibody
Anti-CCP	anti-cyclic citrullinated peptide
Anti-dsDNA	anti-double stranded DNA (antibodies)
AP	anteroposterior
APACHE	acute physiology and chronic health evaluation
ARDS	acute respiratory distress syndrome
ARF	acute renal failure

AROM	active range of movement
AS	ankylosing spondylitis
ASD	atrial septal defect
ATN	acute tubular necrosis
AV	atrioventricular
AVF	arteriovenous fistula
AVR	aortic valve replacement
AVSD	atrioventricular septal defect
AXR	abdominal X-ray
b.d./b.i.d.	twice a day (Latin)
BCC	basal cell carcinoma
BEA	below elbow amputation
BKA	below knee amputation
BLS	basic life support
BM	blood glucose monitoring
BMI	body mass index
BMR	basal metabolic rate
BNO	bowels not opened
BO	bowels opened
BOS	base of support
BP	blood pressure
BPM	beats per minute
BS	bowel sounds/breath sounds
BSA	body surface area
BVHF	bi-ventricular heart failure
c.c	with meals/food (Latin)
c/o	complains of
Ca	carcinoma, cancer
CABG	coronary artery bypass graft
CAD	coronary artery disease
CAH	chronic active hepatitis
CAL	chronic airflow limitation
CAO	chronic airways obstruction
CAPD	continuous ambulatory peritoneal dialysis
CAT	coaxial or computed axial tomography
CAVG	coronary artery vein graft
CAVHF	continuous arterial venous haemofiltration
CBT	cognitive behavioural therapy
CCB	calcium channel blocker
CCF	congestive cardiac failure
CCU	coronary care unit
CDH	congenital dislocation of the hip
CF	cystic fibrosis
CFI	cardiac function index
CFS	chronic fatigue syndrome
CHD	coronary heart disease/congenital heart disease
CHF	chronic heart failure
CI	chest infection/confidence interval
CK	creatinine kinase
CLD	chronic lung disease/chronic liver disease

CML	chronic myeloid leukaemia
CNS	central nervous system
CO	cardiac output
COAD	chronic obstructive airways disease
COPD	chronic obstructive pulmonary disease
COT	continuous oxygen therapy
CP	cerebral palsy
CPAP	continuous positive airway pressure
CPPD	calcium pyrophosphate dihydrate
CPK	creatine phosphokinase
CPM	continuous passive movements
CPN	community psychiatric nurse
CPR	cardiopulmonary resuscitation
Cr	creatinine
CRF	chronic renal failure/corticotropin-releasing factor
CRP	C-reactive protein
CRPS	complex regional pain syndrome
CSF	cerebrospinal fluid
CSU	catheter specimen of urine
CT	computed tomography
CT	cerebral tumour/coronary thrombosis/computed tomography
CT	computed axial tomography
CTD	connective tissue diseases
CTEV	congenital talipes equinovarus
CTG	cardiotocograph
CV	cardiovascular
CVA	cerebrovascular accident
CVD	cardiovascular disease
CVS	cardiovascular system
Cx	cervix
CXR	chest X-ray
D&C	dilation and curettage
D&V	diarrhoea and vomiting
DBP	diastolic blood pressure
DC	discharge
DDH	developmental dysplasia of the hips
DEXA	dual-energy X-ray absorptiometry
DH	drug history
DHS	dynamic hip screw
DIC	disseminated intravascular coagulopathy
DIOS	distal intestinal obstruction syndrome
DIP	distal interphalangeal joints
DLE	discoid lupus erythematosus
DM1	dystrophic myotonica/myotonic dystrophy
DM	diabetes mellitus
DMARD	disease-modifying anti-rheumatic drug
DMD	Duchenne muscular dystrophy
DN	district nurse
DNA	deoxyribonucleic acid/did not attend
DNAR	do not attempt resuscitation

DOB	date of birth
DPP4	dipeptidyl peptidase-4
DS	disseminated sclerosis
DSA	digital subtraction angiography
DU	duodenal ulcer
DVT	deep vein thrombosis
Dx	diagnosis
DXT	deep X-ray therapy
EBV	Epstein-Barr virus
ECF	extracellular fluid
ECG	electrocardiogram/electrocardiography
EDM	early diastolic murmur
EEG	electroencephalogram
EIA	exercise-induced asthma
EMG	electromyography
ENA	extractible nuclear antigens
ENT	ear, nose and throat
EOR	end of range
ESR	erythrocyte sedimentation rate
ESRF	end-stage renal failure
ET	endotracheal
ETT	endotracheal tube/exercise tolerance test
EUA	examination under anaesthetic
FB	foreign body
FBC	full blood count/fluid balance chart
FBG	fasting blood glucose
FES	functional electrical stimulation
FFD	fixed flexion deformity
FGF	fibroblast growth factor
FH	family history
FH	family history
FHF	fulminant hepatic failure
FITT	frequency, intensity, time and type
fMRI	functional magnetic resonance imaging
FROM	full range of movement
FSH	facioscapulohumeral muscular dystrophy
FUO	fever of unknown origin
FWB	full weight-bearing
GA	general anaesthetic
GAP	gravity-assisted positioning
GBS	Guillain-Barré syndrome
GC	general condition
GCA	giant cell arteritis
GCS	Glasgow coma scale
GH	general health
GI	gastrointestinal
GIS	gastrointestinal system
GIT	gastrointestinal tract
GOR	gastro-oesophageal reflux
GP	general practitioner

GTN	glyceryl trinitrate
GTT	glucose tolerance test
GU	gastric ulcer/genitourinary
GUM	genitourinary medicine
GUS	genitourinary system
Gyn	gynaecology
H+	hydrogen ion
HAART	highly active anti-retroviral therapy
HASO	hip abduction spinal orthosis
Hb/Hgb	haemoglobin
HCP	healthcare professional
HCT	haematocrit
HD	haemodialysis/Huntington's disease
HDU	high dependency unit
HEP	home exercise programme
HF	heart failure/haemofiltration
HH	hiatus hernia/home help
HHV-8	herpes virus 8
HI	head injury
HIB	haemophilus influenzae B
HIV	human immunodeficiency virus
HLA	human leukocyte antigen
HNPU	has not passed urine
HPC	history of presenting condition
HPOA	hypertrophic pulmonary osteoarthropathy
HPV	human papilloma virus
HR	heart rate
HS	heart sounds
HT	hypertension
Hx	history (of complaint)
IBS	irritable bowel syndrome
ICF	intracellular fluid
ICP	intracranial pressure
ICS	intercostal space
ICU	intensive care unit
IDC	indwelling catheter
IDDM	insulin-dependent diabetes mellitus
Ig	immunoglobulin
IGF	insulin growth factor
IGT	impaired glucose tolerance
IHD	ischaemic heart disease
IL	interleukin
ILD	interstitial lung disease
IM	intramuscular/intramedullary
IP	in-patient/interphalangeal
IQ	intelligence quotient
ISQ	no change (in status quo)
ITU	intensive therapy unit
IUCD	intrauterine contraceptive device
IV	intravenous

IVB	intervertebral block
IVF	*in vitro* fertilisation
IVH	intraventricular haemorrhage
IVI	intravenous infusion
IVOX	intravenacaval oxygenation
IVP	intravenous pyelogram
IVP	intravenous pyelogram
IVUS	intravascular ultrasound
Ix	investigations
JVP	jugular venous pressure
K	potassium
KAFO	knee-ankle-foot orthosis
KO	knee orthosis
KUB	kidney, ureter and bladder
LA	local anaesthetic
LBP	low back pain/low blood pressure
LDH	lactate dehydrogenase
LE	lupus erythematosus
LED	light-emitting diode
LFT	liver function test/lung function test
LIF	left iliac fossa
LIH	left inguinal hernia
LKS	liver, kidney and spleen
LL	lower limb/lower lobe
LLQ	left lower quadrant
LMN	lower motor neurone
LN	lymph node
LOC	level of consciousness
LOS	length of stay
LP	lumbar puncture
LUQ	left upper quadrant
LUT	lower urinary tract
MANE	in the morning
MAP	mean airway pressure/mean arterial pressure
MAS	minimal access surgery
MAU	medical admissions unit
MCH	mean corpuscular haemoglobin
MCL	mid-clavicular line
MCPJ	metacarpophalangeal joint
MCV	mean corpuscular volume
MD	muscular dystrophy
MDM	mid-diastolic murmur
MDT	multidisciplinary team
ME	myalgic encephalomyelitis
METS	metastases
mg	milligram
MGUS	monoclonal gammopathy of uncertain significance
MI	myocardial infarction
MIP	maximal inspiratory pressure
ml	millilitre

MM	muscle
mmol/L	millimoles per litre
MMR	measles, mumps & rubella
MND	motor neurone disease
MOP	medical outpatient
MOW	meals on wheels
MRI	magnetic resonance imaging
MRSA	methicillin-resistant staphylococcus aureus
MS	mitral stenosis/multiple sclerosis
MSE	mental state examination
MSK	musculoskeletal system
MSU	midstream urine
MTX	methotrexate
MUA	manipulation under anaesthetic
MVR	mitral valve replacement
N/S	nursing staff
N&V	nausea and vomiting
NA	not applicable
NAD	nothing abnormal detected
NAI	non-accidental injury
NBI	no bony injury
NBM	nil by mouth
NE	not engaged
NFR	not for resuscitation
NG	nasogastric
NH	nursing home
NICU	neonatal intensive care unit
NIDDM	non-insulin-dependent diabetes mellitus
NITU	neonatal intensive care unit
NIV	non-invasive ventilation
Nocte	at night
NOF	neck of femur
NOH	neck of humerus
NOS	not otherwise specified
NP	nasopharyngeal
NP	not palpable/nasal passage
NPA	nasopharyngeal airway
NPO	nothing by mouth
NPU	not passed urine
NR	nodal rhythm
NREM	non-rapid eye movement
NS	nervous system
NSA	no significant abnormality
NSAID	non-steroidal anti-inflammatory drug
NSR	normal sinus rhythm
NWB	non-weight-bearing
NYD	not yet diagnosed
O.d.	daily/once a day
O/E	on examination
OA	oral airway/osteoarthritis/on admission

Obs.	obstetrics
OCD	obsessive-compulsive disorder
OD	overdose
OGD	oesophagogastroduodenoscopy
OGTT	oral glucose tolerance test
OLT	orthotopic liver transplantation
OM	otitis media
OOH	out of hours
OPD	outpatient department
ORIF	open reduction and internal fixation
OSA	obstructive sleep apnoea
OT	occupational therapist
OTC	over-the-counter (bought medication)
PA	pernicious anaemia/posteroanterior/pulmonary artery
PACO2	partial pressure of carbon dioxide in alveolar gas
PAD	peripheral arterial disease
PADL	personal activities of daily living
PaO2	partial pressure of oxygen in arterial blood
PAP	pulmonary artery pressure
PAT	paroxysmal atrial tachycardia
PAWP	pulmonary artery wedge pressure
PBC	primary biliary cirrhosis
PC	presenting condition/pressure control
PCA	patient-controlled analgesia
PCB	post-coital bleeding
PCD	primary ciliary dyskinesia
PCP	pneumocystis carinii pneumonia
PD	Parkinson's disease/peritoneal dialysis
PD&P	postural drainage and percussion
PDA	patent ductus arteriosus
PE	pulmonary embolus
PEG	percutaneous endoscopic gastrostomy
PERLA	pupils equal and reactive to light accommodation
PET	positron emission tomography
PET	pre-eclamptic toxaemia
PH	past history
PHC	pulmonary hypertension crisis
PICC	peripherally inserted central catheter
PICU	paediatric intensive care unit
PID	pelvic inflammatory disease/prolapsed intervertebral disc
PIE	pulmonary interstitial emphysema
PIFR	peak inspiratory flow rate
PIP	proximal interphalangeal joint
PM	post mortem
PMB	postmenopausal bleeding
PMH	past medical history
PMR	percutaneous myocardial revascularisation/polymyalgia rheumatica
PN	percussion note; postnatal
PND	paroxysmal nocturnal dyspnoea/postnatal depression
PNS	peripheral nervous system

PO	by mouth
PO2	partial pressure of oxygen
POMR	problem-oriented medical record
POP	plaster of Paris
POP	progesterone-only pill
PPH	postpartum haemorrhage
PR	by rectum
PRN	as required
PROM	passive range of movement
PS	pulmonary stenosis
PTB	pulmonary tuberculosis
PTCA	percutaneous transluminal coronary angioplasty
PTH	parathyroid hormone
PTHrp	parathyroid hormone-related peptide
PTSD	post-traumatic stress disorder
PTT	partial thromboplastin time
PU	passed urine; peptic ulcer
PUO	pyrexia of unknown origin
PV	per vagina
PVD	peripheral vascular disease
PVT	paroxysmal ventricular tachycardia
PWB	partial weight-bearing
Qds/qid	four times a day
QOL	quality of life
R	right
R/O	removal of
RA	rheumatoid arthritis/right atrium
RBC	red blood cell
RBS	random blood sugar
RCA	right coronary artery
RDS	respiratory distress syndrome
REM	rapid eye movement
RF	rheumatoid factor
RFT	respiratory function test
RH	residential home
Rh	Rhesus factor
RI	respiratory infection
RIF	right iliac fossa
RIH	right inguinal hernia
RIP	rest in peace
RLL	right lower lobe
RLQ	right lower quadrant
RMT	respiratory muscle training
ROM	range of movement/motion
RPE	rating of perceived exertion
RPP	rate pressure product
RR	respiratory rate
RR	respiration rate
RS	respiratory system
RSI	repetitive strain injury

RTA	road traffic accident
RTC	return to clinic/road traffic crash
RTI	respiratory tract infection
RUA	right upper arm
RUQ	right upper quadrant
RVE	right ventricular enlargement
RVF	right ventricular failure
RVH	right ventricular hypertrophy
Rx	prescription or treatment
SA	sinoatrial
SAH	subarachnoid haemorrhage
SALT	speech and language therapist
Sao2	arterial oxygen saturation
SB	sinus bradycardia/spina bifida/still-born
SBE	subacute bacterial endocarditis
SBE	subacute bacterial endocarditis
SBG	serum blood glucose
SBP	systolic blood pressure
SC	subcutaneous
SCI	spinal cord injury
SDH	subdural haematoma
SGLTI	selective sodium glucose co-transporter-2 inhibitor
SH	social history
SHO	senior house officer
SIJ	sacroiliac joint
SIMV	synchronised intermittent mandatory ventilation
SIRS	systemic inflammatory response syndrome
SL	sublingual
SLAP	superior labrum, anterior and posterior
SLE	systemic lupus erythematosus
SLR	straight leg raise
SM	systolic murmur
SMA	spinal muscle atrophy
SMR	sub-mucous resection
SNS	sympathetic nervous system
SOA	swelling of ankles
SOAP	subjective, objective, assessment, plan (notes)
SOB	shortness of breath
SOBAR	short of breath at rest
SOBOE	short of breath on exertion
SOOB	sit out of bed
SOP	surgical outpatients
Spo2	pulse oximetry arterial oxygen saturation
Spr	special registrar
SR	sinus rhythm
SROM	spontaneous rupture of membranes
SS	social services
SSRIs	selective serotonin reuptake inhibitors
ST	sinus tachycardia
Stat	immediately

STD	sexually transmitted disease
STI	sexually transmitted infection
SVC	superior vena cava
SVD	spontaneous vaginal delivery
SVG	saphenous vein graft
SVT	supraventricular tachycardia
SW	social worker
SWD	short wave diathermy
T&A	tonsils and adenoids
T3	triiodothyronine
T4	thyroxine
T21	trisomy 21 (Down's syndrome)
TAA	thoracic aortic aneurysm
Tabs	tablets
TAH	total abdominal hysterectomy
TAVR	tissue atrial valve repair
TB	tuberculosis
TBI	traumatic brain injury
TCA	tricyclic antidepressants
Tcco2	transcutaneous carbon dioxide
TCI	to come in
Tco2	transcutaneous oxygen
tds/tid	three times a day
TENS	transcutaneous electrical nerve stimulation
TFA	transfemoral arteriogram
TFT	thyroid function test
THR	total hip replacement
TIA	transient ischaemic attack
TKA	through knee amputation
TKR	total knee replacement
TLC	total lung capacity
TLSO	thoracolumbar spinal orthosis
TMJ	temporo-mandibular joint
TMVR	tissue mitral valve repair
TNFα	tumour necrosis factor-alpha
TNS	transcutaneous nerve stimulator
TOP	termination of pregnancy
TPN	total parenteral nutrition
TPO	thyroid peroxidase antibodies
TPR	temperature, pulse and respiration
TSH	thyroid-stimulating hormone
TSR	total shoulder replacement
TT	tetanus toxoid/tuberculin tested
TURBT	transurethral resection of bladder tumour
TURP	transurethral resection of prostate
TV	tidal volume
TV	trichomonas vaginalis
TWB	touch weight-bearing
Tx	transplant

U	urea/unit
U&E	urea and electrolytes
UAO	upper airway obstruction
UAS	upper abdominal surgery
UC	ulcerative colitis
UGS	urogenital system
UL	upper limb/upper lobe
UMN	upper motor neurone
URTI	upper respiratory tract infection
USS	ultrasound scan
UTI	urinary tract infection
UV	ultraviolet light
VAS	visual analogue scale
VATS	video-assisted thoracoscopy surgery
VBG	venous blood gas
VD	venereal disease
VE	vaginal examination
VEGF	vascular endothelial growth factor
VER	visual evoked response
VF	ventricular fibrillation/vocal fremitus
VI	virgo intacta
VR	venous return/vocal resonance
VRE	vancomycin-resistant enterococcus
VSD	ventricular septal defect
VT	tidal volume
VT	ventricular tachycardia
VTE	venous thromboembolism
VV	varicose vein(s)
W/R	ward round
WBC	white blood count/white blood cell
WCC	white cell count
WNL	within normal limits
WOB	work of breathing
Wt	weight
XR	X-ray

Prefixes and Suffixes

Prefix/Suffix	Definition	Example
adeno-	gland	adenoma
-aemia	blood	hyperglycaemia
-algia	pain	neuralgia
angio-	vessel	angiogram
ante-	before	antenatal
arteri-	artery	arteriosclerosis
arthro-	joint	arthroscopy
-asis	condition	homeostasis
atel-	imperfect	atelectasis
athero-	fatty	atherosclerosis
auto-	self	autoimmunity
baro-	pressure	barotrauma
bi-	two, twice or double	bilateral, biconcave
bili-	bile	bilirubin
-blast	cell	osteoblast
brachi-	arm	brachial artery
brady-	slow	bradycardia
carcin-	cancer	carcinogen
cardio-	heart	cardiology
carpo-	wrist	carpal tunnel
-centesis	to puncture	amniocentesis
cephal-	head	cephalad
cerebro-	brain	cerebrospinal fluid
cervic-	neck	cervical fracture
chol-	bile	cholestasis
chondro-	cartilage	chondromalacia
contra-	against	contraindicated
costo-	rib	costochondral junction
cranio-	skull	craniotomy
cryo-	cold	cryotherapy

Prefix/Suffix	Definition	Example
cut-	skin	cutaneous
cyano-	blue	cyanosis
cysto-	bladder	cystoscopy
cyto-	cell	cytoplasm
dactyl-	finger	dactylomegaly
derm-	skin	dermatome
diplo-	double	diplopia
dors-	back	dorsum
dys-	difficult	dyspnoea
-ectasis	dilatation	bronchiectasis
ecto-	outside	ectoplasm
-ectomy	excision	appendectomy
encephalo-	brain	encephalitis
endo-	within	endochondral
entero-	intestine	enterotomy
erythro-	red	erythrocyte
extra-	outside	extrapyramidal
ferro-	iron	ferrous sulphate
gastro-	stomach	gastroenteritis
-genic	producing	iatrogenic
haem-	blood	haematoma
hepato-	liver	hepatectomy
hetero-	dissimilar	heterosexual
homo-	same	homosexual
hydro-	water	hydrotherapy
hyper-	excessive	hyperactive
hypo-	deficiency	hypoxaemia
iatro-	medicine, doctors	iatrogenic
idio-	one's own	idiopathic
infra-	beneath	infrapatellar
inter-	among	interrater
intra-	inside	intrarater
iso-	equal	isotonic
-itis	inflammation	tendinitis
laparo-	loins, abdomen	laparotomy
lipo-	fat	liposuction
-lysis	breakdown	autolysis
macro-	large	macrodactyly

Continued on following page

Prefix/Suffix	Definition	Example
mal-	bad, abnormal	malignant
-malacia	softening	osteomalacia
mammo-	breast	mammogram
mast-	breast	mastectomy
-megalo	enlarged	cardiomegaly
mening-	membranes	meninges
-morph	form or shape	ectomorph
myel-	spinal cord, marrow	myelitis
myo-	muscle	myotonic
naso-	nose	nasopharyngeal
necro-	death	necrosis
nephr-	kidney	nephritis
oculo-	eyes	monocular
-oid	resembling	marfanoid
oligo-	deficiency	oliguria
-oma	tumour	lymphoma
oophoro-	ovaries	oophorectomy
-opsy	examine	biopsy
-osis	state, condition	nephrosis
osseo-	bone	osseous
osteo-	bone	osteolysis
-ostomy	to form an opening	colostomy
oto-	ear	otalgia
-otomy	to make a cut	osteotomy
para-	beside	paraspinal
-penia	deficiency	thrombocytopenia
peri-	around	periosteum
phago-	eat, destroy	phagocytosis
pharyngo-	throat	pharyngoscope
-philia	love of	hydrophilia
phleb-	vein	phlebitis
-phobia	fear of	hydrophobia
-plasia	formation	hyperplasia
-plasty	moulding	rhinoplasty
-plegia	paralysis	hemiplegia
pneum-	breath, air	pneumothorax
-pnoea	breathing	dyspnoea

Prefix/Suffix	Definition	Example
poly-	many	polymyositis
pseud-	false	pseudoplegia
pyelo-	kidney	pyeloplasty
reno-	kidneys	renography
retro-	behind	retrograde
rhino-	nose	rhinitis
-rrhagia	abnormal flow	haemorrhage
salping-	fallopian tube	salpingostomy
sarco-	flesh	sarcoma
sclero-	hardening	scleroderma
-scopy	examination	endoscopy
somat-	body	somatic
spondyl-	vertebrae	spondylosis
-stasis	stagnation	haemostasis
steno-	narrow	stenosis
-stomy	surgical opening	colostomy
supra-	above	suprapubic
syn-	united with	syndesmosis
tachy-	swift	tachycardia
thoraco-	chest	thoracotomy
thrombo-	clot	thrombolytic
-tomy	incision	gastrostomy
trans-	across	transection
-trophy	growth	hypertrophy
uro-	urine	urology
vaso-	vessel	vasospasm
veno-	vein	venography

Laboratory Values

Biochemistry

Alanine aminotransferase (ALT)	10–40 U/L
Albumin	36–47 g/L
Alkaline phosphatase	40–125 U/L
Amylase	90–300 U/L
Aspartate aminotransferase (AST)	10–35 U/L
Bicarbonate (arterial)	22–28 mmol/L
Bilirubin (total)	2–17 mmol/L
C–reactive protein	<7 mg/L
Caeruloplasmin	150–600 mg/L
Calcium	2.1–2.6 mmol/L
Chloride	95–105 mmol/L
Cholesterol (total)	Desirable level <5.2 mmol/L
Cholesterol (HDL)	
Males	0.5–1.6 mmol/L
Females	0.6–1.9 mmol/L
Copper	13–24 mmol/L
Creatine kinase (total)	
Males	30–200 U/L
Females	30–150 U/L
Creatinine	55–150 mmol/L
Globulins	24–37 g/L
Glucose (venous blood, fasting)	3.6–5.8 mmol/L
Iron	
Males	14–32 μmol/L
Females	10–28 μmol/L
Iron-binding capacity total (TIBC)	45–70 μmol/L
Lactate (arterial)	0.3–1.4 mmol/L
Lactate dehydrogenase (total)	230–460 U/L
Lead (adults, whole blood)	<1.7 μmol/L
Magnesium	0.7–1.0 mmol/L
Osmolality	275–290 mmol/kg
Phosphate (fasting)	0.8–1.4 mmol/L
Potassium (serum)	3.6–5.0 mmol/L
Protein (total)	60–80 g/L
Sodium	136–145 mmol/L
Transferrin	2–4 g/L
Triglycerides (fasting)	0.6–1.8 mmol/L

Urate	
Males	0.12–0.42 mmol/L
Females	0.12–0.36 mmol/L
Urea	2.5–6.5 mmol/L
Uric acid	
Males	0.1–0.45 mmol/L
Females	0.09–0.36 mmol/L
Vitamin A	0.7–3.5 μmol/L
Vitamin C	23–57 μmol/L
Zinc	11–22 μmol/L

Haematology

Activated partial thromboplastin time (APTT)	30–40 s
Bleeding time (Ivy)	2–8 min
Erythrocyte sedimentation rate (ESR)	
Adult males	1–10 mm/h
Adult females	3–15 mm/h
Fibrinogen	1.5–4.0 g/L
Folate (serum)	4–18 mg/L
Haemoglobin	
Males	130–180 g/L
	(13–18 g/dL)
Females	115–165 g/L
	(11.5–16.5 g/dL)
International normalised ratio (INR)	0.89–1.10
Mean cell haemoglobin (MCH)	27–32 pg
Mean cell haemoglobin concentration (MCHC)	30–35 g/dL
Mean cell volume (MCV)	78–95 fL
Packed cell volume (PCV or haematocrit)	
Males	0.40–0.54 (40–54%)
Females	0.35–0.47 (35–47%)
Platelets (thrombocytes)	$150–400 \times 10^9$/L
Prothrombin time (PT)	12–16 s
Red cells (erythrocytes)	
Males	$4.5–6.5 \times 10^{12}$/L
Females	$3.85–5.30 \times 10^{12}$/L
Reticulocytes	$4.5–6.5 \times 10^{12}$/L
White cell count (leukocytes)	$4.0–11.0 \times 10^9$/L

Values vary from laboratory to laboratory, depending on the testing methods used. These reference ranges should be used as a guide only. All reference ranges apply to adults only; they may differ in children.

Conversions and units

Pounds/kg

lb	kg
1	0.45
2	0.91
3	1.36
4	1.81
5	2.27
6	2.72
7	3.18
8	3.63
9	4.08
10	4.54
11	4.99
12	5.44
13	5.90
14	6.35

Stones/kg

Stones	kg
1	6.35
2	12.70
3	19.05
4	25.40
5	31.75
6	38.10
7	44.45
8	50.80
9	57.15
10	63.50
11	69.85
12	76.20
13	82.55
14	88.90
15	95.25
16	101.60
17	107.95
18	114.30

MASS

1 kilogram (kg) = 2.205 pounds (lb)
1 pound (lb)   = 454 milligrams (mg)
              = 16 ounces (oz)
1 ounce   = 28.35 grams (g)

LENGTH

1 inch (in)   = 2.54 centimetres (cm)
1 metre (m) = 3.281 feet (ft)
              = 39.37 in
1 foot (ft)   = 30.48 cm
              = 12 in

VOLUME

1 litre (L) = 1000 millilitres (mL)
1 pint   ≈ 568 mL

PRESSURE

kPa	mmHg
1	7.5
2	15
4	30
6	45
8	60
10	75
12	90
14	105

1 millimetre of mercury (mmHg) = 0.133 kilopascal (kPa)
1 kilopascal (kPa)   = 7.5 mmHg

7.4

National Early Warning Score for the Acutely Ill or Deteriorating Patient

National early warning score (NEWS2) is a clinical assessment tool used in acute and ambulance settings to improve the detection of acute clinical illness, risk of deterioration and clinical response in adult patients, including those with sepsis.

The NEWS2 is based on a simple aggregate scoring system in which a score is allocated to physiological measurements when patients present to or are being monitored in hospital. The NEWS2 should not be used for children (under 16 years), pregnant women and those with spinal cord injury.

Six physiological parameters form the basis of the scoring system:

1. Respiration rate
2. Oxygen saturation
3. Systolic blood pressure
4. Pulse rate
5. Level of consciousness or new confusion*
6. Temperature

*The patient has new-onset confusion, disorientation and/or agitation, where previously, their mental state was normal. The patient may respond to questions coherently, but there is some confusion, disorientation and/or agitation. This would score three or four on the Glasgow coma scale (rather than the normal five for verbal response) and three on the NEWS system.

Physiological parameter	Score						
	3	2	1	0	1	2	3
Respiration rate (per minute)	≤8		9–11	12–20		21–24	≥25
SpO$_2$ Scale 1 (%)	≤91	92–93	94–95	≥96			
SpO$_2$ Scale 2 (%)	≤83	84–85	86–87	88–92 ≥93 on air	93–94 on oxygen	95–96 on oxygen	≥97 on oxygen
Air or oxygen?		Oxygen		Air			
Systolic blood pressure (mmHg)	≤90	91–100	101–110	111–219			≥220
Pulse (per minute)	≤40		41–50	51–90	91–110	111–130	≥131
Consciousness				Alert			CVPU
Temperature (°C)	≤35.0		35.1–36.0	36.1–38.0	38.1–39.0	≥39.1	

The **ACVPU** is a scale used to assess and track a patient's neurological status and level of consciousness.

ACVPU stands for:

- **A**lert
- **C**onfusion
- **V**oice
- **P**ain
- **U**nresponsive

Clinical Response to the NEWS2 Trigger Thresholds

NEW score	Frequency of monitoring	Clinical response
0	Minimum 12 hourly	• Continue routine NEWS monitoring
Total 1–4	Minimum 4–6 hourly	• Inform registered nurse, who must assess the patient • Registered nurse decides whether increased frequency of monitoring and/or escalation of care is required
3 in single parameter	Minimum 1 hourly	• Registered nurse caring for the patient to inform medical team, who will review and decide whether escalation of care is necessary
Total 5 or more Urgent response threshold	Minimum 1 hourly	• Registered nurse caring for the patient to immediately inform the medical team • Registered nurse to request urgent assessment by a clinician or team with core competencies in the care of acutely ill patients • Provide clinical care in an environment with monitoring facilities
Total 7 or more Emergency response threshold	Continuous monitoring of vital signs	• Registered nurse caring for the patient to immediately inform the medical team - this should be at least at specialist registrar level • Emergency assessment by a team with critical care competencies, including practitioner(s) with advanced airway management skills • Consider transfer of care to a level 2 or 3 clinical care facility (ie, higher-dependency unit or ICU) • Clinical care in an environment with monitoring facilities

NEWS2 Observation Chart

NEWS key			FULL NAME			
0 1 2 3			DATE OF BIRTH		DATE OF ADMISSION	

			Score
	DATE		
	TIME		
A+B Respirations Breaths/min	≥25		3
	21–24		2
	18–20		
	15–17		
	12–14		
	9–11		1
	≤8		3
A+B SpO₂ Scale 1 Oxygen saturation (%)	≥96		
	94–95		1
	92–93		2
	≤91		3
SpO₂ Scale 2† Oxygen saturation (%) Use Scale 2 if target range is 88–92% (e.g. in hypercapnic respiratory failure) †ONLY use Scale 2 under the direction of a qualified clinician	≥97 on O₂		3
	95–96 on O₂		2
	93–94 on O₂		1
	≥93 on air		
	88–92		
	86–87		1
	84–85		2
	≤83		3
Air or oxygen?	A=Air		
	O₂ L/min		2
	Device		
C Blood pressure mmHg Score uses systolic BP only	≥220		3
	201–219		
	181–200		
	161–180		
	141–160		
	121–140		
	111–120		
	101–110		1
	91–100		2
	81–90		
	71–80		
	61–70		3
	51–60		
	≤50		
C Pulse Beats/min	≥131		3
	121–130		2
	111–120		
	101–110		1
	91–100		
	81–90		
	71–80		
	61–70		
	51–60		
	41–50		1
	31–40		3
	≤30		
D Consciousness Score for NEW onset of confusion (no score if chronic)	Alert		
	Confusion		
	V		3
	P		
	U		
E Temperature °C	≥39.1°		2
	38.1–39.0°		1
	37.1–38.0°		
	36.1–37.0°		
	35.1–36.0°		1
	≤35.0°		3
NEWS TOTAL			
Monitoring frequency			
Escalation of care Y/N			
Initials			

7.5

Adult Basic Life Support

7.5.1 Adult Basic Life Support in Community Settings

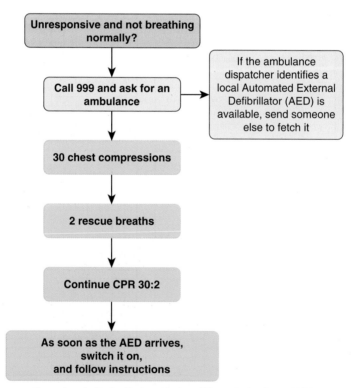

Reproduced with the kind permission of Resuscitation Council UK.

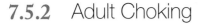

7.5.2 Adult Choking

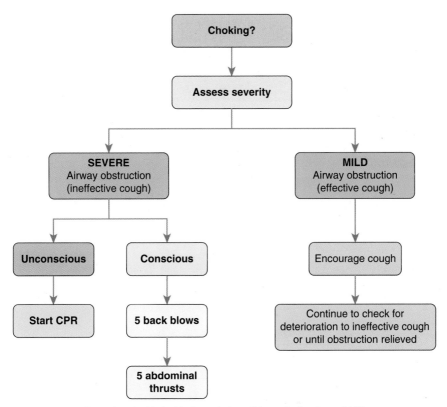

Reproduced with the kind permission of Resuscitation Council UK.

7.6

Paediatric Basic Life Support

7.6.1 Paediatric Basic Life Support (Hospital)

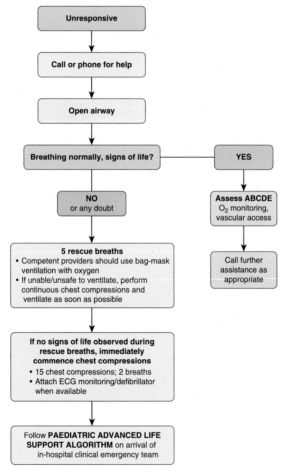

Reproduced with the kind permission of Resuscitation Council UK.

7.6.2   Paediatric Out-of-Hospital Basic Life Support

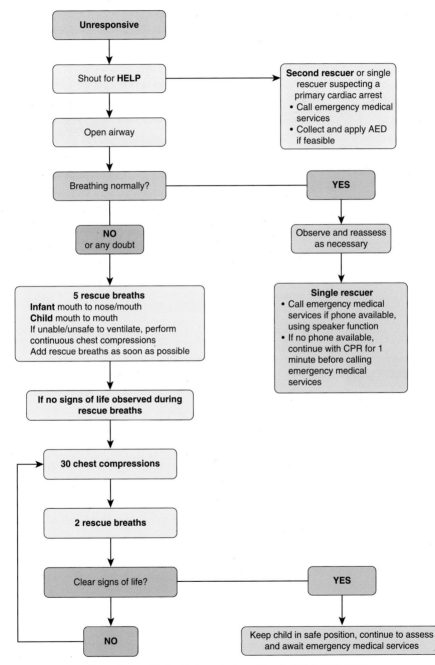

Reproduced with the kind permission of Resuscitation Council UK.

7.6.3   Paediatric Foreign Body Airway Obstruction

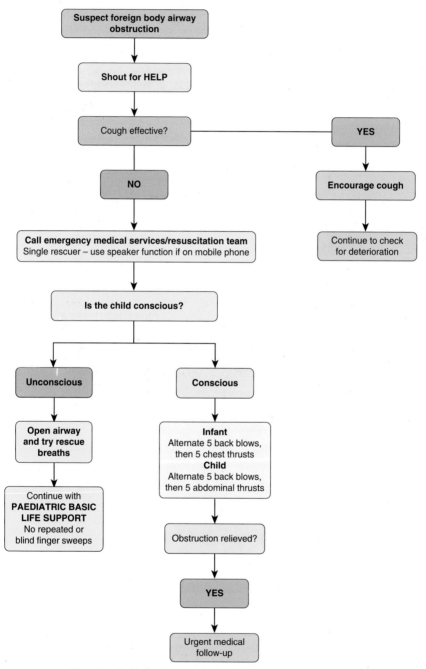

Reproduced with the kind permission of Resuscitation Council UK.

Body Mass Index Chart

Legend: ☐ Underweight   ■ Normal weight   ☐ Overweight   ■ Obese   ■ Extreme obesity

inch	cm	120	130	140	150	160	170	180	190	200	210	220	230	240	250
4'6	137	29	31	34	36	39	41	43	46	48	51	53	56	58	60
4'8	142.2	27	29	31	34	36	38	40	43	45	47	49	52	54	56
4'10	147.3	25	27	29	31	34	36	38	40	42	44	46	48	50	52
5'0	152.4	23	25	27	29	31	33	35	37	39	41	43	45	47	49
5'2	157.4	22	24	26	27	29	31	33	35	37	38	40	42	44	46
5'4	162.5	21	22	24	26	28	29	31	33	34	36	38	40	41	43
5'6	167.6	19	21	23	24	26	27	29	31	32	34	36	37	39	40
5'8	172.7	18	20	21	23	24	26	27	29	30	32	34	35	37	38
5'10	177.8	17	19	20	22	23	24	26	27	29	30	32	33	35	36
6'0	182.8	16	18	19	20	22	23	24	26	27	28	30	31	33	34
6'2	187.9	15	17	18	19	21	22	23	24	26	27	28	30	31	32
6'4	193	15	16	17	18	20	21	22	23	24	26	27	28	29	30
6'6	198.1	14	15	16	17	19	20	21	22	23	24	25	27	28	29
6'8	203.2	13	14	15	17	18	19	20	21	22	23	24	25	26	28
kg		54.5	59	63.5	68	72.6	77.1	81.6	86.2	90.7	95.3	99.8	104.3	108.9	113
lb		120	130	140	150	160	170	180	190	200	210	220	230	240	250

Suspected Cancer – Recognition and Referral

Suspected Cancer	Symptoms	Action Suggested
Osteosarcoma (in adults)	Unexplained bone swelling and pain	• X-ray (within 48 h) if symptoms suggestive • Referral under 2WW [two week wait (i.e. urgent)] pathway if X-ray suggests osteosarcoma
Soft tissue sarcoma (in adults)	Unexplained lump increasing in size	• Urgent ultrasound (within two weeks) if symptoms suggestive of sarcoma • Refer under 2WW pathway if ultrasound findings suggestive of sarcoma (or uncertain/clinical concern persists)

Prostate	Lower urinary tract symptoms
	• Nocturia
	• Urinary frequency
	• Hesitancy
	• Urinary urgency
	• Retention
	• Erectile dysfunction
	• Visible haematuria
		• Consider PSA and digital rectal examination if symptoms
		• Refer anyone with a malignant feeling prostate under 2WW
		• Consider referral under 2WW if symptoms and raised PSA for age
		  • age 40 – 49 >2.5
		  • age 50 – 59 >3.5
		  • age 60 – 69 >4.5
		  • age 70 – 79+ >6.5

Bladder/renal	• >45 with unexplained visible haematuria (with no UTI) • >45 with visible haematuria that persists after treating UTI • >60 with unexplained microscopic haematuria + dysuria or raised WCC	• Refer under 2WW if presence of relevant symptoms • Consider non-urgent referral if age >60 with recurrent or persistent UTI
Testicular cancer	• Non-painful enlargement of testis • Change in shape or texture of testes	• Refer under 2WW if symptoms present • Consider ultrasound scan if other unexplained or persistent testicular symptoms

Malignant melanoma	Use the seven-point checklist for a pigmented lesion
	• Two points for each of
	  • Change in size
	  • Irregular shape
	  • Irregular colour
	• One point each for
	  • >7 mm diameter
	  • Inflammation
	  • Oozing
	  • Change in sensation
		Refer under 2WW pathway if a pigmented lesion with checklist score of three or more
		Consider 2WW referral if appearance under dermoscopy suggests melanoma or if appearance suggests nodular melanoma

Suspected Cancer	Symptoms	Action Suggested
Squamous cell carcinoma	• Commonly in sun-exposed areas of skin • Enlarging scaly red lesions with thickened, wart-like growths – may crust, bleed or itch	Refer under 2WW pathway if features suggestive of SCC
Basal cell carcinoma	• Usually slow growing • May be non-ulcerated nodule on the skin or an ulcerated lesion with a raised, rolled edge, with prominent fine blood vessels around it	• Routine referral for people with suspected BCC • Refer more urgently if concerns about size/location of site
Acute leukaemia	• Pale • Persistent fatigue • Unexplained fever • Unexplained persistent or recurrent infection • Generalised lymphadenopathy (>1 cm persisting more than six weeks) • Unexplained bleeding • Unexplained petechia • Enlarged liver/spleen	• Organise FBC within 48 h – looking for elevated WCC, low RCC and presence of immature white cells (blasts) • Discuss with haematologist and consider admission if blood tests suggestive of acute leukaemia
Myeloma	• Age 60 and over with persistent bone pain (back/ribs) and/or an un-explained fracture Also consider if • Unexplained bleeding (e.g. nosebleeds) • Recurrent/persistent infections	• Offer FBC, calcium, ESR/PV first, and if low WCC/raised calcium, **then** offer myeloma screen (serum protein electrophoresis/urine BJP or serum free light chain assay) • Refer under 2WW pathway if myeloma screen results are suggestive of myeloma
Lymphoma	• Unexplained lymphadenopathy (>1 cm persisting more than six weeks) • Enlarged spleen • Fever • Weight loss • Night sweats • Shortness of breath • Itching • Weight loss	• Consider referral under 2WW pathway
Lung cancer and me-sothelioma	Minor symptoms • Cough • Fatigue • Shortness of breath • Chest pain • Weight loss • Appetite loss Major symptoms • Persistent or recurrent chest infections • Finger clubbing • Supraclavicular lymphadenopathy or persistent cervical lymphadenopathy • Chest signs (e.g. wheeze/stridor, reduced air entry [possible lobar collapse/effusion/abscess], focal crepitations [bronchiectasis/pneumonia])	• Offer urgent chest X-ray (within two weeks) if age >40 and two or more minor symptoms or one or more and they have ever smoked or been exposed to asbestos • Offer urgent chest X-ray if age >40 and *any* of the major symptoms • Refer under 2WW if chest X-ray is suggestive of lung cancer OR if aged >40 and have unexplained haemoptysis

Continued on following page

Suspected Cancer	Symptoms	Action Suggested

Oesophageal cancer	• Dysphagia (difficulty swallowing – usually for solids first before liquids)
	• Upper abdominal pain
	• Reflux
	• Dyspepsia (discomfort/pain after eating/drinking)
		• Refer for endoscopy under 2WW if
		  • Dysphagia
		  • age >55 with weight loss and any abdominal pain, reflex or dyspepsia
		• Refer for non-urgent endoscopy if history of haematemesis (vomited blood)
		• Refer for non-urgent endoscopy if age >55 with
		  • Dyspepsia not responding to treatment
		  • Upper abdominal pain and anaemia
		  • Raised platelet count with any of the following
		    ◦ Nausea
		    ◦ Vomiting
		    ◦ Weight loss
		    ◦ Reflux
		    ◦ Dyspepsia
		    ◦ Upper abdominal pain
		  • Nausea and vomiting with
		    ◦ Weight loss
		    ◦ Reflux
		    ◦ Dyspepsia
		    ◦ Upper abdominal pain

Stomach cancer	• Nausea
	• Vomiting
	• Weight loss
	• Reflux
	• Dyspepsia
	• Upper abdominal pain
		• Refer under 2WW if there is a palpable upper abdominal mass
		• Refer under 2WW for urgent endoscopy if
		  • Dysphagia
		  • age >55 with weight loss and any of the following
		    ◦ Upper abdominal pain
		    ◦ Reflux
		    ◦ Dyspepsia
		• Refer for non-urgent endoscopy if history of haematemesis (vomited blood)
		• Refer for non-urgent endoscopy if age >55 with
		  • Dyspepsia not responding to treatment
		  • Upper abdominal pain and anaemia
		  • Raised platelet count with any of the following
		    ◦ Nausea
		    ◦ Vomiting
		    ◦ Weight loss
		    ◦ Reflux
		    ◦ Dyspepsia
		    ◦ Upper abdominal pain
		  • Nausea and vomiting with any of the following
		    ◦ Weight loss
		    ◦ Reflux
		    ◦ Dyspepsia
		    ◦ Upper abdominal pain

Suspected Cancer	Symptoms	Action Suggested
Colorectal cancer	• Change in bowel habit • Blood in faeces • Rectal bleeding • Unexplained weight loss • Abdominal pain • Rectal mass • Iron deficiency anaemia	• Refer using 2WW pathway if 　• age >40 with unexplained weight loss and abdominal pain 　　OR 　• age >50 with unexplained rectal bleeding 　　OR 　• age >60 with 　　○ Iron deficiency anaemia or change in bowel habit 　　　OR 　　○ Test shows occult blood in faeces • Also consider referral under 2WW pathway if 　○ Rectal or abdominal mass 　○ age >50 with rectal bleeding and any of the following 　　○ Abdominal pain 　　○ Change in bowel habit 　　○ Weight loss 　　○ Iron deficiency anaemia • FIT (faecal immunochemical tests) should be offered to adults who are 　○ age >50 with unexplained abdominal pain or weight loss 　○ age <60 with change in bowel habit or iron deficiency anaemia 　○ age >60 with anaemia, even if not iron deficiency anaemia
Breast cancer	• Breast lump (with or without pain) • Nipple discharge, retraction • Axillary lymphadenopathy • Skin-dimpling, peau d'orange (skin similar to skin of orange), nipple eczema, visible mass and ulceration in late stage	• Refer under 2WW pathway if 　• age >30 with unexplained breast lump 　• age >50 with unilateral nipple changes (discharge, retraction) or changes of concern 　• Skin changes suggestive of breast cancer 　• age >30 with unexplained lump in axilla • Consider non-urgent referral if age <30 with unexplained breast lump with or without pain

Continued on following page

Suspected Cancer	Symptoms	Action Suggested

Ovarian cancer	• Persistent bloating or abdominal distention
	• Feeling full early (early satiety) and/or loss of appetite
	• Pelvic or abdominal pain
	• Increased urinary frequency/urgency
	• Weight loss
	• Fatigue
	• Change in bowel habit
	• Pelvic or abdominal mass (not known to be fibroids)
		• Refer urgently under 2WW pathway if there is ascites and/or pelvic or abdominal mass (not uterine fibroids)
		• Measure CA125 if the following symptoms are persistent or frequent (especially if >12/month)
		  • Persistent bloating or abdominal distention
		  • Feeling full early (early satiety) and/or loss of appetite
		  • Pelvic or abdominal pain
		  • Increased urinary frequency/urgency
		• If CA125 is 35 IU/mL or greater – arrange ultrasound of abdomen and pelvis
		• If ultrasound suggestive of cancer, refer under 2WW pathway
		• If CA125 <35 IU/mL or ultrasound normal, advise further assessment and advise to return to GP if symptoms become more frequent/persistent

Endometrial cancer	• Vaginal discharge
	• Vaginal bleeding
	• Blood in urine
	• Pelvic pain is rare, usually a late sign
		• Refer using 2WW pathway if age >55 with post-menopausal bleeding (unexplained vaginal bleeding more than 12 months after menstruation has stopped due to the menopause)
		• age <55 with post-menopausal bleeding
		• Consider urgent ultrasound if age >55 with
		  • Unexplained vaginal discharge for the first time or if accompanied by either thrombocytosis or haematuria
		  • Visible haematuria with low haemoglobin, thrombocytosis or high blood glucose levels

Notes: clinical opinions may vary on what is considered clinically 'significant' when describing some signs, but a rough guide is as follows:

• 'Significant' lymphadenopathy is lymph nodes >1 cm in size persisting for more than six weeks that cannot be explained by local/systemic infection
• 'Significant' weight loss – the definition of this varies, and any unintentional weight loss is cause for concern, but some quote >5% of body weight in 6/12 as a benchmark[1]

[1]Nicholson, B. D., Aveyard, P., Hamilton, W., Hobbs, F. R. (2019). When should unexpected weight loss warrant further investigation to exclude cancer? *British Medical Journal, 366*.

FURTHER READINGS

Section 1

Cyriax, J. (1982). *Textbook of orthopaedic medicine* (8th ed., Vol. 1). Diagnosis of soft tissue lesions. London: Baillière Tindall.

Drake, R. L. & Vogl, W., Mitchell, A. W. M. (2019). *Gray's anatomy for students* (4th ed.). Philadelphia: Churchill Livingstone.

Kenyon, K. & Kenyon, J. (2018). *The physiotherapist's pocketbook: essential facts at your fingertips.* Elsevier.

Magee, D. J. & Manske, R. C. (2021). *Orthopedic physical examination* (7th ed.). St. Louis: Elsevier.

O'Brien, M. D. (2010). *Guarantors of 'Brain' 2009–2010. Aids to the examination of the peripheral nervous system* (5th ed.). Edinburgh: W B Saunders.

Soames, R., & Palastanga, N. (2018). *Anatomy and human movement: structure and function* (7th ed.). Edinburgh: Churchill Livingstone.

Standring, S. (2020). *Gray's anatomy: the anatomical basis of clinical practice* (42nd ed). Elsevier.

Thompson, J. C. (2016). *Netter's concise orthopaedic anatomy* (2nd ed.). Philadelphia: Saunders.

Section 2

Beighton, P., Solomon, L., & Soskolne, C. L. (1973). Articular mobility in an African population. *Annals of the Rheumatic Diseases*, 32, 413–418.

Brukner, P., Khan, K., Clarsen, B., Cools, A., Crossley, K., Hutchinson, M., McCory, P., Bahr, R. & Cook, J. (2016). *Bruckner and Khan's clinical sports medicine: injuries* (5th ed., Vol. 1). Sydney: McGraw-Hill.

Compston, A. (2010). Aids to the investigation of peripheral nerve injuries. Medical Research Council: Nerve Injuries Research Committee. His Majesty's Stationery Office: 1942; 48 (iii) and 74 figures and 7 diagrams; with aids to the examination of the peripheral nervous system. By Michael O'Brien for the Guarantors of Brain. Saunders Elsevier: 2010;[8] 64 and 94 Figures. *Brain.* 133(10), 2838–2844.

Cyriax, J. (1982). *Textbook of orthopaedic medicine* (8th ed., Vol. 1). Diagnosis of soft tissue lesions. London: Baillière Tindall.

Day, R., Fox, J. & Paul-Taylor, G. (2009). *Neuromusculoskeletal clinical tests: a clinician's guide.* : Edinburgh: Churchill Livingstone.

Finucane, L. M., Downie, A., Mercer, C., Greenhalgh, S. M., Boissonnault, W. G., Pool-Goudzwaard, A. L., Beneciuk, J. M., Leech, R. L. & Selfe, J. (2020). International framework for red flags for potential serious spinal pathologies. *Journal of Orthopaedic & Sports Physical Therapy*, 50(7), 350–372.

Glattacker, M., Heyduck, K., Jakob, T. (2018). Yellow flags as predictors of rehabilitation outcome in chronic low back pain. *Rehabilitation Psychology*, 63(3), 408–417.

Grahame, R., Bird, H. A., & Child, A. (2000). The British society special interest group on heritable disorders of connective tissue criteria for the benign joint hypermobility syndrome. The revised (Brighton 1998) criteria for the diagnosis of the BJHS. *Journal of Rheumatology*, 27 (7), 1777–1779.

Gray, H., Adefolarin, A. T. & Howe, T. E. (2011). A systematic review of instruments for the assessment of work-related psychosocial factors (Blue Flags) in individuals with non-specific low back pain. *Manual Therapy*, 16(6), 531–543.

Hakim, A.J. & Grahame, R. (2003). A simple questionnaire to detect hypermobility: an adjunct to the assessment of patients with diffuse musculoskeletal pain. *International Journal of Clinical Practice*, 57, 163–166.

Hallett, M. (1993). National Institute of Neurological Disorders and Stroke myotatic reflex scale. *Neurology*, 43(12), p. 2723.

Hallner, D. & Hasenbring, M. (2004). Classification of psychosocial risk factors (yellow flags) for the development of chronic low back and leg pain using artificial neural network. *Neuroscience Letters*, 361(1-3), 151–154.

Hamblen, D. L. & Simpson, H. W. (2009). *Adams's Outline of Orthopaedics* (14th ed.). Edinburgh: Churchill Livingstone.

Harden, R. N., Bruehl, S., Stanton-Hicks, M. & Wilson, P. R. (2007). Proposed new diagnostic criteria for complex regional pain syndrome. *Pain Medicine*, 8(4), 326–331

Harding, M. M., Kwong, J., Roberts, D., Hagler, D. & Reinisch, C. (2020). *Lewis's medical-surgical nursing: assessment and management of clinical problems* (11th ed.). St. Louis: Elsevier.

Hattam, P. & Smeatham, A. (2020). *Handbook of special tests in musculoskeletal examination: an evidence-based guide for clinicians*. Elsevier.

Hayden, J. A., Dunn, K. M., van der Windt, D. A., & Shaw, W. S. (2010). What is the prognosis of back pain? *Best Practice & Research. Clinical Rheumatology*, 24, 167–179.

Innes, J. A., Doverm A, R. & Fairhurst, K. (2018). Macleod's clinical examination (14th ed.). Edinburgh: Elsevier.

Levy, H.P. Hypermobile Ehlers-Danlos Syndrome Synonyms: Benign Joint Hypermobility Syndrome, EDS Hypermobility Type, EDS Type III, Ehlers-Danlos Syndrome Hypermobility Type, Ehlers-Danlos Syndrome Type III, hEDS, Joint Hypermobility Syndrome.

Magee, D. J. & Manske, R. C. (2021). *Orthopedic Physical Examination* (7th ed.). St Louis: Elsevier.

Malanga, G. A. & Mautner, K. (2016). *Musculoskeletal Physical Examination: an evidence based approach* (2nd ed.). Philadelphia: Elsevier.

Medical Research Council. (1976). *Aids to the investigation of peripheral nerve injuries*. London: HMSO.

Nicholas, M. K., Linton, S. J., Watson, P. J. & Main, C. J. (2011). "Decade of the Flags" Working Group. Early identification and management of psychological risk factors ("yellow flags") in patients with low back pain: a reappraisal. *Physical Therapy*, 91(5), 737–753.

Petty, N. J. & Dionne, R. (2018). *Neuromusculoskeletal examination and assessment: a handbook for therapists* (5th ed.). Elsevier.

Reese, N. B. & Bandy, W. D. (2016). *Joint range of motion and muscle length testing* (3rd ed.). Philadelphia: W B Saunders.

Shacklock, M. (2005). *Clinical neurodynamics: A new system of musculoskeletal treatment*. Edinburgh: Butterworth Heinemann.

Simons, D. G., Travell, J. G. & Simons, L. S. (1998). *Travell and Simon's myofascial pain and dysfunction: the trigger point manual volume 1. upper half of body* (2nd ed.). Baltimore: Lippincott Williams & Wilkins.

Stiell, I. G., McKnight, R. D., Greenberg, G. H., McDowell, I., Nair, R. C., Wells, G. A., Johns, C., & Worthington, J. R. (1994). Implementation of the Ottawa ankle rules. *Journal of the American Medical Association,* 271, 827–832,

Tortora, G. J. & Derrickson, B. H. (2017). *Principles of anatomy and physiology* (15th ed.). Singapore: John Wiley & Sons.

Travell, J. G. & Simons, D. G. (1991). *Myofascial Pain and Dysfunction: The Trigger Point Manual Volume 2. The lower extremities*. Baltimore: Lippincott Williams & Wilkins.

Wippert, P. M., Fliesser, M. & Krause, M. (2017). Risk and protective factors in the clinical rehabilitation of chronic back pain. *Journal of Pain Research*, 10, 1569–1579.

Wolfe, F., Clauw, D. J., Fitzcharles, M. A., Goldenberg, D. L., Katz, R. S., Mease, P., Russell, A. S., Russell, I. J., Winfield, J. B., & Yunus, M. B. (2010). The American College of Rheumatology preliminary diagnostic criteria for fibromyalgia and measurement of symptom severity. *Arthritis Care & Research (Hoboken)*, 62(5), 600–610.

Section 3

Alentado, V. J., Lubelski, D., Steinmetz, M. P., Benzel, E. C., & Mroz, T. E. (2014). Optimal duration of conservative management prior to surgery for cervical and lumbar radiculopathy: a literature review. *Global Spine Journal*, 4(4), 279–286.

Alfredson. H. & Cook, J. (2007). A treatment algorithm for managing Achilles tendinopathy: new treatment options. *British Journal of Sports Medicine*, 41, 211–216.

Amin, N. H., Kumar, N. S., & Schickendantz, M. S. (2015). Medial epicondylitis: evaluation and management. *The Journal of the American Academy of Orthopaedic Surgeons*, 23(6), 348–355.

Ansok, C. B., & Muh, S. J. (2018). Optimal management of glenohumeral osteoarthritis. *Orthopedic Research and Reviews*, 10, 9–18.

Ariens, G.A., Van Mechelen, W., Bongers, P.M., Bouter, L.M. & Van Der Wal, G. (2000). Physical risk factors for neck pain. *Scandinavian Journal of Work, Environment & Health*, 7–19.

Battié, M. C., Videman, T., Kaprio, J., Gibbons, L. E., Gill, K., Manninen, H., Saarela, J., & Peltonen, L. (2009). The Twin Spine Study: contributions to a changing view of disc degeneration. *The Spine Journal : Official Journal of the North American Spine Society*, 9(1), 47–59.

Brinkji, W., Luetnmer, P. H., Comstock, B., Bresnahan, B. W., Chen, L.E., Deyo, R. A., Halabia, S., Turner, J. A., Avins, A. L., James, K. & Wald, J. T. (2015). Systemic literature review of imaging features of spinal degeneration in asymptomatic populations. *American Journal of Neuroradiology*, 36(4), 811–816.

Brownson, P., Donaldson, O., Fox, M., Rees, J. L., Rangan, A., Jaggi, A., Tytherleigh-Strong, G., McBernie, J., Thomas, M., & Kulkarni, R. (2015). BESS/BOA Patient Care Pathways: Traumatic anterior shoulder instability. *Shoulder & Elbow*, 7(3), 214–226.

Brukner, P., Khan, K., Clarsen, B., Cools, A., Crossley, K., Hutchinson, M., McCory, P., Bahr, R. & Cook, J. (2016). *Brukner and Khan's clinical sports medicine: injuries* (5th ed. Vol. 1). Sydney: McGraw-Hill.

Bubra, P. S., Keighley, G., Rateesh, S. & Carmody, D. (2015). Posterior tibial tendon dysfunction: an overlooked cause of foot deformity. *Journal of Family Medicine and Primary Care*, 4(1), 26–29.

Bytomski, J. & Moorman, C. T. (2010). *Oxford American handbook of sports medicine*. Oxford University Press, New York.

Caridi, J. M., Pumberger, M. & Hughes, A. P. (2011). Cervical radiculopathy: a review. *Musculoskeletal Journal of Hospital for Special Surgery*, 7(3), 265–272.

Charis, G. N., Rotator cuff disease. (2020). In *Ferri FF. Ferri's clinical advisor: 5 books in 1*. Elsevier; 1217. e5–1217.e10

Cohen, S.P., Bhaskar, A., Bhatia, A., Buvanendran, A., Deer, T., Garg, S., Hooten, W.M., Hurley, R.W., Kennedy, D.J., McLean, B.C. & Moon, J.Y. 2020. Consensus practice guidelines on interventions for lumbar facet joint pain from a multispecialty, international working group. *Regional Anesthesia & Pain Medicine*, 45(6), 424–467.

Davda, K., Malhotra, K., O'Donnell, P., Singh, D., & Cullen, N. (2017). Peroneal tendon disorders. *EFORT Open Reviews*, 2(6), 281–292.

Dwivedi, S., Paxton, E. S. (2020). In *Ferri FF. Ferri's clinical advisor: 5 books in 1*. Elsevier; 77.e2–77.e3

Ekedahl, H., Jönsson, B., Annertz, M. & Frobell, R. B., (2018). Accuracy of clinical tests in detecting disk herniation and nerve root compression in subjects with lumbar radicular symptoms. *Archives of Physical Medicine and Rehabilitation*, 99(4), 726–735.

Ferguson, A., Christophersen, C., Elattar, O. & Farber, D. C. (2009). *Achilles Tendinopathy and Associated Disorders. Foot & Ankle Orthopaedics*.

Ferrari, J. (2009). Bunions. *British Medical Journal Clinical Evidence*, 1112.

Ferrari, R. & Russell, A. S. (2003). Neck pain. *Best Practice & Research Clinical Rheumatology*, 17(1), 57–70.

Finucane, L.M., Downie, A., Mercer, C., Greenhalgh, S.M., Boissonnault, W.G., Pool-Goudzwaard, A.L., Beneciuk, J.M., Leech, R.L. & Selfe, J. (2020). International framework for red flags for potential serious spinal pathologies. *Journal of Orthopaedic & Sports Physical Therapy*, 50(7), 350–372.

Fongemie, A. E., Buss, D. D. & Rolnick, S. J. (1998). Management of shoulder Impingement syndrome and rotator cuff tears. *American Family Physician*, 57(4), 667–674.

Gil, J. A., DeFroda, S. & Owens, B. D. (2017). Current Concepts in the Diagnosis and Management of Traumatic, Anterior Glenohumeral Subluxations. *Orthopaedic Journal of Sports Medicine*, 5(3), 2325967117694338.

Guerrero, P., Busconi, B., Deangelis, N., & Powers, G. (2009). Congenital instability of the shoulder joint: assessment and treatment options. *The Journal of Orthopaedic and Sports Physical Therapy*, 39(2), 124–134.

Hamblen, D. L, Simpson, H. W. (2009). *Adams's Outline of Orthopaedics* (14th ed.). Edinburgh: Churchill Livingstone.

Hankins, D. A., Korcek, L., & Richter, D. L. (2021). Femoroacetabular Impingement and Management of Labral Tears in the Athlete. *Clinics in Sports Medicine*, 40(2), 259–270.

Harding, M. M., Kwong, J., Roberts, D., Hagler, D. & Reinisch, C. (2020). Lewis's medical-surgical nursing: assessment and management of clinical problems (11th ed.). St. Louis: Elsevier.

Heiderscheit B., & McClinton S. (2016). Evaluation and Management of Hip and Pelvis Injuries. *Physical Medicine and Rehabilitation Clinics of North America*. 27(1), 1–29.

Hicks B.L., Lam J.C., & Varacallo M. Piriformis Syndrome. In: *StatPearls*. Treasure Island (FL): StatPearls Publishing; April 21, 2022.

Huang, J.H. and Zager, E.L., 2004. Thoracic outlet syndrome. *Neurosurgery*, 55(4), 897–903.

Hudson Z., & Small C. (2011). Managing the injured athlete: assessment, rehabilitation and return to play. Churchill Livingston, Elsevier

Ibounig T., Simons T., Launonen A., & Paavola M. (2021). Glenohumeral osteoarthritis: an overview of etiology and diagnostics. *Scandinavian Journal of Surgery*, 110(3), 441–451.

Innes J.A., Dover A.R., & Fairhurst K. (2018). *Macleod's clinical examination* (14th ed.). Edinburgh: Elsevier.

Ishøi, L., Nielsen, M. F., Krommes, K., Husted, R. S., Hölmich, P., Pedersen, L. L., & Thorborg, K. (2021). Femoroacetabular impingement syndrome and labral injuries: grading the evidence on diagnosis and non-operative treatment-a statement paper commissioned by the Danish Society of Sports Physical Therapy (DSSF). *British Journal of Sports Medicine*, 55(22), 1301–1310.

Jaggi, A., & Alexander, S. (2017). Rehabilitation for Shoulder Instability - Current Approaches. *The Open Orthopaedics Journal*, 11, 957–971.

Jankovic, D., Peng, P., & van Zundert, A. (2013). Brief review: piriformis syndrome: etiology, diagnosis, and management. *Canadian Journal of Anaesthesia*, 60(10), 1003–1012.

Johnson, K. A., & Strom, D. E. (1989). Tibialis posterior tendon dysfunction. *Clinical Orthopaedics and Related Research*, (239), 196–206.

Kelsey, J. L., Githens, P. B., Walter, S. D., Southwick, W. O., Weil, U., Holford, T. R., Ostfeld, A. M., Calogero, J. A., O'Connor, T., & White, A. A., 3rd (1984). An epidemiological study of acute prolapsed cervical intervertebral disc. *The Journal of Bone and Joint Surgery. American volume*, 66(6), 907–914.

Kuisma, M., Karppinen, J., Haapea, M., Niinimäki, J., Ojala, R., Heliövaara, M., Korpelainen, R., Kaikkonen, K., Taimela, S., Natri, A., & Tervonen, O. (2008). Are the determinants of vertebral endplate changes and severe disc degeneration in the lumbar spine the same? A magnetic resonance imaging study in middle-aged male workers. *BMC musculoskeletal disorders*, 9, 51.

Kulkarni, R., Gibson, J., Brownson, P., Thomas, M., Rangan, A., Carr, A. J., & Rees, J. L. (2015). Subacromial shoulder pain. *Shoulder & elbow*, 7(2), 135–143.

Laprade RF, Wijdicks CA, (2012). The management of injuries to the medial side of the knee. *Journal of Orthopaedic Sports Physical Therapy*, 42(3), 221–233.

Lareau EM. Tendinitis and bursitis. (2013). In Adams JG ed. Emergency Medicine Clinical Essentials (2nd ed., 756-762). Philadelphia: Saunders.

Le, H. V., Lee, S. J., Nazarian, A., & Rodriguez, E. K. (2017). Adhesive capsulitis of the shoulder: review of pathophysiology and current clinical treatments. Shoulder & elbow, 9(2), 75–84.

Lespasio, M. J., Sultan, A. A., Piuzzi, N. S., Khlopas, A., Husni, M. E., Muschler, G. F., & Mont, M. A. (2018). Hip osteoarthritis: a primer. *The Permanente journal*, 22, 17–084.

Lewis, A., Kitamura, T. & Bayley, J.I.L. (2008). Mini symposium: shoulder instability (ii) the classification of shoulder instability: new light through old windows! *Current Orthopaedics*, 18, 97–108.

Linscott, M. *Injuries to the shoulder girdle and humerus*. In Adams JG ed. Emergency Medicine Clinical Essentials (2nd ed.). Philadelphia: Saunders.

Luoma, K., Riihimäki, H., Raininko, R., Luukkonen, R., Lamminen, A., & Viikari-Juntura, E. (1998). Lumbar disc degeneration in relation to occupation. *Scandinavian Journal of Work, Environment & Health*, 24(5), 358–366.

Majlesi, J., Togay, H., Unalan, H., & Toprak, S. (2008). The sensitivity and specificity of the Slump and the Straight Leg Raising tests in patients with lumbar disc herniation. *Journal of Clinical Rheumatology: Practical Reports on Rheumatic & Musculoskeletal Diseases*, 14(2), 87–91.

Malliaras, P., Cook, J., Purdam, C., & Rio, E. (2015). Patellar Tendinopathy: Clinical Diagnosis, Load Management, and Advice for Challenging Case Presentations. *The Journal of Orthopaedic and Sports Physical Therapy*, 45(11), 887–898.

Magee, D. J., & Manske, R. C. (2021). *Orthopedic Physical Examination* (7th ed.). St. Louis: Elsevier.

McNamee, J., Flynn, P., O'Leary, S., Love, M., & Kelly, B. (2013). Imaging in cauda equina syndrome—a pictorial review. *The Ulster Medical Journal*, 82(2), 100–108.

Millett, P.J., Gobezie, R., Boykin, R.E. (2008). Shoulder osteoarthritis: diagnosis and management. *American Family Physician*, 78(5), 605–611.

Monahan, F.D., Neighbours, M., & Green, C.J. (2011). *Swearingen's Manual of Medical Surgical Nursing: A Care Planning Approach* (7th ed.). Elsevier.

Mora, J. C., Przkora, R., & Cruz-Almeida, Y. (2018). Knee osteoarthritis: pathophysiology and current treatment modalities. *Journal of Pain Research*, 11, 2189–2196.

Musick, S.R., Varacallo, M. Snapping Hip Syndrome. In: *StatPearls*. Treasure Island (FL): StatPearls Publishing; May 1, 2022.

Myerson, M.S. (1997). Adult acquired flatfoot deformity: treatment of dysfunction of the posterior tibial tendon. *Instructional Course Lectures*, 46, 393–405.

Nakano, N., & Khanduja, V. (2018). Femoroacetabular impingement: the past, current controversies and future perspectives. *The Physician and Sports Medicine*, 46(3), 270–272.

Nho, S. J., Strauss, E. J., Lenart, B. A., Provencher, M. T., Mazzocca, A. D., Verma, N. N., & Romeo, A. A. (2010). Long head of the biceps tendinopathy: diagnosis and management. *The Journal of the American Academy of Orthopaedic Surgeons*, 18(11), 645–656.

Noorani, A., Goldring, M., Jaggi, A., Gibson, J., Rees, J., Bateman, M., Falworth, M., & Brownson, P. (2019). BESS/BOA patient care pathways: Atraumatic shoulder instability. *Shoulder & Elbow*, 11(1), 60–70.

Nutall C., & Winters B.A. (2015). Understanding anterior knee pain: patellofemoral pain syndrome. *The Journal for Nurse Practitioner*. 11(10), 1032–1035.

Petersen, T., Laslett, M. and Juhl, C. (2017). Clinical classification in low back pain: best-evidence diagnostic rules based on systematic reviews. *BioMed Central Musculoskeletal Disorders*, 18(1), 1–23.

Radhakrishnan, K., Litchy, W. J., O'Fallon, W. M., & Kurland, L. T. (1994). Epidemiology of cervical radiculopathy. A population-based study from Rochester, Minnesota, 1976 through 1990. *Brain: A Journal of Neurology*, 117 (Pt 2), 325–335.

Raney, E. B., Thankam, F. G., Dilisio, M. F., & Agrawal, D. K. (2017). Pain and the pathogenesis of biceps tendinopathy. *American Journal of Translational Research*, 9(6), 2668–2683.

Rangan, A., Goodchild, L., Gibson, J., Brownson, P., Thomas, M., Rees, J., & Kulkarni, R. (2015). Frozen Shoulder. *Shoulder & Elbow*, 7(4), 299–307.

Rees H.W. (2020). Management of Osteoarthritis of the Hip. *The Journal of the American Academy of Orthopaedic Surgeons*, 28(7), e288–e291.

Rockwood CA., Jr. (1984). Fractures and dislocations of the shoulder. In: Rockwood CA Jr, Green DP, editors. Fractures in Adults (860–910). Philadelphia, PA: Lippincott.

Roquelaure, Y., Bodin, J., Ha, C., Le Marec, F., Fouquet, N., Ramond-Roquin, A., Goldberg, M., Descatha, A., Petit, A., & Imbernon, E. (2014). Incidence and risk factors for thoracic spine pain in the working population: the French Pays de la Loire study. *Arthritis Care Research*, 66(11), 1695–1702.

Ross, M. H., Smith, M. D., Mellor, R., & Vicenzino, B. (2018). Exercise for posterior tibial tendon dysfunction: a systematic review of randomised clinical trials and clinical guidelines. *BMJ Open Sport & Exercise Medicine*, 4(1), e000430.

Sampath, P., Bendebba, M., Davis, J. D., & Ducker, T. (1999). Outcome in patients with cervical radiculopathy. Prospective, multicenter study with independent clinical review. *Spine*, 24(6), 591–597.

Sanders, R. J., Hammond, S. L., & Rao, N. M. (2007). Diagnosis of thoracic outlet syndrome. *Journal of Vascular Surgery*, 46(3), 601–604.

Singh, A., Tetreault, L., Fehlings, M. G., Fischer, D. J., & Skelly, A. C. (2012). Risk factors for development of cervical spondylotic myelopathy: results of a systematic review. *Evidence-based spine-Care Journal*, 3(3), 35–42.

Speers, C. J., & Bhogal, G. S. (2017). Greater trochanteric pain syndrome: a review of diagnosis and management in general practice. *The British journal of general practice : the journal of the Royal College of General Practitioners*, 67(663), 479–480.

Steuri, R., Sattelmayer, M., Elsig, S., Kolly, C., Tal, A., Taeymans, J., & Hilfiker, R. (2017). Effectiveness of conservative interventions including exercise, manual therapy and medical management in adults with shoulder impingement: a systematic review and meta-analysis of RCTs. *British Journal Of Sports Medicine*, 51(18), 1340–1347.

Tannast, M., Siebenrock, K. A., & Anderson, S. E. (2007). Femoroacetabular impingement: radiographic diagnosis—what the radiologist should know. *American Journal of Roentgenology*, 188(6), 1540–1552.

Terrell, S. L., Olson, G. E., & Lynch, J. (2021). Therapeutic exercise approaches to nonoperative and postoperative management of femoroacetabular impingement syndrome. *Journal of Athletic Training*, 56(1), 31–45.

Thomas, M., Bidwai, A., Rangan, A., Rees, J. L., Brownson, P., Tennent, D., Connor, C., & Kulkarni, R. (2016). *Glenohumeral Osteoarthritis. Shoulder & Elbow*, 8(3), 203–214.

Thorborg, K., Reiman, M. P., Weir, A., Kemp, J. L., Serner, A., Mosler, A. B., & HÖlmich, P. (2018). Clinical Examination, Diagnostic Imaging, and Testing of Athletes With Groin Pain: An Evidence-Based Approach to Effective Management. *The Journal of Orthopaedic and Sports Physical Therapy*, 48, 4, 239–249.

Todd, N.V., & Dickson, R.A., 2016. Standards of care in cauda equina syndrome. *British Journal of Neurosurgery*, 30(5), 518–522.

Van der Windt, D.A., Simons, E., Riphagen, I.I., Ammendolia, C., Verhagen, A.P., Laslett, M., Devillé, W., Deyo, R.A., Bouter, L.M., de Vet, H.C., & Aertgeerts B. (2010). Physical examination for lumbar radiculopathy due to disc herniation in patients with low-back pain. *Cochrane Database Systematic Reviews*, (2), CD007431.

Weir, A., Brukner, P., Delahunt, E., Ekstrand, J., Griffin, D., Khan, K. M., Lovell, G., Meyers, W. C., Muschaweck, U., Orchard, J., Paajanen, H., Philippon, M., Reboul, G., Robinson, P., Schache, A. G., Schilders, E., Serner, A., Silvers, H., Thorborg, K., Tyler, T., Geoffrey V., Robert-Jan de V., Zarko V., & Hölmich, P. (2015). Doha agreement meeting on terminology and definitions in groin pain in athletes. *British Journal of Sports Medicine*, 49(12), 768–774.

White, A.E., Patel, N.K., Hadley, C.J., & Dodson C.C. (2019). An algorithmic approach to the management of shoulder Instability. *Journal of the American Academy of Orthopaedic Surgeons Global Research and Reviews*, 3(12), e19.00168.

Willy, R.W., Hoglund, L.T., Barton, C.J., Bolgla, L.A., Scalzitti, D.A., Logerstedt, D.S., Lynch, A.D., Snyder-Mackler, L., & McDonough, C.M. (2019). Patellofemoral Pain: Clinical practice guidelines linked to the international classification of functioning, disability and health from the Academy of Orthopaedic Physical Therapy of the American Physical Therapy Association. *Journal of Orthopaedic & Sports Physical Therapy*, 49, 9, CPG1-CPG95.

Section 4

Alpay-Kanıtez, N., Çelik, S., & Bes, C. (2019). Polyarthritis and its differential diagnosis. *European Journal of Rheumatology*, 6(4), 167-173.

Bailey, S. E., Ukoumunne, O. C., Shephard, E. A., & Hamilton, W. (2017). Clinical relevance of thrombocytosis in primary care: a prospective cohort study of cancer incidence using English electronic medical records and cancer registry data. *British Journal of General Practice*, 67(659), e405–e413.

Beronius, M., Bergman, B., & Andersson, R. (2001). Vertebral Osteomyelitis in Göteborg, Sweden: A Retrospective Study of Patients During 1990-95. *Scandinavian Journal of Infectious Diseases*, 33(7), 527–532.

Bird, J. M., Owen, R. G., D'Sa, S., Snowden, J. A., Pratt, G., Ashcroft, J., Yong, K., Cook, G., Feyler, S., Davies, F., Morgan, G., Cavenagh, J., Low, E., Behrens, J., & Haemato-oncology Task Force of British Committee for Standards in Haematology (BCSH) and UK Myeloma Forum. (2011). Guidelines for the diagnosis and management of multiple myeloma. *British Journal of Haematology*, 154(1), 32–75.

Boulton, A. J., Gries, F. A., & Jervell, J. A. (1998). Guidelines for the diagnosis and outpatient management of diabetic peripheral neuropathy. *Diabetic Medicine*, 15, 508–514.

Brinkji, W., Luetnmer, P. H., Comstock, B., Bresnahan, B. W., Chen, L. E., Deyo, R. A., Halabia, S., Turner, J. A., Avins, A. L., James, K. & Wald, J.T. (2015). Systemic literature review of imaging features of spinal degeneration in asymptomatic populations. *American Journal of Neuroradiology*, 36(4), 811–816.

Buttgereit, F., Dejaco, C., Matteson, E. L., & Dasgupta, B. (2016). Polymyalgia Rheumatica and Giant Cell Arteritis: A Systematic Review. *Journal of the American Medical Association*, 315(22), 2442–2458.

Cojocaru, M., Cojocaru, I. M., Silosi, I., & Vrabie, C. D. (2011). Manifestations of systemic lupus erythematosus. *Maedica*, 6(4), 330–336.

Cooper, A., Brew, S., & de Lusignan, S. (2002). The effectiveness of blood tests in detecting secondary osteoporosis or mimicking conditions in postmenopausal women. *British Journal of General Practice*, 52(477), 311–313.

Coury, F., Peyruchaud, O., & Machuca-Gayet, I. (2019). Osteoimmunology of bone loss in inflammatory rheumatic diseases. *Frontiers in Immunology*, 10, 679.

Cylwik, B. & Chrostek, L. (2011). Zaburzenia metabolizmu kwasu foliowego i homocysteiny w warunkach naduzywania alkoholu [Disturbances of folic acid and homocysteine metabolism in alcohol abuse]. *Polski Merkuriusz Lekarski*, 30(178), 295–299.

Dasgupta, B., Borg, F. A., Hassan, N., Barraclough, K. Bourke, B., Fulcher, J., Hollywood, J., Hutchings, A., Kyle, V., Nott, J., Power, M., Samanta, A., on behalf of the BSR and BHPR Standards. (2010). Guidelines and Audit Working Group, BSR and BHPR guidelines for the management of polymyalgia rheumatica. *Rheumatology*, 49(1), 186–190.

Davenport, G. (2004). Rheumatology and musculoskeletal medicine. *British Journal of General Practice*, 54(503), 457–464.

Dougados, M. & Baeten, D. (2011). Spondyloarthritis. *The Lancet*, 377(9783), 2127–2137.

Duyff, R.F., Van den Bosch, J., Laman, D.M., van Loon, B.J.P. & Linssen, W.H. (2000). Neuromuscular findings in thyroid dysfunction: a prospective clinical and electrodiagnostic study. *Journal of Neurology, Neurosurgery & Psychiatry*, 68(6), 750–755.

Escadafal, C., Incardona, S., Fernandez-Carballo, B. L., & Dittrich, S. (2020). The good and the bad: using C reactive protein to distinguish bacterial from non-bacterial infection among febrile patients in low-resource settings. *BMJ Global Health*, 5, e002396.

Eslick, R. & Talaulikar, D. (2013). Multiple myeloma: from diagnosis to treatment. *Australian Family Physician*, 42(10), 684.

Goldner, W. (2016). Cancer-related hypercalcemia. *Journal of Oncology Practice*, 12(5), 426–432.

Gruys, E., Toussaint, M.J.M., Niewold, T.A. & Koopmans, S.J. (2005). Acute phase reaction and acute phase proteins. *Journal of Zhejiang University. Science. B*, 6(11), 1045.

Hamad, H. & Mangla, A. (2019). Lymphocytosis. StatPearls Publishing.

Hamilton, F., Carroll, R., Hamilton, W. & Salisbury, C. (2014).The risk of cancer in primary care patients with hypercalcaemia: a cohort study using electronic records. *British Journal of Cancer*, 111(7), 1410–1412.

Hamilton, W., Lancashire, R., Sharp, D., Peters, T.J., Cheng, K.K. & Marshall, T. (2008). The importance of anaemia in diagnosing colorectal cancer: a case–control study using electronic primary care records. *British Journal of Cancer*, 98(2), 323–327.

Helliwell, T., Muller, S. & Hider, S. (2012). ESR can be normal in giant cell arteritis and polymyalgia rheumatica. *British Medical Journal*, 344, e1408.

Hernandez, R.K., Wade, S.W., Reich, A., Pirolli, M., Liede, A. & Lyman, G.H. (2018). Incidence of bone metastases in patients with solid tumors: analysis of oncology electronic medical records in the United States. *BioMed Central Cancer*, 18(1), 44.

Hopkins, R., Bailey, S.E., Hamilton, W.T. & Shephard, E.A. (2020). Microcytosis as a risk marker of cancer in primary care: a cohort study using electronic patient records. *British Journal of General Practice*, 70(696), e457–e462.

Hsu, D.C., Wilkenfeld, P. & Joshua, D.E. (2012). Easily missed? Multiple myeloma. *Praxis*, 101(13), 857–861.

Hughes, R. (2010). Investigation of peripheral neuropathy. *British Medical Journal*, 341, c6100.

Ingegnoli, F., Castelli, R. & Gualtierotti, R. (2013). Rheumatoid factors: clinical applications. *Disease Markers*, 35(6), 727–734.

Kaferle, J., & Strzoda, C.E. (2009). Evaluation of macrocytosis. *American family physician*, 79(3), 203–208.

Katzmann, J.A. (2009). Screening panels for monoclonal gammopathies: time to change. *The Clinical Biochemist Reviews*, 30(3), 105-111.

Koshiaris, C., Van den Bruel, A., Oke, J.L., Nicholson, B.D., Shephard, E., Braddick, M. & Hamilton, W. (2018). Early detection of multiple myeloma in primary care using blood tests: a case–control study in primary care. *British Journal of General Practice*, 68(674), e586–e593.

Kuriakose, E., Cheppayil, S. N. U., Narayanan, S. K. & Vasudevan, A. (2019). A study on free light chain assay and serum immunofixation electrophoresis for the diagnosis of monoclonal gammopathies. *Indian Journal of Clinical Biochemistry*, 34(1), 76–81.

Lee, J. K., Chuang, M. J., Lu, C. C., Hao, L. J., Yang, C. Y., Han, T. M. & Lam, H. C. (1997). Parathyroid hormone and parathyroid hormone related protein assays in the investigation of hypercalcemic patients in hospital in a Chinese population. *Journal of Endocrinological Investigation*, 20(7), 404–409.

Lin, R. J., Afshar-Kharghan, V. & Schafer, A.I. (2014). Paraneoplastic thrombocytosis: the secrets of tumor self-promotion. *Blood, The Journal of the American Society of Hematology*, 124(2), 184–187.

Litao, M. K. S. & Kamat, D. (2014). Erythrocyte sedimentation rate and C-reactive protein: how best to use them in clinical practice. *Pediatric Annals*, 43(10), 417–420.

Macedo, F., Ladeira, K., Pinho, F., Saraiva, N., Bonito, N., Pinto, L. & Gonçalves, F. (2017). Bone metastases: an overview. *Oncology Reviews*, 11(1), 321.

Marcinowska-Suchowierska, E., Kupisz-Urbańska, M., Łukaszkiewicz, J., Płudowski, P. & Jones, G. (2018). Vitamin D toxicity–a clinical perspective. *Frontiers in Endocrinology*, 9, 550.

Markanday A. (2015). Acute Phase Reactants in Infections: Evidence-Based Review and a Guide for Clinicians. *Open Forum Infectious Diseases*, 2(3), ofv098.

Mazziotti, G., Canalis, E. & Giustina, A. (2010). Drug-induced osteoporosis: mechanisms and clinical implications. *The American Journal of Medicine*, 123(10), 877–884.

McAllister, K., Goodson, N., Warburton, L. & Rogers, G. (2017). Spondyloarthritis: diagnosis and management: summary of NICE guidance. *British Medical Journal*, 356, j839.

Mease, P., Clauw, D., Fitzcharles, M., Goldenberg, D., Hauser, W., Katz, R. et al. (2010). Development of the fibromyalgia survey diagnostic criteria, a modification of the American College of Rheumatology (ACR, 2010) preliminary diagnostic criteria for fibromyalgia to the ACR 2010 fibromyalgia diagnostic criteria (FDC). MYOPAIN 2010 Abstracts Book, 23. 2010.

Merriel, S.W., Carroll, R., Hamilton, F. & Hamilton, W. (2016). Association between unexplained hypoalbuminaemia and new cancer diagnoses in UK primary care patients. *Family Practice*, 33(5), 449–452.

Nau, K,C. & Lewis, W.D. (2008). Multiple myeloma diagnosis and treatment. *American Family Physician*, 78 (7), 853–859

NOGG Guidelines found at: www.sheffield.ac.uk/NOGG/NOGG%20Guideline%202017.pdf

Palumbo, A. & Anderson K. (2011). Multiple myeloma. *The New England Journal of Medicine*, 364(11), 1046–1060

Putto, A., Meurman, O. & Ruuskanen, O. (1985). C-reactive protein in viral and bacterial infections. *Pediatric Research*, 19, 1103.

Rosenblum, M. D., Remedios, K. A. & Abbas, A. K. (2015). Mechanisms of human autoimmunity. *The Journal of Clinical Investigation*. 125(6), 2228–2233.

Royal Osteoporosis Society guidelines found at theros.org.uk/healthcare-professionals/tools-and-resources/clinical-guidance/

Rudwaleit, M., Metter, A., Listing, J., Sieper, J. & Braun, J. (2006). Inflammatory back pain in ankylosing spondylitis: a reassessment of the clinical history for application as classification and diagnostic criteria. *Arthritis & Rheumatism: Official Journal of the American College of Rheumatology*, 54(2), 569–578.

Rutka, K., Garkowski, A., Karaszewska, K. & Łebkowska, U. (2021). Imaging in Diagnosis of Systemic Sclerosis. *Journal of Clinical Medicine*, 10(2), 248.

Sadowski, A. & Houck, R.C. (2020). Alcoholic neuropathy. StatPearls [Internet]. Available at https://www.ncbi.nlm.nih.gov/books/NBK499856/

Sampson, H.W., 2002. Alcohol and other factors affecting osteoporosis risk in women. *Alcohol Research & Health*, 26(4), 292–298.

Sanvisens, A., Zuluaga, P., Pineda, M., Fuster, D., Bolao, F., Juncà, J., Tor, J., & Muga, R. (2017). Folate deficiency in patients seeking treatment of alcohol use disorder. *Drug and Alcohol Dependence*, 180, 417–422.

Shephard, E. A., Neal, R. D., Rose, P., Walter, F. M., Litt, E. J. & Hamilton, W.T. (2015). Quantifying the risk of multiple myeloma from symptoms reported in primary care patients: a large case–control study using electronic records. *British Journal of General Practice*, 65(631), e106–e113.

Siao-Pin, S., Damian, L.O., Muntean, L.M. & Rednic, S. (2016). Acroosteolysis in systemic sclerosis: An insight into hypoxia-related pathogenesis. *Experimental and Therapeutic Medicine*, 12(5), 3459–3463.

Singer, S. & Eberlein, T. J. (1997). Surgical management of soft tissue sarcoma. *Advances in Surgery*, 31, 395–420.

Singh, A. G., Kermani, T. A., Crowson, C. S., Wey, C. M., Matteson, E. L., & Warrington, K. J. (2015). Visual manifestations in giant cell arteritis: trend over 5 decades in a population-based cohort. *The Journal of Rheumatology*, 42(2), 309–315.

Sokka, T. & Pincus, T. (2009). Erythrocyte sedimentation rate, C-reactive protein, or rheumatoid factor are normal at presentation in 35%–45% of patients with rheumatoid arthritis seen between 1980 and 2004: analyses from Finland and the United States. *The Journal of Rheumatology*, 36(7), 1387–1390.

Steinman, J. & Shibli-Rahhal, A. (2019). Anorexia nervosa and osteoporosis: pathophysiology and treatment. *Journal of Bone Metabolism*, 26(3), 133–143.

Tarp, S., Bartels, E. M., Bliddal, H., Furst, D. E., Boers, M., Danneskiold-Samsøe, B., Rasmussen, M., & Christensen, R. (2012). Effect of nonsteroidal antiinflammatory drugs on the C-reactive protein level in rheumatoid arthritis: a meta-analysis of randomized controlled trials. *Arthritis and Rheumatism*, 64(11), 3511–3521.

Tasnim, N., Dutta, P., Nayeem, J., Masud, P., Ferdousi, A., Ghosh, A.S., Hossain, M., Rajia, S., Kubra, K.T., Sakibuzzaman, M. & Khan, A.T. (2021). Osteoporosis, an inevitable circumstance of chronic kidney disease: A systematic review. *Cureus*, 13(10), e18488.

The International Myeloma Working Group. (2003). Criteria for the classification of monoclonal gammopathies, multiple myeloma and related disorders: a report of the International Myeloma Working Group. *British Journal of Haematology*, 121, 749–757.

Themistocleous, A.C., Ramirez, J.D., Serra, J., Bennett, D.L. (2014). The clinical approach to small fibre neuropathy and painful channelopathy. *Practical Neurology*, 14(6), 368–379.

Tsantes, A. G., Papadopoulos, D. V., Vrioni, G., Sioutis, S., Sapkas, G., Benzakour, A., Benzakour, T., Angelini, A., Ruggieri, P. & Mavrogenis, A.F. (2020). Spinal infections: an update. *Microorganisms*, 8(4), 476.

Tuchendler, D. & Bolanowski, M. (2014). The influence of thyroid dysfunction on bone metabolism. *Thyroid Research*, 7(1), 12.

Udovcic, M., Pena, R. H., Patham, B., Tabatabai, L. & Kansara, A. (2017). Hypothyroidism and the heart. *Methodist DeBakey Cardiovascular Journal*, 13(2), 55.

Walter, E. J., Hanna-Jumma, S., Carraretto, M. & Forni, L. (2016). The pathophysiological basis and consequences of fever. *Critical Care*, 20(1), 200.

Watson, J., Jones, H. E., Banks, J., Whiting, P., Salisbury, C. & Hamilton, W. (2019). Use of multiple inflammatory marker tests in primary care: using Clinical Practice Research Datalink to evaluate accuracy. *British Journal of General Practice*, 69(684), e462–e469.

Watson, J., Mounce, L., Bailey, S. E., Cooper, S. L. & Hamilton, W. (2019). Blood markers for cancer. *British Medical Journal*, 367, l5774.

Watson, J., Salisbury, C., Banks, J., Whiting, P. & Hamilton, W. (2019). Predictive value of inflammatory markers for cancer diagnosis in primary care: a prospective cohort study using electronic health records. *British Journal of Cancer*, 120(11), 1045–1051.

Watson, J., Salisbury, C., Whiting, P., Banks, J., Pyne, Y. & Hamilton, W. (2019). Added value and cascade effects of inflammatory marker tests in UK primary care: a cohort study from the Clinical Practice Research Datalink. *British Journal of General Practice*, 69(684), e470–e478.

Werhun, A. & Hamilton, W., 2013. Are we overusing thyroid function tests. *British Journal of General Practice*, 63(613), 404.

Hutchinson, W. L., Koenig, W., Fröhlich, M., Sund, M., Lowe, G. D. O. & Pepys, M. B. (2000). Immuno-radiometric assay of circulating c-reactive protein: age-related values in the adult general population. *Clinical Chemistry*, 46(7), 934–938.

Wong, A. Y., Karppinen, J. & Samartzis, D. (2017). Low back pain in older adults: risk factors, management options and future directions. *Scoliosis and Spinal Disorders*, 12(1), 14.

Yan, Y., Guo, T. M. & Zhu, C. (2018). Effects of nonsteroidal anti-inflammatory drugs on serum proinflammatory cytokines in the treatment of ankylosing spondylitis. *Biochemistry and Cell Biology*, 96(4), 450–456.

Young, P. J., Saxena, M., Beasley, R., Bellomo, R., Bailey, M., Pilcher, D., Finfer, S., Harrison, D., Myburgh, J. & Rowan, K. (2012). Early peak temperature and mortality in critically ill patients with or without infection. *Intensive Care Medicine*, 38, 437–444.

Section 6

Derry, S., Bell, R. F., Straube, S., Wiffen, P. J., Aldington, D. & Moore, R. A. (2019). Pregabalin for neuropathic pain in adults. *The Cochrane Database Of Systematic Reviews*, 1(1), CD007076.

Moore, R. A., Derry, S., Aldington, D., Cole, P. & Wiffen, P. J. (2015). Amitriptyline for neuropathic pain in adults. *The Cochrane Database Of Systematic Reviews*, 2015(7), CD008242.

Wiffen, P. J., Derry, S., Bell, R. F., Rice, A. S., Tölle, T. R., Phillips, T. & Moore, R. A. (2017). Gabapentin for chronic neuropathic pain in adults. *The Cochrane Database Of Systematic Reviews*, 6(6), CD007938.

Joint Formulary Committee. *British National Formulary (online) London: BMJ Group and Pharmaceutical Press* <http://www.medicinescomplete.com> [Accessed on 12 March 2022].

Hitchings, A., Lonsdale, D., Burrage, D. & Baker, E. (2018). *The top 100 drugs: clinical pharmacology and practical prescribing* (2nd ed.). Elsevier.

O'Shaughnessy, K. M. (2021). *New Guide to Medicine and Drugs: The complete home reference to over 3,000 medicines* (11th ed.). DK.

Ritter, J. M., Flower, R. J., Henderson, G., Loke, Y. K., MacEwan, D. & Rang, H. P. (2020). *Rang and Dale's pharmacology* (9th ed.). Elsevier.

Kizior, R. J. & Hodgson. (2022). *Saunders nursing drug handbook.* St Louis: Elsevier.